HARDCORE BODYBUILDING

A SCIENTIFIC APPROACH

Frederick C. Hatfield, Ph.D.

Foreword by TOM PLATZ

CB

CONTEMPORARY
BOOKS

CHICAGO

Library of Congress Cataloging-in-Publication Data

Hatfield, Frederick C.
    Hardcore bodybuilding : a scientific approach / Frederick C.
Hatfield.
       p.   cm.
    Includes bibliographical references (p.).
    ISBN 0-8092-3728-8
    1. Bodybuilding.   I. Title.
GV546.5.H386   1993
646.7′5—dc20   93-23960
                                            CIP

Portions of this book are excerpted from *Fitness: The Complete Guide*, copyright © 1991 by Frederick C. Hatfield, published by the International Sports Sciences Association (ISSA). All rights reserved.

Front-cover photo of Eddie Robinson used by permission of *WBF* magazine

"In the days when science was weak and religion was strong, man mistook magic for medicine. Now that science is strong and religion weak, man mistakes medicine for magic."

Author Unknown

"When the day comes that both science and religion are strong, all of mankind will turn their backs on drugs as an archaic measure of desperate men and turn instead to bodybuilding; and God be praised!"

Dr. Squat

Frederick C. Hatfield is the Director of Research and Development for **ICOPRO**, Inc., and cofounding Director of Sports and Fitness Sciences for the International Sports Sciences Association (**ISSA**). He has written more than fifty books and hundreds of articles in the general areas of sports training, fitness, bodybuilding, and nutrition. A three-time winner of the world championship of powerlifting, Hatfield has served as the national coach of the U.S. Powerlifting Team and has been coach and training consultant to scores of world-ranked and professional athletes as well as sports governing bodies and professional sports teams worldwide.

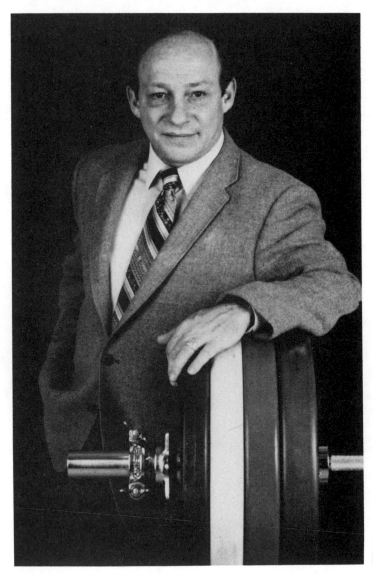

**Frederick C.
Hatfield, Ph.D.**

DEDICATION

To the great professional bodybuilders of the World Bodybuilding Federation. They, together with Tom Platz (who wrote the Foreword for this book), took a profoundly important step for the sport of bodybuilding. With financial and marketing backing afforded by Vince McMahon, they formed the WBF. Together they made the decision to train and compete totally drug-free. The members of WBF, in collaboration with Dr. Mauro DiPasquale, instituted the most stringent and broad-based drug-testing program the sports world had ever seen.

Their contributions to bodybuilding will be remembered well. Each chapter in this book is dedicated to one of them, and most of the exercises are illustrated by them.

These were true men of iron.

TABLE OF CONTENTS

Foreword   xiii

Preface   xvi

Acknowledgments   xix

Part One: Introduction to Bodybuilding   1

   1 Bodybuilding Is Unique   2

   2 Strength: Your Foundation   3

   3 Some Training Terms You Should Be Familiar With   7

   4 The Factors Contributing to Muscle Mass   13

   5 Principles of Training   20

Part Two: Bodybuilding Systems   29

   6 The Bodybuilding Lifestyle   30

   7 The ABCs of Hard-Core Bodybuilding   33

   8 Testing the Effectiveness of ABC Training: A Research Report   64

Part Three: Bodybuilding Exercise Techniques   71

   9 Introduction to Exercise Technique   72

   10 Bodybuilding Exercises   76

Part Four: Special Forms of Strength Training   136

   11 Anaerobic Strength   137

   12 Strength with Mass for Sports   142

   13 Aerobic or Anaerobic?   146

   14 An Example of an Integrated Training Regimen for Aerobic and Anaerobic Sports   150

Part Five: Integrated Nutrition for Bodybuilding   160

15 Maximum Nutrition for Maximum Bodybuilding Results   161

16 Zigzag Your Way to Muscular Weight Gain   167

17 Losing Fat and Keeping it Off   180

18 Easy Methods of Determining Your Body-Fat Percentage   196

19 You Are What You Eat   205

20 Fad Diets and Bodybuilding   228

21 Your Metabolic Rate   231

22 The Glycemic Index   234

23 Supplements   237

Part Six: Bodybuilding and the Endocrine System   244

24 Your Hormones   245

25 The Growth Hormone Response   254

26 Your Muscles' Hypertrophy Process   258

Part Seven: Drugs and Other Substances   264

27 Substances to Look Out For   265

28 Aspirin: The Best Supplement of All?   269

29 Other Drugs   272

30 Herbs: Nature's Sports Pharmacy   279

31 Antioxidants: Mother Nature's Ultimate Ergogen   285

Part Eight: Advanced Techniques and Theories   293

32 Forced Reps   294

33 Cheating Movements   298

34 To Be Great, Get Lazy!   300

35 Computers Can Integrate Training Technologies Best   303

36 Sauna   308

37 New Training Techniques and Technologies   311

Part Nine: Problem Areas for Bodybuilders   316

    38 Overtraining and Avoiding Injury   317

    39 Bodybuilding Burnout   322

    40 A Thumbnail Sketch of the Factors Involved in Recovery   329

    41 Your Tolerance to Exercise   331

    42 Symmetry   336

    43 Getting a Competition Tan Safely   341

Part Ten: Psychological Strategies for Success   345

    44 Conditioning Your Mind   346

    45 Your Emotional State   351

    46 Depression   355

Part Eleven: Contest Preparation   363

    47 Precontest Preparation   364

    48 Carbohydrate Supercompensation ("Carbo Loading") Strategies for Looking Your Best at Prejudging   369

Part Twelve: Mythic Concepts in Bodybuilding   372

    49 Myths about Drugs, Nutrition, and Training   373

Postscript   381

    A Brother's Saga   382

Glossary   385
Bibliography   412
Index   417

FOREWORD

A GREAT WORKOUT FOR YOUR BODY OF KNOWLEDGE

A lot of bodybuilders in years past mistakenly believed that the best way to get big muscles was to use a class of drugs, both dangerous and illegal, called anabolic steroids. Sure, that's one way. But it's certainly not the best way.

As a two-time winner of the Mr. Universe bodybuilding championship, I know a thing or two about getting big muscles, believe me! There are a lot of good bodybuilding methods. Some are better than others. But I can tell you that there's only one best way to get massive—through hard, disciplined, focused, scientific, integrated training coupled with state-of-the-art nutrition. For all other athletes wishing to excel in their respective sports, it's the same.

Every sport has its own unique requirements. But it's also true that all sports (especially bodybuilding) share one requirement that is by far the most important—muscular strength. Where does the strength for producing great force output come from? Of course, it comes from muscle.

Wait a minute, though! Marathon runners can't have massive muscles or they'd never make it through twenty-six miles. Featherweight boxers or wrestlers can't have huge muscles, either—they'd have to compete at a higher weight division if they put on too much muscle. The answer again lies in science. Sometimes you have to know how to produce great strength without the encumbrance of massive muscles. On the other hand, in some sports it will be to your advantage to get bigger muscles. It all depends on the requirements of your sport. In the sport of bodybuilding, getting huge, ripped, and massively strong is the ultimate objective.

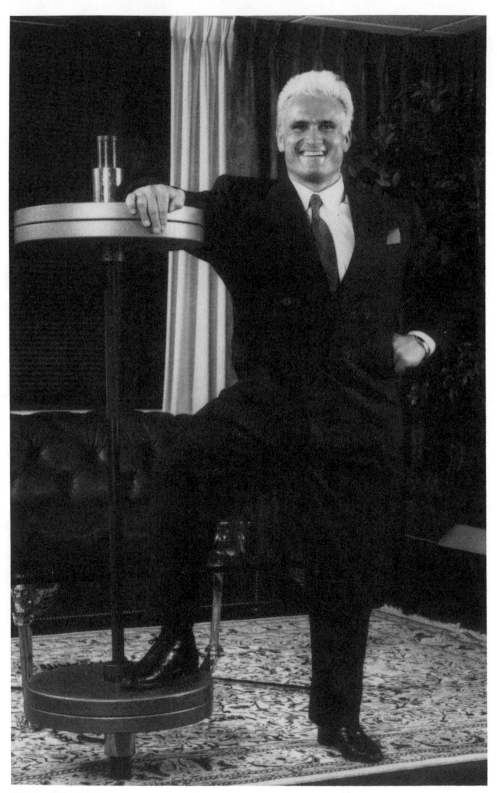

Tom Platz

I've had the pleasure of working with Dr. Hatfield (better known as Dr. Squat) for several years. He has assisted me in several aspects of my own training and nutrition program. While collaborating with eight-time Mr. Olympia bodybuilding champion Lee Haney (whom he also advised on bodybuilding science), Dr. Hatfield developed the winning training and nutrition program used by former heavyweight boxing champion Evander Holyfield to prepare for his title fight against Buster Douglas. Dr. Hatfield has worked with dozens of world-class athletes and bodybuilders in a similar fashion.

In case you didn't know it, Dr. Hatfield has broken dozens of world records in the premier sport of strength—powerlifting. He lifted more weight in competition than any man in the history of the world. He knows what strength as well as big muscles are all about.

If you're really into the great sport of bodybuilding, getting massively huge and "shredded" is great. If you're an athlete from any other sport, getting as big as you need to be in order to improve your total sports performance capabilities is the name of the game. Dr. Hatfield has given you the ultimate bible of bodybuilding greatness.

Listen to him and learn. Knowledge *is* power. And always remember—you *can* do it without drugs.

Tom Platz
Two-Time Mr. Universe

PREFACE

This book is about the intricacies of integrated bodybuilding science. You will learn how to get big and get cut without having to resort to dangerous drugs. But like anything that's worth having, there's a price you must be willing to pay. You've got to want to do things right. You've got to work at it long enough for it to pay you the dividends you seek.

WHY BODYBUILD IN THE FIRST PLACE?

Who cares about getting big, healthy, good-looking muscles? Only a pencilneck would ask such a question. *You* do! But do you have the guts to do what it takes to make it happen? Find the guts! I'll show you the best, most efficient way you can, based on what science has to offer.

Let's start with the obvious question. Why build your body? What are, or what should, your objectives be? First, bodybuilding promotes health. All of your body's systems benefit, not just your muscles. Your heart, your lungs, your self-esteem, even your sex life all become healthier when you live the bodybuilding lifestyle.

Second, with better health comes improved strength, muscle size, and general fitness. Strength, muscle mass, and fitness are hard to come by if all you're doing is lifting weights, though. You must truly believe in and live the bodybuilding lifestyle. With optimum health and fitness, you are ready to begin pushing the limits of your total body strength and size upward to a level of muscle mass that few dare dream about, let alone achieve. If you can visualize yourself growing lean and massive beyond mere convention, that is where you must go.

WHAT IS "INTEGRATED BODYBUILDING TRAINING"?

If you had to put a name to something that greatly surpassed anything that has gone before it, what would you call it? Something that was so profoundly superior to its relatively paltry predecessors, so utterly complete and powerful in its unique assemblage of both manmade and natural forces that nothing could possibly surpass it?

Many things come to mind. Whatever it is, it represents the nth degree of man's technological inventiveness, the nth degree of nature's awesome power. Something that has progressed by multiplicative power beyond the comprehension of mere corporate marketeers, into the passionate, dedicated domain of hard-core bodybuilders who aspire to greatness, to a state of being wherein only the strong survive.

No, fellow iron freaks, it's not the twilight zone, and it's not merely rhetoric. It's real and it's explained in this book. It's the natural outcome of the aggregate genius of creative athletes and bodybuilders getting together and understanding that what the greats of yesterday did to become great is no longer enough. You, my friend, will have to do battle with men infinitely wiser than those greats of yesterday ever encountered.

Get this, and get it good. If you wanna play with the big boys, you're gonna have to be willing to pay the price. You'll never become a Mr. Olympia contender, let alone beat any serious competitors in the elite ranks of bodybuilding, by approaching your training as though it were a hobby.

Yes, champions *can* be made without drugs. The answer is scientific, integrated training . . . and a good measure of passion.

Frederick C. Hatfield, Ph.D.
"Dr. Squat"

ACKNOWLEDGMENTS

TitanSports, Inc., the parent company of the World Wrestling Federation, World Bodybuilding Federation, and ICOPRO, Inc. (Integrated Conditioning Programs), is acknowledged for its support and encouragement in this major endeavor. All of the posing and exercise photographs in this book were provided by TitanSports and were taken by bodybuilding photographer Robert Reiff of Los Angeles.

The International Sports Sciences Association (ISSA) has worked diligently over the past few years to establish a credible, comprehensive, and comprehensible curriculum for certifying personal fitness trainers and sports conditioning specialists (strength coaches). Much of the information in this book originated with my efforts on ISSA's behalf while fulfilling its mission to bring integrated science into the gyms.

PART ONE

INTRODUCTION TO BODYBUILDING

DEDICATED TO GARY STRYDOM

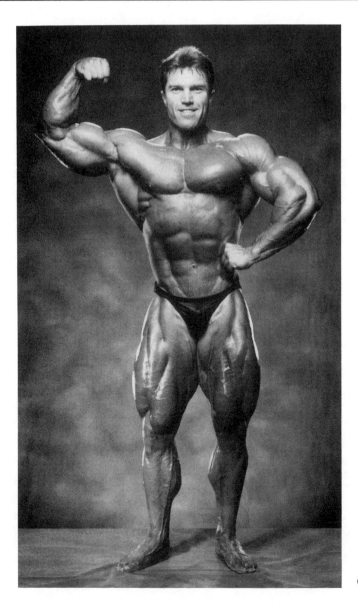

Gary Strydom

1

BODYBUILDING IS UNIQUE

Bodybuilding is the only sport wherein developing an aesthetically pleasing appearance by selectively maximizing your muscles' mass is the ultimate objective. Bodybuilders do not have to perform skilled movements or display great speed, strength, or stamina during competition in the same sense as other athletes.

Bodybuilding's uniqueness doesn't end there. The methods of training used to become a great bodybuilder are also radically different. Consider, for example, that a shot putter's objective is to put a 16-pound chunk of iron as far out from a seven-foot circle as possible. That requires great explosive and starting strength. The shot putter's methods of training reflect his ultimate objective. The same holds true for a powerlifter and a wrestler. All athletes key in on competition objectives when they choose their training methods.

Bodybuilders, however, must train for the explosiveness of the shot putter, the strength endurance of a wrestler, and the limit strength of a powerlifter. Bodybuilders must use a broad array of training techniques in order to get each and every muscle cell—and each of the subcellular elements of each muscle cell—to increase in size or number. That's where great muscular size comes from.

To understand this concept fully, and to put it into practice in your own bodybuilding efforts, you will have to understand the very essence of human movement. What makes humans able to move? Muscles. What gives our muscles the wherewithal to move us? Their inherent ability to contract—their strength. What is strength? Read on.

2

STRENGTH: YOUR FOUNDATION

Strength. It's a word you've grown comfortable with because of your intimate relationship with it. Most of you use this word every day. But it's an infinitely complex concept that cannot be adequately defined in a single fleeting thought or sentence. So many factors interrelate to produce it, and it can be physically expressed in a multitude of ways and under a vast array of metabolic and environmental circumstances.

If there were a single definition of strength, it would be as follows: "Your ability to contract your muscles with maximum force, given constraints stemming from: structural/anatomical factors, physiological/biochemical factors, psychoneural/psychosocial factors, and external/environmental factors."

Putting it into bodybuilding or sports-related terms, strength is your ability to exert musculoskeletal force against an external object such as a barbell, the ground, or an opponent. It comes from four main sources:

1. How your body is put together as a machine
2. How your internal systems work to create energy and to promote repair, remodeling, and growth in response to training
3. How your skills, attitudes, beliefs, and tolerance to pain all interrelate to allow your body to function at peak efficiency
4. How factors external to your body—weather, gravity, equipment, for example—can be manipulated to produce greater force output

As you read this book, you will begin to understand strength and how its various forms relate to successful bodybuilding. You will learn how to manipulate them at will as part of an integrated approach to scientific bodybuilding.

Strength is the universal requirement of all athletes in every sport. But you have to be careful to distinguish exactly what kind of strength you're talking about. There are at least five different categories of strength, and all sports require more or less of each and every kind. Problem is, which of the thirty-nine factors which affect strength do you need as a bodybuilder? Of those, which are most important? Look at Figure 2-1.

FIGURE 2-1

A Partial List of the Factors Affecting Strength

STRUCTURAL/ANATOMICAL

1. Muscle fiber arrangement
2. Musculoskeletal leverage
3. Tissue leverage (interstitial and intracellular leverage stemming from fat deposits, sarcoplasmic content, satellite cell proliferation, and the accumulation of fluid)
4. Freedom of movement between fibers and between gross muscles (scar tissue and adhesions can limit muscles' contractile strength)
5. Tissue viscoelasticity
6. Intramuscular/intracellular friction
7. Ratio of fast-, intermediate-, and slow-twitch fibers
8. Range of motion (must be normal)
9. Freedom from injury
10. Connective tissue (tendinous/ligamentous) mass and structural characteristics

PHYSIOLOGICAL/BIOCHEMICAL

11. Stretch reflex (muscle spindles)
12. Sensitivity of the Golgi tendon organ
13. Endocrine system functions (hormones)
14. Extent of conversion of Type IIb muscle fibers to Type IIa
15. Extent of myofibrillarization
16. Motor unit recruitment capacity
17. Energy transfer systems' efficiency
18. Extensiveness of capillarization
19. Mitochondrial growth and proliferation

20. Stroke volume of the left ventricle
21. Ejection fraction of the left ventricle
22. Pulmonary (ventilatory) capacity
23. Efficiency of gas exchange in the lungs
24. Heart rate
25. Max VO_2 uptake (volume of oxygen taken into your working muscles) (mil/kg bwt/min)
26. Freedom from disease
27. Extent of fusion of satellite cells with contractile cells (controlled by insulinlike growth factors I and II)

PSYCHONEURAL/PSYCHOSOCIAL

28. Arousal level ("psych")
29. Tolerance to pain (pain of effort, stress, or lactic acid accumulation in the cells and blood)
30. Ability to concentrate ("focus")
31. Incentive system installed (motivation)
32. Social learning (effectiveness of deinhibitory efforts in overcoming learned inhibitory responses)
33. Coordination ("skill" involving the efficient sequencing of activation/inhibition of prime movers, stabilizers, and synergists; sequencing efforts involve factors of position, direction, timing, rate, speed, and effect of force application)
34. Spiritual factors (acknowledged but unexplained)
35. The "placebo" effect

EXTERNAL/ENVIRONMENTAL

36. Equipment (use of the best available tools)
37. External environment (temperature, humidity, precipitation, wind, altitude)
38. Effect of gravity
39. Opposing and assisting forces (e.g., opponent's efforts may add to your force output vis-à-vis Newton's three laws of motion)

All of these factors can be augmented, manipulated, or in some way made more efficient through various and timely applications of one or more of the eight technologies of training (defined in Chapter Three). Bear in mind that many of the factors affecting strength are inextricably interrelated and may be directly or indirectly, positively or negatively, affected by your attempts to augment any of them, regardless of which technologies are employed in training.

From Figure 2-2, it's clear that only certain of the thirty-nine factors are most germane to your bodybuilding interests. We'll explore all the methods science has to offer to increase each of these factors and others of interest to you.

First, let's establish some working definitions for words and phrases commonly used in bodybuilding. Most of them are listed in the glossary of this book. The most important ones, however, are listed in the following chapter. Understanding each of these words and terms will allow you to read this book intelligently.

FIGURE 2-2

Factors Affecting Each Category of Strength and Factors Influencing Muscle Mass

TYPE OF STRENGTH	CRITICAL FACTORS	SOMETIMES IMPORTANT	RARELY IMPORTANT
Absolute and Limit Strength	1–4, 7, 9, 10, 12, 13, 15, 16, 26, 27, 30–32, 36, 38	5, 6, 8, 11, 14, 17, 18, 29, 33–35, 37–39	19–25
Speed-Strength	1, 2, 4, 5, 7, 9, 10–13, 15, 16, 26, 28, 30–32, 36	8, 14, 17–19, 28, 29, 33–35, 37–39	3, 6, 20–25, 27
Anaerobic Strength	2, 4, 7, 9, 14, 15, 17–19, 26, 29, 31, 32, 36	1, 5, 8, 10–13, 16, 20–25, 28, 30, 33–35, 37–39	3, 6, 27
Aerobic Strength	4, 7, 9, 14, 17–26, 29, 31, 32, 36	1, 2, 8, 13, 15, 16, 30, 33–35, 37, 38	3, 5, 6, 10–12, 27, 29, 39
Muscle Mass for Bodybuilding	3, 13, 15, 18, 19, 26, 27, 29	4, 7, 9, 10, 16, 17, 28, 30–32, 34, 35, 37	1, 2, 5, 6, 8, 11, 12, 14, 20–25, 33, 36, 38, 39

3

SOME TRAINING TERMS YOU SHOULD BE FAMILIAR WITH

LIMIT STRENGTH

How much musculoskeletal force you can generate for one all-out effort, limit strength is your bodybuilding foundation. All of your muscles should have a good level of limit strength. It's like building your house on a rock instead of the sand. While it's important for bodybuilders, only powerlifters need to maximize their limit strength for competition. There are three kinds of limit strength:

1. Eccentric strength: how much weight you can lower without losing control
2. Static strength: how much weight you can hold stationary without losing control
3. Concentric strength: how much weight you can lift one time with an all-out muscle contraction

ABSOLUTE STRENGTH

Absolute strength is the same as limit strength with one important distinction. Limit strength is achieved while under the influence of some form of work-producing aid (supplements, hypnosis, therapeutic techniques, etc.), while absolute strength is achieved through training alone—au naturel. That makes limit strength more important for your purposes. All bodybuilders should take every available advantage science has to offer, short of using drugs or other illegal techniques or strategies against the rules of the sport. Absolute strength is still an important concept for fitness enthusiasts, kids, and weekend warriors however. Usually, they aren't as scientific or as dedicated to excellence as competitive bodybuilders and may wish to train au naturel for their fitness or sports goals.

SPEED-STRENGTH

You may have heard this kind of strength referred to as power. Speed-strength, however, is a more descriptive term. There are two types of strength under the general heading of speed-strength: starting strength and explosive strength. Speed-strength is how well you apply force with speed. Its importance in bodybuilding cannot be overemphasized, as this kind of movement is what it takes to stimulate your fast-twitch muscle fibers to respond. Slow movements just won't do it.

Starting Strength

Your ability to turn on as many muscle fibers (muscle cells) as possible instantaneously is known as starting strength. Firing a 100-mph fastball requires tremendous starting strength, as does each footfall in a 100-meter sprint or throwing a quick knockout punch in boxing.

Explosive Strength

Once your muscle fibers are turned on, your ability to leave them turned on for a measurable period is referred to as *explosiveness*. A football lineman pushing his opponent or a shot putter putting the shot as far as possible is an example of explosive strength in action. Olympic-style weightlifting (snatch and clean and jerk) is perhaps the best example of maximum explosive strength in action. The ultimate form in which explosive strength is displayed is called *acceleration*.

Bodybuilding movements done with explosive, accelerative force is an advanced technique discussed in Part Eight of this book under the heading of Cheating Movements.

ANAEROBIC STRENGTH

The word *anaerobic* means without oxygen. If your activity is performed without your muscles having to be supplied with oxygen, it's anaerobic. Of course, you need oxygen to stay alive, and you'll have to repay your muscles the oxygen debt you owe after performing anaerobically. You do this by breathing hard once you stop. Scientists classify movements in sports as being driven by the ATP/CP energy pathway, the glycolytic pathway, or the oxidative pathway. The first two categories do not involve oxygen and are therefore considered anaerobic. ATP/CP refers to the biochemicals inside your muscles that produce energy for your muscles to work (adenosine triphosphate and creatine phosphate). Glycolytic refers to the sugar stored inside your muscles (glycogen). When you run out of ATP and CP, you have to begin using that glycogen to resynthesize the ATP and CP so work can continue. Neither of these two muscle energy processes need oxygen for them to work.

Linear Anaerobic Strength Endurance

Your ability to sustain all-out, maximum running speed is an example of linear anaerobic strength endurance. Believe it or not, even Carl Lewis begins to slow down during the last 40 meters of a 100-meter race! The extent to which he is forced to slow down because of fatigue during the last half of the race is his measure of linear anaerobic strength endurance. The word *linear* simply means that the same movement is repetitively performed, such as running strides or doing reps in bodybuilding. Marathon running, then, is an example of linear aerobic strength endurance.

Nonlinear Anaerobic Strength Endurance

Your ability to play with exceeding explosiveness for four quarters is an example of nonlinear anaerobic strength endurance. A powerlifter in competition must perform 9 maximum lifts on the lifting platform and perhaps as many as 20 near-maximum warm-up lifts during a three- or four-hour competition. That also requires tremendous anaerobic strength endurance. Because the lifts are performed between intervals of time (as opposed to rowing, running, or other linear sports movements), it's nonlinear anaerobic strength endurance. Playing a particularly fast-paced basketball game or soccer match for an hour or two would be examples of nonlinear aerobic strength endurance, and also intermittent bursts of speed-strength (jumping, starting, dodging, etc.).

AEROBIC STRENGTH

The word *aerobic* means with oxygen. The efficiency with which you get oxygen to your working muscles and remove the metabolic wastes that are building up there is called cardiovascular endurance, which is the key to exerting force under aerobic conditions.

There are two kinds of aerobic strength: linear and nonlinear. These two terms are described above in the discussion of anaerobic strength. Measures of your cardiovascular efficiency are a low heart rate (how many times your heart beats each minute), a high stroke volume (how much blood you pump out of your heart with each beat), a high ejection fraction of the left ventricle (the percentage of blood in the left ventricle of your heart muscle that's pushed out with each beat), and a high maximum oxygen uptake ability (how much oxygen your muscles use during exercise).

Bodybuilders have little need for a high level of aerobic strength. In fact, it would be counterproductive for them to acquire it.

THE EIGHT TECHNOLOGIES OF TRAINING

The eight technologies of weight training are branches of science of greatest consequence to bodybuilders. Each represents a different approach to getting bigger and more cut up. Remember that there are only so many hours in the day, so make prudent use of the technologies that will yield the greatest returns to you.

The basic rule of thumb in choosing the technologies that will give you the most "bang for your buck" is to zero in on the most important training objectives for the training mesocycle you're in. Then, through a multiplicative approach that incorporates the concepts of integration and synergy (that's what this book is all about), you choose the methods that will get you to your goals most quickly and to the greatest extent possible.

Weight Training

Dumbbells, barbells, fluids, pressurized air, elastic devices, springs, and the host of devices designed to provide heavy external resistance to one's musculoskeletal effort all constitute resistance training.

Tradition has it that exercises designed to be performed with dumbbells and barbells (and the technologies designed to simulate traditional dumbbell and barbell movements) constitutes weight training. The existing categories of weight training technologies are constant resistance devices, variable resistance devices, accommodating resistance devices, and static resistance devices. New technologies will be developed in time.

Special Forms of Resistance Training

Running, swimming, calisthenics, aerobic dance, and plyometrics are among the special forms of light resistance training. Body weight alone is the source of resistance. Cycling, rowing, stair-climbers, and similar forms of training which utilize light external resistance collectively constitute a second category of light resistance training.

Psychological Techniques

Self-hypnosis, mental imagery training, transcendental meditation, and a lot of other "mind games" can help improve your strength-output capabilities in training. Perhaps most important are the methods at your disposal for maintaining motivation, incentive, and self-image.

Therapeutic Modalities

Whirlpools, heat, ice, electrical muscle stimulation, massage, ultra-sound, music, intense light, and a host of other therapies can have a very positive effect on your strength training efforts, both indirectly (how quickly you can recover from your previous workout) and directly (greater force output).

Medical Support

Periodic checkups, preventive care, chiropractic adjustments, and even clinical use of prescription drugs are sometimes indicated for

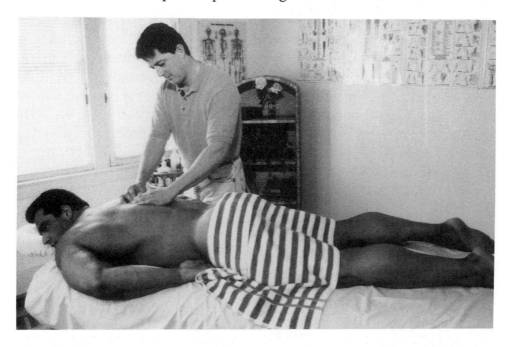

Chiropractic care is elemental to bodybuilding longevity.

bodybuilders in heavy training when medical problems arise. Only qualified sports-medicine specialists are able to prescribe such support.

Biomechanics (Skill) Training

Performing your skill perfectly will almost always result in greater force being applied, whether it is applied to an object, an opponent, or the ground. Good skills execution involves the efficient sequencing of activation/inhibition of prime-mover, stabilizer, and synergistic muscles. Your sequencing efforts involve factors of position, direction, timing, rate, speed, and effect of force application.

Dietary Manipulation Techniques

Athletes don't eat only to stay alive and healthy; they eat to excel at their sport. Their eating is designed to assist in achieving specific sports/training objectives. Many nutritional techniques will ensure greater force output capabilities both immediately as well as over time, thereby improving your training and competition efforts. Despite your most dedicated efforts, however, you will not be able to gain ample nutritional support from food alone, a point which has been supported time and time again in sports nutrition research.

Nutritional Supplementation

Most often, eating is not sufficient to give you all the nutrients you need in order to achieve your sports/training objectives. This point is widely disputed among sports scientists and nutritionists alike who would have us believe that eating three square meals per day is ample fare for athletes in heavy training. They overlook at least three important points: many state-of-the-art supplements are designed to take your body beyond normal biochemical functioning, no one on Earth consistently eats square meals, and myriad research reports clearly show that deficiencies exist in athletes' diets for many reasons.

4

THE FACTORS CONTRIBUTING
TO MUSCLE MASS

"Gotta go train" is a phrase heard by bodybuilders' spouses everywhere. What does it mean? It typically means going to a gym to lift weights. Many of the factors affecting mass are augmented in ways other than merely lifting weights.

Tch, tch! Lifting weights is *not* bodybuilding! It's certainly an integral part of bodybuilding training, but there's so much more.

We've identified what strength is and where it comes from. Now we have to lay down some simple guidelines as to how each of the factors affecting strength can be augmented in such a way that muscle mass will be enhanced.

MATCHING TRAINING TECHNOLOGIES
TO TRAINING OBJECTIVES

Now you know which of the various classifications of strength most contribute to muscle mass and the technologies of training you must employ in order to increase mass. Let's explore some of what you'll have to learn how to manipulate in the interests of getting massive.

Some of the factors listed under "sometimes important" in Figure 2-2 may indeed be important some of the time, especially among beginners who have no background in high-level training for muscle mass. But let's concentrate on the critical factors that will give most of us the greatest returns in muscle mass for immediate and long-term bodybuilding excellence.

Your job—which I've done for you throughout the remainder of this book—is always going to be to identify and apply those technologies which best augment each of the important factors and incorporate them into a coherent, integrated training program.

As you read the following discussions on the factors that contribute to muscle mass, bear in mind that the "Factor" numbers in parentheses correspond to the factors listed in Figure 2-1.

FACTORS AFFECTING MUSCULAR GROWTH

Muscle Fiber Arrangement (Factor 1)

Sorry, folks, but there's nothing you can do about this one. You can, however, take advantage of your knowledge about how the fibers of each muscle are arranged. Some are made for speed, some for great limit strength, some for stability, and some for all three. Train them that way (once in a while, at least). The theory is that by training a muscle the way Mother Nature intended for it to be used, you will experience growth that you otherwise might not have achieved. The technologies of choice: weight training, special forms of resistance training, and biomechanics (skill) training.

Musculoskeletal Leverage (Factor 2)

Again, nothing you can do short of radical surgical procedures will change your leverage. But, by knowing how best to take advantage of your leverage systems' structures, efficiency in lifting techniques (and thus your strength output) will optimize your training efficiency. The technology of choice: weight training and biomechanics (skill) training.

Tissue Leverage (Factor 3)

Interstitial and intracellular leverage stemming from fat deposits (both subcutaneous and intramuscular), sarcoplasmic content, satellite cell proliferation (see Factor 27), and the accumulation of intra- and extracellular fluid can, to a degree, augment both force output and gross size. Aside from ingesting certain illegal and potentially dangerous androgens or sheer gluttony, the best way to improve tissue leverage is through careful training, dietary manipulation, and supplementation.

Freedom of Movement Between Fibers (Factor 4)

Adhesions and scar tissue between muscle fibers and between gross muscles can limit your muscles' ability to contract fully. They can also limit your muscles' ability to grow. Neuromuscular reeducation, postworkout rolfing, and other forms of deep fiber massage (often called *sports massage*) are the best therapies. Postworkout ultrasound treatments, a postworkout whirlpool, or a hard-beating shower on your just-trained muscles also helps tremendously in eliminating or avoiding these strength- and size-limiting adhesions and scar tissue. The technologies of choice: biomechanics (skill) training, various therapeutic modalities, and medical support systems.

Ratio of Fast-, Intermediate-, and Slow-Twitch Fibers (Factor 7)

It used to be believed that heredity controlled your fiber ratios. True, to a large degree. However, as you will see (in Factor 27), some conversion within the Type II fiber category can take place. Remember that your white muscle fibers (the ones that contract explosively) have a greater capacity to hypertrophy than do your red (slow-twitch) fibers. Engaging in *very* explosive training will selectively stress your white muscle fibers (fast-twitch fibers). The technologies of choice: biomechanics (skill) training, weight training, and various other forms of light resistance training.

Freedom from Injury (Factor 9)

Obviously, an injury can keep you from your goal of greatness. Even minuscule ones can nag you enough to prevent you from training effectively. What's the best way to treat injuries? Avoid them! That means following excellent technique and integrated training principles. The technologies of choice: medical support systems, various therapeutic modalities, biomechanics (skill) training, weight training, and various other forms of light resistance training.

Connective Tissue Structure (Factor 10)

Tendinous and ligamentous mass and their structural characteristics all contribute to your potential strength level. Did you know, for example, that the collagenous matrix comprising various ligaments and tendons is susceptible to change through highly specialized training? Check into it!

You know that maximum limit strength will increase your ability to inflict maximum adaptive stress upon your muscles. A serendipitous outcome is that you will have injury-proofed yourself in the process. The technologies of choice: various therapeutic modalities, biomechanics (skill) training, weight training, and various other forms of light resistance training.

Endocrine System Functions (Hormones) (Factor 13)

Your hormones ebb and flow according to your body's little-understood circadian rhythms or in response to internal and external stimuli. You can indeed control many of them, and doing so requires a full understanding of circadian rhythmicity and the host of stimulatory factors. Many of the factors of interest to bodybuilders are covered in Part Six. The technologies of choice: dietary and nutritional supplementation strategies, various therapeutic modalities, weight training, and various other forms of light resistance training. Of greatest influence is the precise scheduling of the appropriate technologies of training in such a way that they coincide with, or in some way enhance, your circadian rhythm.

Extent of Myofibrillarization (Factor 15)

Myofibrils are the actual contractile elements within your working muscles. Old technology had it that all you had to do was increase the number of myofibrils inside each cell to increase your limit strength. Sure—if you want to remain in the also-ran group. For bodybuilders, increased myofibrillarization will give you that much sought-after appearance of muscular density. The technologies of choice: dietary and nutritional supplementation strategies, biomechanics (skill) training, weight training, and various other forms of light resistance training.

Motor Unit Recruitment (Factor 16)

Firing as many muscle fibers as possible instantly is the name of the game in speed-strength (both starting strength and explosive strength). It's also the name of the game in limit strength. For bodybuilders, achieving maximum fiber recruitment will ensure maximum myofibrillarization spoken of in Factor 15. The technologies of choice: several psychological and psychosocial strategies, biomechanics (skill) training, "controlled" ballistic weight training, and various other forms of light resistance training.

Energy Transfer Systems' Efficiency (Factor 17)

Understanding how your muscles produce energy and learning how to manipulate the biochemical processes hold an important key to maximizing training efficiency. The only substance that will cause your muscles to contract is ATP (adenosine triphosphate), and you run out of it within 2–3 seconds of training. CP (creatine phosphate) is broken down to produce more ATP, and you run out of it quickly as well. Sugar stored in your muscles (glycogen) has to be metabolized in order to make more CP. Lactic acid is formed by the metabolic process of glycogen utilization and is the nasty stuff that causes fatigue and forces your muscles to stop contracting. The best way to get rid of lactic acid is by getting some oxygen to the working muscles. At that point, continued training is called aerobic training because oxygen is involved. Until oxygen became involved, your training energy was purely anaerobic (without oxygen).

Got all that? It's not important for you to remember all the particulars, but it *is* of critical importance for you to learn how best to manipulate your muscles' abilities to get rid of lactic acid and replace oxygen. The training technologies of choice: special forms of resistance training, various therapeutic modalities, dietary manipulation, and nutritional supplementation.

Extensiveness of Capillarization (Factor 18)

Capillaries, as you know, are what bring nutrients and oxygen to your working muscles. They also get rid of metabolic wastes formed as a result of energy expenditure during training stress. The amazing thing about capillaries is that you can radically increase their extensiveness in a muscle. What does that result in? Obviously, if you can get more nutrients in and wastes out, you can support greater muscle growth. The technology of choice: high rep, continuous tension weight training.

Mitochondrial Growth and Proliferation (Factor 19)

Mitochondria are tiny organelles inside your muscle cells that manufacture ATP and perform all of the oxidative functions inside the cell. They are often referred to as your muscle cells' powerhouses. Not only will your gut-busting training sessions become easier by increasing the number of them each cell has (so you can bust your gut more), but these little critters take up space. They have mass and they can contribute to greater overall muscle mass. High rep training is the technology of choice.

Freedom from Disease (Factor 26)

'Nuff said! The technologies of choice: dietary and nutritional strategies, various therapeutic modalities, and medical intervention.

Extent of Fusion of Satellite Cells with Contractile Cells (Controlled by IGF-I and IGF-II) (Factor 27)

During eccentric contraction (i.e., "lowering" the weight), damage is inflicted upon your fast-twitch fibers that have a low resistance to fatigue (type IIb fibers). The microtrauma to these fibers causes certain biochemicals to be released into the interstitial spaces, causing the adjacent "satellite" cells (noncontractile cells) to fuse with the damaged contractile cells, thereby giving it greater resistance to damage—and greater size.

Arousal Level ("Psych") (Factor 28)

'Nuff said! The technology of choice: psychological and psychosocial strategies.

Tolerance to Pain (Factor 29)

The buildup of lactic acid inside your working muscles causes sensations of pain because nerve endings in the area are irritated. Microtrauma (tiny tears in your muscle cells caused by lifting heavy weights) causes a caustic biochemical called hydroxyproline to irritate surrounding nerve endings as well. Macrotrauma (caused by either cumulative microtrauma or a high volume of trauma suddenly inflicted on tissue) causes pain because of massive destruction of tissue and surrounding nerve endings.

The first two types of pain—lactic acid buildup and microtrauma—are not considered dangerous and, in fact, are desirable. But the frequency and extent of damage must be controlled through periodizing your training. In the case of macrotrauma, the third kind of pain, well, seek medical attention. Better still, avoid it in the first place.

Ability to Concentrate ("Focus") (Factor 30)

Your mind is said to be the master of your body. My experience tells me that with a great majority of bodybuilders the reverse holds true. Tch, tch! The technologies of choice: psychological and psychosocial techniques, dietary and nutritional supplementation strategies, and biomechanics (skill) training.

Incentive System Installed (Motivation) (Factor 31)

In short, you've gotta *want* it! The technologies of choice: psychological and psychosocial strategies.

Social Learning (Effectiveness of Deinhibitory Efforts in Overcoming Learned Inhibitory Responses) (Factor 32)

Overcoming learned inhibitory responses can be a monumental undertaking, especially in light of the fact that your mama scolded you for years not to lift something, run too fast, or whatever, because it'd hurt you. The technologies of choice: psychotherapy and hypnotherapy.

Coordination (Skill) (Factor 33)

The skills of bodybuilding, to be sure, are not the sort normally required by athletes in any other sport. However, the ability to manipulate weights and other forms of resistance in such a way that maximum benefit is derived does take some learning. Skill can be defined as the efficient sequencing of muscles (all of them) with body position, timing, and movement's direction, speed, and force. Learning to choose the best exercises is crucial; this factor is discussed body part per body part in Part Four.

Equipment (Use of the Best Available Tools) (Factor 36)

Are you able to take full advantage of your body's leverage with crummy shoes? A bent bar? Poor equipment? A cold gym? The list is endless. These external factors render your force output efforts less than efficient, and it's time you did something about it! That is, *if* you aspire to greatness!

5

PRINCIPLES OF TRAINING

All forms of training are based on the principle that the body adapts to the type and amount of stress placed upon it. Both the amount and type of stress are easily varied to accommodate any training or fitness goal.

The various forms of weight training are well suited to impose precise types of stress on your muscles and other body systems in such a way that they are forced to respond by adapting to that stress. They do this through anabolism (growth and development) and catabolism (breaking down). These two terms are collectively referred to as your metabolism.

Several collections of principles have been espoused by various fitness authors over the years. Two popular and very good ones for beginners and intermediates getting into bodybuilding training are the FITT principle and the five Rs principle.

THE FITT PRINCIPLE

The FITT principle applies to any type of resistance training, whether it be for limit strength, speed-strength, anaerobic strength, or aerobic strength. FITT is the acronym for Frequency, Intensity, Time, and Type of Exercise. It is especially suited to a beginner's efforts because it spells out exactly what he or she should do to get started. Applying the FITT principle will ensure that your training is reasonably effective. There are four components to this principle:

Frequency of Exercise

How often should you exercise each week? Answer: Twice for maintenance, three times for beginners, five times for serious fitness enthusiasts, and up to fourteen or more times for dedicated and elite bodybuilders.

Intensity of Exercise

How hard should you exercise? Answer: If training two or three times weekly, train with high intensity; if training five or more times weekly, periodize your program into macrocycles, mesocycles, and microcycles, with microcyclic intensity variations applied to each body part to avoid undertraining and overtraining.

Time To Exercise

How long should you exercise each session? Answer: For anaerobic objectives, train for about an hour or so each workout; for aerobic objectives, train for up to two hours each session.

Type of Exercise

What exercises are best? Answer: Beginners training two or three times weekly should choose an array of exercises and exercise methods to reverse the processes of disuse in all major muscle groups and bodily systems. Athletes do likewise, but only during their off-season. Pre- and in-season training must be highly specific to the tasks/skills of their respective sports.

THE FIVE Rs PRINCIPLE

The five Rs are important parts of any beginner's or intermediate's fitness training program. While similar in scope to FITT, the five Rs key on slightly different elements of training technique. The reasonable answer as to which of the two principles is best is that both are good, and either may be applied to your early training career as a bodybuilder. These R principles do not always apply to elite bodybuilders' training because of the often severe and highly specialized objectives and techniques they must incorporate in their training.

Range of Motion

When we speak of range of motion, we mean the complete movement capability of a joint. Each and every exercise a beginning bodybuilder does should be performed through the complete range of motion, in other words, from a fully stretched position of the targeted muscle(s) to a fully contracted position.

As important, each and every muscle spanning (or acting upon) a given joint should be exercised in order to fully maintain or improve that joint's range of movement.

Resistance

The resistance (that is, the weight moved, or the air pressure you're pushing against on Keiser equipment) must be just enough so that the exercise can be performed through its full range of motion without cheating, or using body swing. Yet, the resistance must be such that it taxes your muscles for the desired number of repetitions.

Repetitions

When choosing the number of repetitions (how many times the exercise is to be done), you must first decide what results you want from the program. Generally, low repetitions (3–8) produce absolute strength. Medium repetitions (10–20) produce anaerobic strength endurance. High repetitions (30–40) produce aerobic strength endurance.

As a bodybuilder who is training for increased muscle mass, you should do many sets of many different weights, speeds, and repetitions in order to get as many elements of your muscles to adapt. This sort of variation in your training is the key to maximum size increases.

Despite your muscular size increases from such varied training, you will not have the same absolute or limit strength, as, for example, a powerlifter who trains strictly for absolute or limit strength. This R relates to the fact that your training efforts will yield more generalized results because you are applying stress to your muscles in several different ways. Athletes in other sports must train in a far more specific way depending upon the requirements of their respective sports.

Rest

The fourth R is rest. Your body needs about two to four minutes of rest between each set of repetitions before it is ready to function near full capacity again. For example, several repetitions of the curl would constitute one set of curls. A second set of repetitions should begin after about two to four minutes of rest. The first set will have depleted the cells' adenosine triphosphate (ATP) and creatine phosphate (CP), your muscles' energy for contraction. ATP and CP cannot be replenished in less than about two minutes.

Recovery

The last R, recovery, is very important. Adequate time must be allowed between one workout and the next so the exercised muscles can complete their recovery processes. As a general rule, you should not exercise the same muscle group two days in a row, and usually not more than three times a week. Otherwise, your body will eventually become fatigued and reach a stale, or overtrained, state. If you do not give your muscles a rest, they will take one on their own—you'll get overtrained or, worse, injured. In sports-medicine circles, this phenomenon is commonly called the overuse syndrome and results from cumulative microtrauma.

THE OVERLOAD PRINCIPLE

In order to gain increased fitness from any training, you must exercise against a resistance greater than that normally encountered. For example, overload is using a resistance that is heavier than you've already adapted to. If you use the same amount of resistance for the same number of repetitions every workout, there will be no continued improvement. This doesn't necessarily imply that you are training improperly. In fact, many people are quite happy to follow the same program day in and day out. But it's just not going to increase their muscular performance over their present state. They are merely practicing a maintenance program. As a bodybuilder, the name of the game for you is progressively advancing in your mass and strength increases.

FIGURE 5-1

A Schematic Representation of the Recovery Process

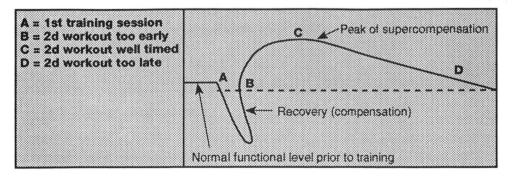

A = 1st training session
B = 2d workout too early
C = 2d workout well timed
D = 2d workout too late

Peak of supercompensation

Recovery (compensation)

Normal functional level prior to training

This progression involves the principles of overload and adaptation. In order to experience continued training benefits, you must continually increase the overload stress as your body adapts to the current overload. You can maintain your current level of muscular fitness with as little as two workouts a week. But, in order to continue your progress, you'll need more than that. Much more.

THE SPECIFICITY PRINCIPLE

Your various bodily systems will adapt in highly specific ways to the demands you impose upon them in your training. Another name for this is the SAID principle, an acronym for Specific Adaptation to Imposed Demands.

If your training objectives include becoming more explosive, then you have to train explosively. If you desire greater limit strength, you must use very heavy weights. If your objectives include deriving cardiovascular benefits, then you must tax the heart muscle as well as the oxygen-using abilities of the working muscles.

And so it goes. For every type of strength, for every training objective, there are specific methods you must employ. Simply running or pumping iron indiscriminately will not bring you to successful goal attainment. Remember this principle as the "good, better, best" principle:

- Doing something is better than doing nothing, and that's *good*
- Training regularly with an appropriate system is *better*
- It's *best*, however, to follow a carefully integrated system which accounts for all of your training goals and which employs all of the various training technologies you have at your disposal

THE USE/DISUSE PRINCIPLE

The principle of use/disuse applies to both training and detraining (cessation of training). If you stress your body and its systems enough, it will adapt to meet the stress. For example, in a bodybuilding program, hypertrophy, or increase in size, occurs in the trained muscle. If you stop stressing it through disuse or detraining, it will adapt to meet the lowered stress. In other words, when you stop your bodybuilding training program, atrophy (decrease in size) occurs in the previously trained muscle. Unfortunately, it takes much less time to become detrained than it does to become trained. The detraining effect is known as the law of reversibility. Fortunately, there is some sort of muscle memory which allows you to regain your strength or size more quickly than it took to gain it in the first place.

SOME GENERAL RULES OF TRAINING

Equipment

Check to see that the resistance level on the exercise station you are about to use is set at a very low resistance level. Before starting an exercise, be sure that you have a feel for the level of resistance on the machine. Never load up the device in an extended body position; increasing the resistance should always be done in the natural position (slightly flexed joint to better feel the resistance being added).

If you are unfamiliar with how the machine you are about to use can be adjusted to your body, check with the certified trainer working at the gym. So many new models of gym equipment are on the market nowadays that you can't know the ins and outs of how to use all of them. Always make certain that each piece of equipment works properly before using it.

Breathing

Two general rules about breathing should be followed when working out on exercise equipment:

1. Do not hold your breath continuously for several consecutive repetitions. Holding your breath during an entire set of repetitions could lead to dizziness and possible fainting, among other more serious complications.
2. Try to develop a rhythmic pattern of breathing that corresponds to the exercise cycle. Exhale during the most strenuous (concentric) portion of each repetition, and inhale during the least strenuous (eccentric) portion.

Here is an example of proper breathing during a military (overhead) press repetition. Inhale as you bring the bar toward your shoulders during the eccentric phase of the repetition. Exhale as your arms extend upward over your head. Exhale slowly and continuously. When you finish the press, you should have no more air in your lungs and should be ready to inhale for the eccentric (down) phase.

Warm-ups

People who train have a tendency to take warming up for granted. Pump a few weights, jog in place, and *wham!* Hit the heavy stuff. Well, it's not that simple.

The theoretical purposes of warm-up exercises include increased muscle temperature associated with enhanced dissociation of oxygen from red blood cells, improved metabolic adjustment to heavy work, increased velocity of nerve conduction, and greater numbers of capillaries opened in the muscles.

There are several psychological factors involved in warm-ups. Skilled performances improve with warm-ups using activity identical or directly related to the sport. Prior physical activity improves the mental set or attitude of the athlete, especially when the activity is identical or directly related to the skill. Warm-ups cause an increased arousal, or enthusiasm, eagerness, and mental readiness. There is one potentially negative effect of warm-ups—fatigue from the prior activity can decrease performance.

Most athletes are told to do their warm-ups faithfully and have accepted the need to do so as dogma. Clinically, there appears to be strong theoretical support for warming up as a deterrent to injury. However, in the real world of training and competition, as well as in research literature, there appears to be little support for the notion that warming up will reduce the incidence of injury.

Several years ago, Dr. B. Don Franks, a sports physiologist, investigated three areas of concern regarding whether warm-ups improve athletic performance: the circumstances under which performance could be enhanced, the circumstances under which performance could be diminished, and circumstances under which no change in performance will occur. Here is my interpretation of Franks's general findings:

1. Athletes engaged in short, explosive types of sports such as powerlifting benefit from warming up vis-à-vis improved performance.
2. Athletes engaged in progressive-type sports or endurance events do not benefit from warming up.
3. Warming up before an endurance-type sport often will decrease performance because of fatigue.
4. Direct warm-ups (exercise directly related or the same as the sport) of moderate intensity and duration prior to explosive sports enhances trained athletes' performance but not necessarily that of untrained athletes.
5. Indirect warm-ups (exercise not directly related to the sport) often can aid performance, as can bicycling for 4–5 minutes and/or flexibility (stretching) exercises.
6. Almost all studies showing a detrimental effect from warm-

ing up used as the subjects untrained people who apparently cannot tolerate high-intensity warm-ups.

7. Heavy, nonrelated warm-ups interfere with one's ability to perform sports skills requiring careful control.

8. Your warm-up should ensure improved performance, and only careful experimenting will yield the best type, intensity, and duration for you.

In general, it seems that the widely held belief in warming up prior to training or competition needs to be carefully considered before a specific warm-up program is adopted.

In bodybuilding, there appears to be little justification for warming up at any vigorous level. Typically, the exercise itself serves as sufficient warm-up. But, unlike other sports, there's probably no good reason *not* to warm up, either. If you do, use light weights for the targeted muscles or a general warm-up until you're lightly sweating.

One final point on warm-ups: *never* do flexibility exercises as a warm-up. Stretching a cold muscle is the easiest way to inflict microtrauma or (worse) macrotrauma.

Cooldown

At the end of each exercise session, cool down for five to ten minutes. This is especially important after high-intensity exercise which contains an anaerobic component (for example, very high-resistance training such as bodybuilding). Anaerobic exercise results in lactic acid accumulation in your bloodstream and muscles. A cooldown period of light aerobic activity and mild stretching will help remove the lactic acid. Also, the muscle soreness that usually follows heavy exercise (resulting not from lactic acid accumulation, as was once believed, but rather from microtrauma at the cellular level) is minimized or eliminated.

The poorest way to recover is to simply fall to the ground or sit around. The rhythmic contractions of your mildly active muscles help return blood to your heart. Many pints of blood are distributed to your working muscles during exercise and will tend to pool there rather than aid in swift removal of wastes and supply needed oxygen and nutrients (especially glucose for replacement of spent energy from muscle glycogen, and amino acids for repair and growth). Give your heart some help with light aerobic cooldown activities.

The cooldown should also contain mild stretching exercises for the muscles you just finished training. This will assist in avoiding postexercise muscle soreness by breaking up tiny adhesions resulting from the microtrauma they've just suffered during training. For all these reasons, it'll also assist your affected muscles' recovery.

CONCLUDING STATEMENT

Strength is the foundation upon which you can build the physique you've always wanted. If you're already an accomplished bodybuilder and have a few wins under your belt, it's the key you'll need to gain access to the circle of Olympians in this sport.

With anything less than supernormal strength, you will never be able to push each and every one of your muscles to the level of adaptive stress that's required for Olympian proportioning. Seek it, live for it. Eat, sleep, and breathe it. It is the very essence of bodybuilding and all other sports as well.

Part Two is your roadmap. But without acquiring strength to continue on your journey, you will never be able to reach your destination.

PART TWO
BODYBUILDING SYSTEMS
DEDICATED TO EDDIE ROBINSON

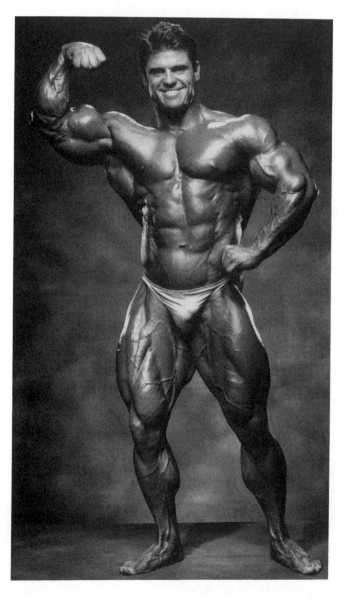

Eddie Robinson

6

THE BODYBUILDING LIFESTYLE

I hate the term *off-season*. Off from what? Sure, it makes a bit of sense to erstwhile athletes who "play" in seasonal sports. But to bodybuilders, there is no off-season. For dedicated athletes in general—even those in the seasonal sports—there is no such thing as an off-season either. If science has taught us anything, it's that bodybuilding, like all other sports endeavors, must be a lifestyle commitment. It must not be merely a precontest commitment—that is, if you aspire to greatness.

Speaking of lifestyle commitment, how can anyone in his right mind commit himself to greatness through the use of drugs? The sad truth is that many modern bodybuilders view drug use (particularly anabolic steroids, but there are many others) as an integral part of the sport of bodybuilding.

In the sport of bodybuilding, steroids are responsible for spawning fully three generations of lazy, poorly trained bodybuilders whose great appearance stemmed from a few short weeks of intensive precontest training, careful diet, and—woefully—prodigious stacks and staggers of steroids.

Imagine! Three generations of bodybuilders who never learned how to train or eat properly—properly, that is, had they never used steroids. Steroids, you see, have been the great equalizer in bodybuilding. With steroids, any pencilneck could get to look great with minimal effort and virtually no dedication to scientific conditioning practices.

30

Tragically, such people seem to have totally forgotten the deep and inspiring, almost religious, exhilarating purity of mind and body which compelled them to begin bodybuilding in the first place. To these generations of bodybuilders, the term *off-season* has traditionally meant cutting back on steroids, gaining a few pounds of ugly fat, and kicking back. They knew they could get away with it because of the steroids' effectiveness in guaranteeing a speedy (if not healthy) comeback in time for the next show.

To these generations of bodybuilders I bid adieu. Sayonara, adios, arrivederci, because they ain't gonna make it in today's world of drug-free training. They don't have the guts, they don't have the knowledge, and they lost the passion. They never acquired the sophistication of disciplined, integrated training because they never needed it. Drug-free bodybuilders need to stay in shape year-round. It's too hard to make comebacks. You should compete three times yearly. That way, you're always getting ready for a contest, and staying in shape will become an elemental part of your lifestyle.

Ever hear of the term *periodicity*? The former Soviets are credited with developing the concept to a keen science. In common parlance, periodicity means cycle training.

It makes scientific sense to construct a training "shell" which will be modified to reflect your uniqueness. Outlined later in this section is that universal shell. Assuming that you've already laid a solid bodybuilding foundation over years of time, it takes about sixteen weeks to really get contest-ready. A detailed, step-by-step guide to contest preparation is presented in Part Eleven.

7

THE ABCS OF
HARD-CORE BODYBUILDING

Most training systems never helped you with the down-and-dirty, nitty-gritty details of precise prescription of

- Reps
- Sets
- Precise poundage to use rep-per-rep or set-per-set
- Precise tonnage ("training load") to use workout-per-workout
- Recovery time
- Variability in cyclic changes in intensity
- What to eat
- When to eat it
- What to use for supplements
- What kind of therapies work best to speed recovery
- What kind of therapies work best to improve performance
- How often to sleep each day
- How long to sleep each time
- Exactly how fast to move each rep
- How to vary the speed of movement based on the muscle's structural characteristics

and the host of other factors important in successful bodybuilding. In short, no training regimen ever developed has given you a road-map through the complex array of training technologies in such a way that your training efforts will pay you the dividends you seek: peak performance, massive muscular size, and extremely low percent bodyfat.

I'd like to do this for you personally, but I can't. Too much info for a single book. These factors all change periodically as you advance in your training, and they're different for every bodybuilder. What I can—and will—do is give you a workable model that's utterly simplistic and quite revolutionary in scope. It's designed to make it totally easy for you to account for all the factors mentioned above in such a way that it fits you like a glove. It's the only way to personalize your training program. Even an ironhead who's hard-core to the bone can master it, because he has the guts, and he has the will. Do you? It isn't an easy row to hoe.

FIGURE 7-1

How to Periodize a Full Year's Training

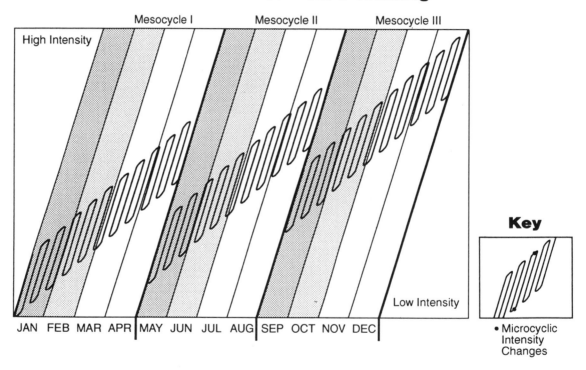

Take a look at Figure 7-1. I've presented a one-year period broken down into three macrocycles lasting four months. Each macrocycle has four mesocycles. For the sake of simplicity we can call this one-year period a *period*. In strict scientific terms, however, a true period is far longer—usually an entire portion of your sports career. Your bodybuilding career is further broken down into phases depending on what level of proficiency you've scheduled yourself to attain within the time frames of each phase of your career.

A macrocycle is an entire training cycle culminating in a competition (or peaking). Macrocycles are divided into mesocycles because as your training progresses and you get closer to a competition, your training objectives change accordingly. Your mesocycles are further reduced in size to fluctuating patterns of light, moderate, and heavy microcycles. These microcycles are the essence of day-to-day training and constitute that "revolutionary" concept of bodybuilding I promised you.

Not so revolutionary? Heard all that before? Guess again! This microcyclic concept is based on the variable rate of recovery for each individual muscle you train. It's based on achievement of at least three (for one-a-day training) to as many as seven (for three-a-day training) growth hormone peaks. And some scientists believe that you could benefit from as many as nine growth hormone peaks per day.

The system of microcycles is also based on carefully planned supplementation of your just as carefully planned meals. It's predicated on maximizing the adaptive overload each muscle receives irrespective of training intensity, and it's designed to allow you to take advantage of your own body's biochemistry and circadian rhythms. What's more, it's based upon my longstanding belief that bodybuilders needn't get cute with their exercise movements—just lift the damned bar! You don't need to twist the bar when curling it, you don't need to variably invert or evert your feet to hit all aspects of the calves, and you need never do umpteen different exercises per muscle. That's all bodybuilding mythology that is agonizingly slow in dying. Somehow, it stays alive because the perpetrators of such mythology feel that it makes them appear smarter to the guys they're trying to impress with their not-so-sage wisdom.

LEARNING YOUR ABCs

Choosing your exercises is as simple as ABC. Simply line up origin with insertion and contract the muscle in that direction while holding a weight.

I admit it's easier to just take the brain-dead advice of the muscular guy in the gym, but, believe me, it's not always the best thing to do. Oh, you'll make progress following his brain-dead advice, but for how long? To what extent? If it's anything less than the best science has to offer, I don't want to hear about it. I'm talkin' hard-core here!

Here are the ABCs:

A. Muscle-specific training (low intensity)
B. Targeted-sets training (medium-to-high intensity)
C. Holistic-sets training (ultrahigh intensity)

FIGURE 7-2

The ABCs of Bodybuilding Periodicity

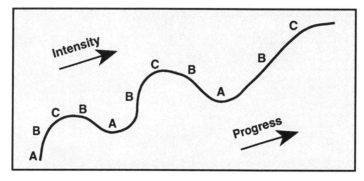

Key
A - Low Intensity
B - Moderate Intensity
C - High Intensity

The higher the intensity, the longer it takes to recover.
These numbers aren't holy. One "A" and three "Cs" for higher
intensity — three "As" and one "C" for lower intensity.

You do "A" training to recuperate a bit as well as to make gains. Why would you ever want an easy day if you were not to benefit? A lot of guys take an easy day because they're gym junkies. They can't stay away. They pump some light iron, call it a workout, and get absolutely nothing from it. There is a better way—"A" training. Your goal during light training days is to limit the amount of microtrauma you inflict on your muscle cells (particularly the fast-twitch fibers, which are prone to being torn because of their low tolerance to fatigue), and to still get significant benefit.

"A" training uses the simple set system. Each exercise is carefully chosen to involve the targeted muscle's major movement pattern (see Figure 7-3). By looking at the type of muscle (fast- or slow-twitch, and unipennate, bipennate, or multipennate) you're able to figure out exactly what kind of movement speed and load Mother Nature intended for that specific muscle. Then, do it.

You do "B" training as your bread-and-butter workouts. Do heavy, moderate, and light sets, targeting each of the important subcellular elements with very specific forms of overload. "B" training provides medium-to-heavy intensity. You target the specific cel-

FIGURE 7-3

Types and Functions of Muscle Fibers

FUNCTIONS

A—Contractile speed
B—Contractile force
C—Contractile force emphasized, with speed
D—Contractile speed emphasized, with force
E and F—Stabilizing force emphasized, short movements

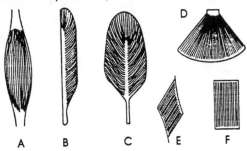

TYPES

A. Fusiform (biceps)
B. Penniform (peroneal muscles, tibialis posterior)
C. Bipenniform (rectus femoris)
D. Triangular or fan-shaped (temporals, latissimus, pectorals)
E. Rhomboidal or quadrilateral (intercostals)
F. Rectangular or quadrilateral (rhomboids, pronator quadratus)

lular elements you wish to stress, thereby forcing highly specific adaptive responses.

You do "C" training—holistic sets—only once each seven to ten days or so. It's an incredibly high intensity experience that goes beyond any form of bodybuilding training intensity you've ever experienced. It flat knocks you out. But it's exquisitely effective in blasting your muscles into a maximum growth mode.

Take a look at Figure 7-2 now. I've taken one mesocycle out of Figure 7-1 and filled in the "A"s, "B"s, and "C"s for you. There are some interesting qualities to this form of microcyclic variability. For instance, there are more "B" days than "A" or "C" days—remember, the "B" days are your bread and butter. You may find that you can recover faster, so more frequent "C" workouts—or fewer "A"s and "B"s—are called for. Maybe you aren't recovering enough in a specific body part between your "C" workouts, so you add an "A" or a "B." That's OK.

The precise pattern is something only personal experience can show you. Also, more for convenience and to better represent how things are most of the time for average bodybuilders, the "A"s, "B"s, and "C"s come in twos. One of the nice things about this system is that you can take a "C" away if it's too tough for you, or you can take an "A" away and add a "C" if it's too easy. Play with it—no schedule is holy.

The ABC table shown here is a good starting place for you. You can adjust it to fit your specific recuperative capabilities as you learn more about how your body responds to the schedule. Remember, each body part has its own unique recovery ability. The secret to integrated bodybuilding is to take advantage of all the safe and effective technologies (discussed in Part One) that can assist you in your quest for muscle mass.

Now comes the really neat stuff! As I noted earlier, each of your muscles has a different microcycle. Remember:

1. Big muscles take longer to recover than smaller ones
2. Fast-twitch muscles (your "explosive" muscles) take longer to recover than slow-twitch muscle fibers ("endurance" muscles)
3. Men recover faster than women (primarily because of hormonal differences)
4. You recover faster from slow movements than from fast movements
5. You recover faster from low-intensity training than from high-intensity training

One thing that's often overlooked is that you can't always train hard. You have to balance periods of high-intensity training with periods of low-intensity training.

WHAT DOES *INTENSITY* MEAN?

Intensity is increased by

- Amplification of mental effort—getting "psyched"
- Approaching your training with a burning passion, as though it were your life
- Adding reps
- Adding weight
- Decreasing rest between reps
- Decreasing rest between sets
- Increasing the number of exercises per body part
- Increasing the total number of exercises or body parts trained at one session
- Increasing the number of training sessions per day
- Increasing the speed of movement
- Increasing the amount of work done at the anaerobic threshold (maximum pain tolerance)

- (Perhaps most importantly) increasing the amount of eccentric work your muscles are required to perform

When you increase the intensity of your workout, a price must be paid. That price, in case you haven't figured it out yet, is discipline in finding methods to improve your recuperative ability. You do this in the following ways.

- Preworkout meal of low-glycemic-index foods
- Preworkout use of appropriate supplements
- During-workout use of appropriate supplements
- Postexercise cooldown (stretching, calisthenics)
- Postcooldown whirlpool of affected muscles
- Postwhirlpool massage of affected muscles
- Postmassage visualization training, autogenic training, TM, or self-hypnosis
- Scheduling 5–6 meals daily
- Ensuring that each meal follows the 1-2-3 rule
- Taking at least one 20–30 minute nap per day
- Working closely with a sports-medicine expert

Sometimes, your muscles need rest, just like your mind does. Perhaps the most important reason for this is that if you continue to apply maximum intensity to your muscles, the level of adaptation they can accommodate will fail. This principle is elaborated upon in Chapter Twenty-Six (Part Six).

Take a look at Figure 7-2 again. Notice that you progress ever upward. That's what you want, but you can't get there by training too hard or too often. I repeat, you have to balance periods of high-intensity training with periods of low-intensity training in order to adequately recuperate.

Each of your muscles requires a different length of rest time between workouts. Your larger muscles need longer recovery time than your smaller ones; short workouts are easier to recover from than long workouts; and your fast-twitch muscles (the ones that give you explosiveness) take longer to recover than your slow-twitch muscles (the ones you use for endurance).

Each muscle has to have its own wavy line with its own unique characteristics. The reasons cited above seem so obvious to me that I just have to scratch my head over some of the dumb stuff I see being done out there—even by top stars! For example, what about the common practice of doing curls on back days and triceps on chest days? On the surface this practice seems to make sense because you tend to use biceps while training the back and triceps while training the chest. However, one of two very bad things

FIGURE 7-4

Variable Split or Variable Double Split Training Program for Elite Bodybuilders

(Rest on Sundays Only)

Note: Be sure to do a gastrointestinal cleanse for three days prior to beginning this mesocycle (see Part Five).

RECOVERY DAYS PER INTENSITY LEVEL

BODY PART	A	B	C
Chest	2	3	4
Shoulders	2	3	4
Back	3	4	5
Biceps	2	3	4
Triceps	2	3	4
Midsection	1	2	3
Legs	3	4	5
Calves	1	2	3
Forearms	1	2	3

DAYS 1–12 OF THE MACROCYCLE

BODY PART	1	2	3	4	5	6	7	8	9	10	11	12
Chest	A	B	B	C		C	—	B		B		
Shoulders				C			—	B			A	
Back	C					B	—			A		
Biceps	A		B			C	—		B	B		
Triceps					C		—		B		C	A
Midsection	B	C	C			B		A	B		C	A
Legs							—					
Calves	B			C				B		A	B	A
Forearms		A	B		C		—	B	B	A	A	B

DAYS 13–31 OF THE MACROCYCLE

BODY PART	13	14	15	16	17	18	19	20	21	22	23	24	25	26	27	28	29	30	31
Chest	A	—	B			C			—	B	A	A	A		B		C	C	
Shoulders	B	—		C	C	C		B	—	A	A	B	B		B	C	C		
Back	B	—		C					—	B			A	A		B			
Biceps	A	—	B		C	C		B	—	B	A	A	A		B		C	C	
Triceps		—	B		C				—		A	B	B		C	B			B
Midsection		—	B		A	B		C	—	B	B	A	A	B	A	C	C		B
Legs		—	B				C		—			B	B		A		B		
Calves	C	—			B	B	A	A	—	C	B	B	C	A	B	C	B	B	B
Forearms		—	C		B	B	A	A	—		C	B	A	B	B		A	A	B

You should notice that the prescribed number of recovery days is not always adhered to. That's because of the rest days. Rather than skipping the body part that falls on a rest day, it's moved forward or backward a day.

Many elite bodybuilders prefer to incorporate a "double-split" system into their routine. That is, they like to work out twice a day. In fact, some even opt for three workouts per day. The benefit of this is that it allows them to spend less time in the gym at each workout, thereby allowing for greater levels of intensity and greater recovery ability. To convert this schedule to a "double-variable split" system, simply do your most important exercises in the morning and the remainder of your exercises in the afternoon. In fact, you should always train your weaknesses first at every workout, whether you're on a single split, double split, or triple split.

An example of a double variable split system is presented in Figure 7-5.

FIGURE 7-5

Double Variable Split Training for Elite Bodybuilders

BODY PART	INTENSITY A	B	C	Recovery Days		1	2	3	4	5	6	7	8	9	10	11	12	13	14	15	16	17	18	19	20	21	22	23	24	25	26	27	28	29	30	31
Chest	2	3	4	2	AM	A		A								C		A		C				B			B			A		A		B		
					PM					B			B									B														B	
Shoulders	2	2½	3	2	AM		C											A		A		B					C			C						
					PM					C					B									B									B		B	
Upper back	2	3	4	2	AM									C					A													A		A		
					PM	A		B			B				B			C				C			B				B							
Lower back	3	4	5	3	AM				A									C	A		B	A	B		B	A		A	B	B		B	C	A	C	
					PM	C					B				C	C																					
Biceps	2	2½	3	2	AM		A		A						C					B						A			A			B		B		
					PM	B		B			B		B					B			B		B		B		B									
Triceps	2	2½	3	2	AM		A		A						C			C			B	A				A		A		B			B			C
					PM	B		B			B									B			B				B						C			
Forearms	1	1½	2		AM			B	C							A	A	B			C		C		B		B	A	A	B		C	C			
					PM	B					C	B	B																							
Midsection	1	1½	2		AM			B	C							A	A	B			C		C		B		B	A	A	B		C	C			
					PM	B					C		B																							
Hips	3	3½	4	3	AM			C					A			A			B			B						B		C				B		
					PM	B				B											C		C			C				C						C
Quads	3	3½	4	3	AM			C							B				B													C			C	
					PM						C											B			B			B								
Hamstrings	3	3½	4	3	AM	B			C				A			A			B										A					B		
					PM	B					C		B		B			B			C		C		B	C	B	A	A	C		B	C		C	
Calves	1	1½	2		AM																								A							
					PM	B		B			C				B					B							B			B		B	C		C	

happens if you do this: you undertrain your back and chest or you overtrain your biceps and triceps.

Why? On the average, it takes your back and chest three or four days to recover but it takes only two or three days for your biceps and triceps to recover. This is a waste of time. Over a year's time—over a career—think about how much time you've lost by doing this. Time's lost both from overtraining (downtime from cumulative microtrauma) and from undertraining.

How do you know how often to train each muscle? Don't worry. I've figured it out for you. Look at Figure 7-4. It lists the average rate of recovery for each of your major muscles for "A" workouts, "B" workouts, and "C" workouts. This is breakthrough stuff, folks! Of course, you may vary a bit from the norm—not to worry. Just change the schedule to meet your own special case. The numbers aren't holy. Only the concept is.

Now for the big one. Take a look at Figure 7-4 again, every muscle's ABC schedule for a full month. Take that and put it together with the guidelines for ABC training in Figure 7-6, along with Figure 7-7's listing of the best exercises for "A", "B", and "C" training, and you have what amounts to the greatest bodybuilding system ever created. The scientific name for this training system is *integrated variable split* training. When more than one workout per day is incorporated, it's called *integrated multiple variable split* training.

The exercises listed in Figure 7-8 aren't holy—you may have some favorites of your own. But I've very carefully chosen those listed, giving consideration to the ease of use in an "A", "B", or "C" system.

GOOD, BETTER, OR BEST?

All this science giving you a headache? Hey, I told you that you'd have to be willing to pay the price, and here's the price! The price is discipline. Discipline in learning the difference between what's good, what's better, and what's best.

It's good to train. It's better to train regularly and practice good nutrition. It's best to take what science has to offer us, and within the scope of human possibility, technological feasibility, and your personal lifestyle commitments, exercise the discipline it takes to become great.

Well! . . . didn't mean to get off on you like that, but this is serious stuff to me, folks. Really, it's as easy as ABC when you approach it systematically.

Ready? OK, let's train!

FIGURE 7-6

Guidelines on
How to Perform the A, B, and C Workouts

"A" Workouts

"A" workouts are characterized by ample rest between sets (usually around 2–3 minutes is sufficient) and total (or as near total as practical) avoidance of eccentric contractions.

For example, after a couple of warm-up sets with a light weight (around 30%–50% of your maximum), you're ready to begin. Start at 10–12 reps for a max effort and stop at 8–10 sets. You will have to reduce the amount of weight you train with in order to complete the required 10 sets. Just make sure that each set is a near-maximum effort. Where feasible, do each exercise in a way that corresponds with the natural function of the muscle(s) involved. And, important, get your training partner to "unload" the weight during the eccentric phase of the movement by giving you a heavy spot on the bar. Alternatively, use a machine that eliminates the eccentric phase of the movement for you.

Average intensity:

- "Speed" muscles: 10 reps/10 sets/60% max
- "Speed and strength" muscles: 12 reps/8 sets/70% max
- "Limit strength" muscles: 8 reps/5 sets/80% max

"B" Workouts

"B" workouts are done with two or three exercises, with the basic exercise done with explosiveness for low reps and heavy weights. The other exercise(s) is/are done for moderate and high reps, respectively. Again, lots of rest between sets (around 2–3 minutes is sufficient). This is a moderate intensity workout.

For example, 3–4 sets of 5–6 explosive reps with heavy weight (85% of max); then do 3–4 sets of 12–15 reps, rhythmic cadence with moderate weight (70%–75% max); then do 3–4 sets of 40 reps, slow, continuous tension with light weights (40%–50% max). It is not generally feasible to perform calf or forearm movements explosively, as these muscle groups involve very short ranges of motion.

Average intensity:

- 5 reps/3 sets/85% max, explosive movements
- 12 reps/3 sets/70% max, rhythmic cadence
- 40 reps/3 sets/40% max, slow, continuous tension

"C" Workouts

"C" workouts are called *holistic* sets. A "C" workout is performed nonstop, combining 2 or more exercises into one giant set. This is a maximum intensity workout.

For example, you'll note that while the exercises you perform in a "C" workout may be the same as in a "B" workout, the holistic set system is in effect. In other words, continuous (nonstop) changing back and forth from explosive, heavy movements to slow, continuous tension movements with lighter weights.

See Figure 7-7 for an example of how a "C" workout is performed. No rest is taken between 5s, 12s, and 40s. Instead, a total of about 200 reps is performed nonstop. Repeat this holistic set once if you feel up to it, but no more than once. It's possible to do this many repetitions because the muscle fibers involved in the explosive movements are not the same ones that are targeted in the slower movements. So, while you're doing slow movements using red (slow-twitch) muscle fibers, for example, the muscle fibers you just got through exercising with explosive reps (white, fast-twitch muscle fibers) are recovering. It is not necessary to perform calf exercises holistically. Instead, "strength shoes" are worn daily in order to keep your calves sufficiently stressed for long periods of time. Also, holistic sets are not used in forearm training, since every time you pick up a weight you're using your forearm muscles for gripping the bar.

Average intensity for one "holistic" set

- 5 reps/85% max, explosive movements
- 12 reps/75% max, rhythmic cadence
- 40 reps/40% max, slow, continuous tension movements

Repeat the above sequence three to five times without resting; reduce weight slightly (i.e., 5–10 pounds) each time as fatigue sets in.

FIGURE 7-7

How to Perform a "C" Workout
Percent Max

| 5 Reps Explosive | 12 Reps Rhythmic | 40 Reps Slow Continuous Tension |

Remember!!!

A "C" workout is one long "giant" set of around 11 or 12 sets. Each set alternates from low reps explosive to medium reps rhythmic with an occasional superlong set of 40 (do at *least* 2 sets of 40).

You must not rest between sets. If you have to wait for a machine then do the exercise with free weights.

Explosive means the concentric movement *must* explode and accelerate like a rocket. For example, on the bench press, lower the weight to your chest. The second it touches your chest, *boom!* Explode it straight up as fast as possible and repeat.

When doing a "C" workout, choose your exercises first (2–4 depending on the body part) then plug them into your "C" giant set where you think appropriate. Some exercises are not suitable for the explosive sets.

FIGURE 7-8

Preferred A, B, and C Exercises for Each Body Part

BODY PART AND INTENSITY LEVEL	PREFERRED EXERCISE	APPROXIMATE REPS, SETS, INTENSITY, AND METHOD
A Chest	bench press	10 reps/10 sets/60% max

Take 1–3 minutes' rest between sets. Use explosive movements. Eliminate eccentric movement (actively lowering the weight).

B Chest	bench press	5 reps/3 sets/85% max; explosive
	dumbbell bench press	12 reps/3 sets/70% max; rhythmic
	cable crossovers	40 reps/3 sets/40% max; slow

Take 1–3 minutes' rest between sets.

C Chest	bench press	5 reps/85% max; explosive
	dumbbell bench press or incline dumbbell bench press	12 reps/75% max; rhythmic
	cable crossovers	40 reps/40% max; slow

Go through above in zigzag fashion without resting (see the "C" workout graph). Wait 3–5 minutes and repeat, reducing the weight slightly each time. Use an array of upper and lower chest exercises for complete chest development, including weighted dips.

A Shoulders	seated dumbbell presses	12 reps/8 sets/70% max

Take 1–3 minutes' rest between sets. Use explosive movements, without resting or pausing between each rep. Bear in mind that you should also mix in some sets of front dumbbell raises in order to achieve total shoulder development. Eliminate eccentric movement (actively lowering the weight).

B Shoulders	seated dumbbell presses	5 reps/3 sets/85% max; explosive
	lateral raises	12 reps/3 sets/70% max; rhythmic
	military presses	40 reps/3 sets/40% max; slow

Bear in mind that you should also mix in some sets of front dumbbell raises in order to achieve total shoulder development. Take 1–3 minutes' rest between sets.

C Shoulders	seated dumbbell presses	5 reps/85% max; explosive
	lateral raises	12 reps/75% max; rhythmic
	military presses	40 reps/40% max; slow

Go through above in zigzag fashion without resting (see the "C" workout graph). Wait 3–5 minutes and repeat, reducing the weight slightly each time. Use an array of shoulder exercises. Bear in mind that you should also mix in some sets of front dumbbell raises in order to achieve total shoulder development.

A Back	back extensions	12 reps/8 sets/70% max
	long cable pulls	12 reps/8 sets/70% max

Take 1–3 minutes' rest between sets. Use explosive movements without resting or pausing between reps. Bear in mind that you should also mix in some sets of lat pulldowns in order to achieve total upper back development. Eliminate eccentric movement (actively lowering the weight).

BODY PART AND INTENSITY LEVEL	PREFERRED EXERCISE	APPROXIMATE REPS, SETS, INTENSITY, AND METHOD
B Back	back extensions	5 reps/3 sets/85% max; explosive
	long cable pulls	12 reps/3 sets/70% max; rhythmic
	one-arm bent rows	40 reps/3 sets/40% max; slow

Take 1–3 minutes' rest between sets. Bear in mind that you should also mix in some sets of lat pulldowns in order to achieve total upper back development.

C Back	back extensions	5 reps/85% max; explosive
	deadlifts	12 reps/75% max; rhythmic
	pulldowns	40 reps/40% max; slow

Go through above in zigzag fashion without resting (see the "C" workout graph). Wait 3–5 minutes and repeat, reducing the weight slightly each time. Use an array of back exercises. Bear in mind that you should also mix in some sets of high pulls (low back and shoulder girdle) and heavy bent rows (posterior deltoids and rhomboids) in order to achieve total back development.

A Biceps	EZ curls or dumbbell curls	10 reps/10 sets/60% max

Take 1–3 minutes' rest between sets. Use explosive movements. Eliminate eccentric movement (actively lowering the weight).

B Biceps	EZ curls	5 reps/3 sets/85% max; explosive
	dumbbell curls	12 reps/3 sets/70% max; rhythmic
	preacher curls	40 reps/3 sets/40% max; slow

Take 1–3 minutes' rest between sets.

C Biceps	EZ curls	5 reps/85% max; explosive
	dumbbell curls	12 reps/75% max; rhythmic
	preacher curls	40 reps/40% max; slow

Go through above in zigzag fashion without resting (see the "C" workout graph). Wait 3–5 minutes and repeat; reducing the weight slightly each time. Use an array of curl exercises throughout the "C" workout.

A Triceps	French presses or nose crushers	8 reps/5 sets/80% max

Take 1–3 minutes' rest between sets. Use explosive movements. Eliminate eccentric movement (actively lowering the weight).

B Triceps	French presses	5 reps/3 sets/85% max; explosive
	nose crushers	12 reps/3 sets/70% max; rhythmic
	pushdowns	40 reps/3 sets/40% max; slow

Take 1–3 minutes' rest between sets.

C Triceps	French presses	5 reps/85% max; explosive
	nose crushers	12 reps/75% max; rhythmic
	pushdowns	40 reps/40% max; slow

Go through above in zigzag fashion without resting (see the "C" workout graph). Wait 3–5 minutes and repeat, reducing the weight slightly each time. Use an array of triceps exercises throughout the "C" workout.

BODY PART AND INTENSITY LEVEL	PREFERRED EXERCISE	APPROXIMATE REPS, SETS, INTENSITY, AND METHOD
A Legs	safety squats	8 reps/5 sets/80% max
	leg extensions	12 reps/8 sets/70% max
	hamstring curls	10 reps/10 sets/60% max

Hamstrings are speed muscles: 10 reps/10 sets/60% max. Do exercise fast without pause between reps.
Quadriceps are speed and strength muscles: 12 reps/8 sets/70% max. Do exercise explosively.
Together, as in squatting, quads and hams are limit strength muscles: 8 reps/ 5 sets/80% max. Do exercise explosively with slight rest pause between reps. Eliminate eccentric movement (actively lowering the weight). Take 1–3 minutes' rest between sets.

B Legs	safety squats	5 reps/3 sets/85% max; explosive
	leg extensions	12 reps/3 sets/70% max; rhythmic
	hack squats	40 reps/3 sets/40% max; slow

Take 1–3 minutes' rest between sets. Stiff-legged deadlifts and leg curls should also be incorporated in order to achieve total upper leg development.

C Legs	safety squats	5 reps/85% max; explosive
	hack squats	12 reps/75% max; rhythmic
	lunge walking with dumbbells	40 reps/40% max; slow

Go through above in zigzag fashion without resting (see the "C" workout graph). Wait 3–5 minutes and repeat, reducing the weight slightly each time. Use an array of upper leg exercises throughout the "C" workout, including stiff-legged deadlifts, leg curls, and glute-ham raises.

A Abs	Russian twists	8 reps/5 sets/80% max

Take 1–3 minutes' rest between sets. Be explosive only coming *out* of twisted position in Russian twists.

B Abs	Russian twists	5 reps/3 sets/85% max
	reverse crunchers	12 reps/3 sets/70% max; rhythmic
	crunchers	40 reps/3 sets/40% max; slow

Take 1–3 minutes' rest between sets. Be explosive only coming *out* of twisted position in Russian twists.

C Abs	Russian twists	5 reps/85% max
	reverse crunchers	12 reps/75% max; rhythmic
	sidebends left and right	40 reps/40% max; slow

Go through above in zigzag fashion without resting (see the "C" workout graph). Wait 3–5 minutes and repeat. Be explosive only coming *out* of twisted position in Russian twists.

A Forearms	regular wrist curls	12 reps/10 sets/70% max

Take 1–3 minutes' rest between sets.

B Forearms	regular wrist curls	5 reps/3 sets/85% max; explosive
	reverse wrist curls	12 reps/3 sets/75% max; rhythmic
	Thor's hammer	40 reps/3 sets/55% max; slow

Take 1–3 minutes' rest between sets.

BODY PART AND INTENSITY LEVEL	PREFERRED EXERCISE	APPROXIMATE REPS, SETS, INTENSITY, AND METHOD
C Forearms	regular wrist curls	5 reps/85% max; explosive
	reverse wrist curls	12 reps/75% max; rhythmic
	Thor's hammer	40 reps/55% max; slow

Go through above in zigzag fashion without resting (see the "C" workout graph). Wait 3–5 minutes and repeat.

CALVES

Unlike other body parts, calves must be severely overloaded in order to force growth. This is because they're so enduring. Remember, you're on them and using them most of the day. The best way to force adaptation is to wear specially built shoes called strength shoes. Begin 5 minutes per day, gradually working over the course of a month up to an hour or two. Don't be afraid to jump around or run while wearing the strength shoes. Just don't let your heels droop to the ground—stay on your toes.

A Calves	standing calf machine	12 reps/12 sets/75% max

Take 1–3 minutes' rest between sets.

B Calves	standing calf machine	12 reps/10 sets/75% max
	seated calf machine	12 reps/10 sets/75% max

Take 1–3 minutes' rest between sets.

C Calves	standing calf	5 sets of 5 reps done explosively; then 5 sets of 12 reps done rhythmically; then 5 sets of 40 reps done with slow, continuous tension

Because calf training isn't likely to interfere with any other body part training, you may want to fit each set in between sets while performing other exercises. This will save a lot of time.

FIGURE 7-9

Variable Split or Variable Double Split Training Program for Elite Bodybuilders

(Allows every fourth day for rest)

RECOVERY DAYS PER INTENSITY LEVEL

BODY PART	A	B	C
Chest	2	3	4
Shoulders	2	3	4
Back	3	4	5
Biceps	2	3	4
Triceps	2	3	4
Midsection	1	2	3
Legs	3	4	5
Calves	1	2	3
Forearms	1	2	3

DAYS 1–12 OF THE MACROCYCLE

BODY PART	1	2	3	4	5	6	7	8	9	10	11	12
Chest	A	B	B	—	C	C	B	—	B	B	A	—
Shoulders		B		—	C	C	B	—		B	A	—
Back	C		B	—		C	B	—		A		—
Biceps	A	B	B	—	C	C	B	—	B	B	A	—
Triceps		B		—				—	B	B		—
Midsection	B	C	C	—		B	B	—	A		A	—
Legs				—				—				—
Calves	B	C	C	—	C	B	B	—	A	B		—
Forearms	A	B	B	—	C			—	B	B	A	—

DAYS 13–31 OF THE MACROCYCLE

BODY PART	13	14	15	16	17	18	19	20	21	22	23	24	25	26	27	28	29	30	31
Chest	A	B	B	—	C	C		—	B	B		—	A	A	B		C	C	B
Shoulders		B		—	C	C		—	B		A	—	B		B	C		C	B
Back	B		B	—	C			—		B		—	A		B				
Biceps	A			—	C	C	A	—		B	A	—		A	B			C	
Triceps		B	B	—	C	C	C	—	B		A	—	B	B		C	C	B	C
Midsection	C		B	—	B		A	—	B	B	C	—	B	B	A	C	B		
Legs	C	B		—			C	—			B	—			A	A		B	
Calves	C		B	—	B	A	A	—	B	C	C	—	B	B		A		B	
Forearms	B		C	—	A	B	B	—	C		A	—	B			C			B

You should notice that the prescribed number of recovery days is not always adhered to. That's because of the rest days. Rather than skipping the body part that falls on a rest day, it's moved forward or backward a day.

Many elite bodybuilders prefer to incorporate a "double split" system into their routine. That is, they like to work out twice a day. In fact, some even opt for three workouts per day. The benefit of this is that it allows them to spend less time in the gym at each workout, thereby allowing for greater levels of intensity and greater recovery ability. To convert this schedule to a "double-variable split" system, simply do your most important exercises in the morning and the remainder of your exercises in the afternoon. In fact, you should always train your weaknesses first at every workout, whether you're on a single split, double split, or triple split.

Be sure to do a gastrointestinal cleanse for three days prior to beginning this mesocycle (see Part Five).

FIGURE 7-10

Variable Split Training Program for Intermediate and Beginning Bodybuilders

(workout four days per week)

RECOVERY DAYS PER INTENSITY LEVEL   **DAYS 1–12 OF THE MACROCYCLE**

BODY PART	A	B	1	2	3	4	5	6	7	8	9	10	11	12
Chest	2	3	—	B	—	A	—	A	B	—	B	—	A	—
Shoulders	2	3	—	B	—	A	—	A	B	—	B	—	A	—
Back	3	4	—	B	—	A	—	A	B	—	B	—	A	—
Biceps	2	3	—	B	—	A	A	B	B	—	B	—	A	—
*Triceps	2	3	—	B	—	A	A	B	B	—	B	—	A	—
Midsection	1	2	—	B	—	A	A	B	B	—	B	—	A	—
*Legs	2	3	—	B	—	A	A	B	B	—	B	—	A	—
Calves	1	2	—	B	—	A	A	B	B	—	B	—	A	—
*Forearms	1	2	—	B	—	A	A	B	B	—	B	—	A	—

DAYS 13–31 OF THE MACROCYCLE

BODY PART	13	14	15	16	17	18	19	20	21	22	23	24	25	26	27	28	29	30	31
Chest	A	B	—	B	—	A	—	A	B	—	B	—	A	—	A	B	—	B	—
Shoulders	A	B	—	B	—	A	—	A	B	—	B	—	A	—	A	B	—	B	—
Back	A	B	—	B	—	A	—	A	B	—	B	—	A	—	A	B	—	B	—
Biceps	B	B	—	B	—	A	—	B	B	—	B	—	A	—	B	B	—	B	—
*Triceps	B	B	—	B	—	A	—	B	B	—	B	—	A	—	B	B	—	B	—
Midsection	B	B	—	B	—	A	—	B	B	—	B	—	A	—	B	B	—	B	—
*Legs	B	B	—	B	—	A	—	B	B	—	B	—	A	—	B	B	—	B	—
Calves	B	B	—	B	—	A	—	B	B	—	B	—	A	—	B	B	—	B	—
*Forearms	B	B	—	B	—	A	—	B	B	—	B	—	A	—	B	B	—	B	—

Notice that "C" workouts are not included for beginning and intermediate bodybuilders. Only you can decide when you're ready to handle the extreme level of intensity afforded by "C" workouts.

Follow a B—A—B—A—B schedule for your weaker body parts and an A—B—A—B schedule for your strongest body parts. This will emphasize the higher-intensity "B" workouts for your weaknesses. In this example chart, I have assumed that the weak body parts are triceps, legs, and forearms. Notice that these three body parts are marked with an asterisk (*). You must adjust this chart to reflect your own individual strengths and weaknesses rather than follow it blindly.

You should notice that the prescribed number of recovery days is not always adhered to. That's because of the rest days. Rather than skipping the body part that falls on a rest day, it's moved forward or backward a day or two.

Be sure to do a gastrointestinal cleanse for three days prior to beginning this mesocycle.

FIGURE 7-11

An example of an integrated conditioning program for bodybuilding competition (for those who work), incorporating a double variable split workout plan.

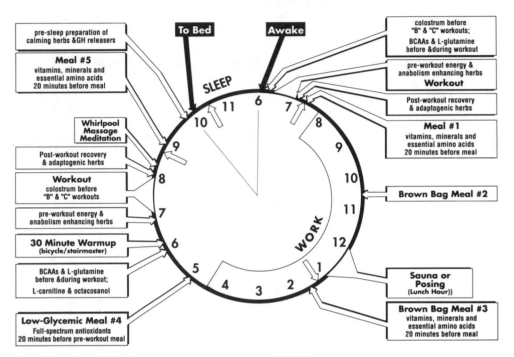

⟹ **Time of significant hGH release; meals also promote a mild hGH response.**

Warning: Food & Drug Administration laws prohibit the sale of L-tryptophan (an essential amino acid) in any form other than its naturally occurring state. Therefore, Peptide-bonded aminos are your only choice. The pure L-form of broad spectrum and essential amino acid supplements on the market today are of little use because they lack L-tryptophan.

Note: High-quality protein powders are available which contain many of the vitamins, minerals, amino acids, and other nutritional supplements you may require. Often, they make excellent (and tasty) additions to your normal meals. Rarely are they suitable as meal replacements.

FIGURE 7-12

An example of an integrated training program for bodybuilders who have jobs, incorporating a double variable split workout plan

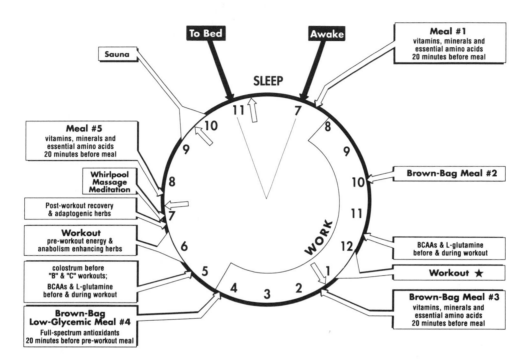

⟹ Time of significant hGH release; meals also promote a mild hGH response.

★ Noon workout can easily be accomplished with a set of dumbbells & other portable devices.

Warning: Food & Drug Administration laws prohibit the sale of L-tryptophan (an essential amino acid) in any form other than its naturally occurring state. Therefore, Peptide-bonded aminos are your only choice. The pure L-form of broad spectrum and essential amino acid supplements on the market today are of little use because they lack L-tryptophan.

Note: High-quality protein powders are available which contain many of the vitamins, minerals, amino acids, and other nutritional supplements you may require. Often, they make excellent (and tasty) additions to your normal meals. Rarely are they suitable as meal replacements.

FIGURE 7-13

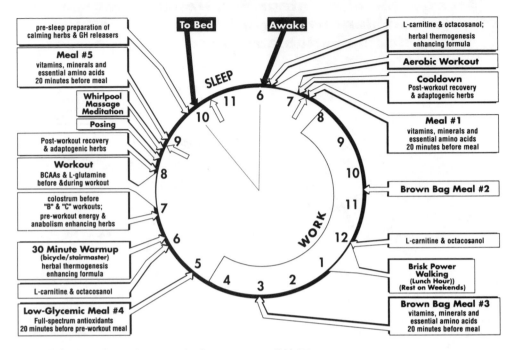

⟹ **Time of significant hGH release; meals also promote a mild hGH response.**

Warning: Food & Drug Administration laws prohibit the sale of L-tryptophan (an essential amino acid) in any form other than its naturally occurring state. Therefore, Peptide-bonded aminos are your only choice. The pure L-form of broad spectrum and essential amino acid supplements on the market today are of little use because they lack L-tryptophan.

Note: High-quality protein powders are available which contain many of the vitamins, minerals, amino acids, and other nutritional supplements you may require. Often, they make excellent (and tasty) additions to your normal meals. Rarely are they suitable as meal replacements.

FIGURE 7-14

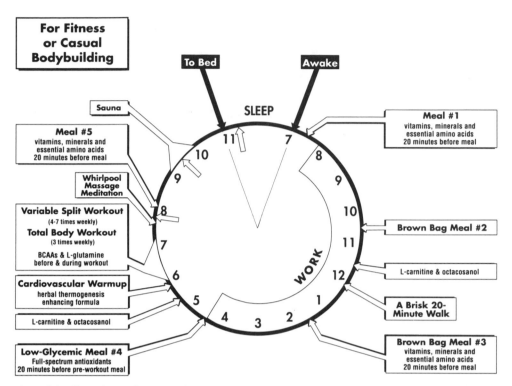

⟹ **Time of significant hGH release; meals also promote a mild hGH response.**

Warning: Food & Drug Administration laws prohibit the sale of L-tryptophan (an essential amino acid) in any form other than its naturally occurring state. Therefore, Peptide-bonded aminos are your only choice. The pure L-form of broad spectrum and essential amino acid supplements on the market today are of little use because they lack L-tryptophan.

Note: High-quality protein powders are available which contain many of the vitamins, minerals, amino acids, and other nutritional supplements you may require. Often, they make excellent (and tasty) additions to your normal meals. Rarely are they suitable as meal replacements.

FIGURE 7-15

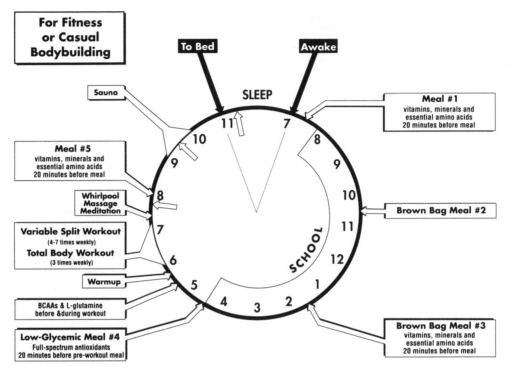

⇒ Time of significant hGH release; meals also promote a mild hGH response.

Warning: Food & Drug Administration laws prohibit the sale of L-tryptophan (an essential amino acid) in any form other than its naturally occurring state. Therefore, Peptide-bonded aminos are your only choice. The pure L-form of broad spectrum and essential amino acid supplements on the market today are of little use because they lack L-tryptophan.

Note: High-quality protein powders are available which contain many of the vitamins, minerals, amino acids, and other nutritional supplements you may require. Often, they make excellent (and tasty) additions to your normal meals. Rarely are they suitable as meal replacements.

FIGURE 7-16

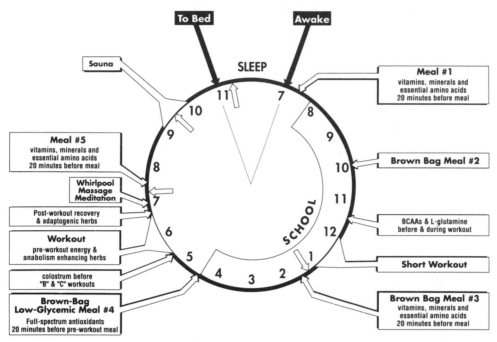

⟹ **Time of significant hGH release; meals also promote a mild hGH response.**

Warning: Food & Drug Administration laws prohibit the sale of L-tryptophan (an essential amino acid) in any form other than its naturally occurring state. Therefore, Peptide-bonded aminos are your only choice. The pure L-form of broad spectrum and essential amino acid supplements on the market today are of little use because they lack L-tryptophan.

Note: High-quality protein powders are available which contain many of the vitamins, minerals, amino acids, and other nutritional supplements you may require. Often, they make excellent (and tasty) additions to your normal meals. Rarely are they suitable as meal replacements.

FIGURE 7-17

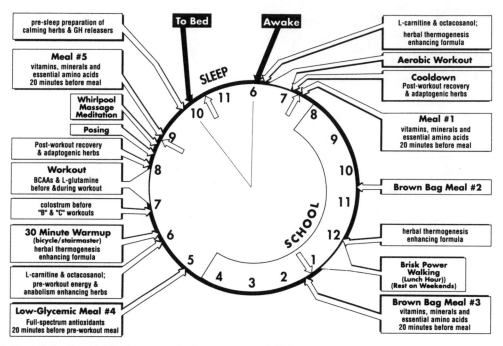

⇒ Time of significant hGH release; meals also promote a mild hGH response.

Warning: Food & Drug Administration laws prohibit the sale of L-tryptophan (an essential amino acid) in any form other than its naturally occurring state. Therefore, Peptide-bonded aminos are your only choice. The pure L-form of broad spectrum and essential amino acid supplements on the market today are of little use because they lack L-tryptophan.

Note: High-quality protein powders are available which contain many of the vitamins, minerals, amino acids, and other nutritional supplements you may require. Often, they make excellent (and tasty) additions to your normal meals. Rarely are they suitable as meal replacements.

FIGURE 7-18

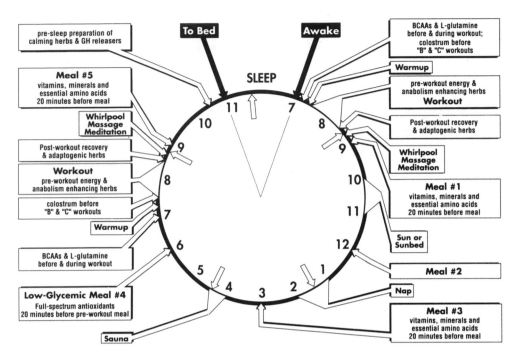

⇒ **Time of significant hGH release; meals also promote a mild hGH response.**

Warning: Food & Drug Administration laws prohibit the sale of L-tryptophan (an essential amino acid) in any form other than its naturally occurring state. Therefore, Peptide-bonded aminos are your only choice. The pure L-form of broad spectrum and essential amino acid supplements on the market today are of little use because they lack L-tryptophan.

Note: High-quality protein powders are available which contain many of the vitamins, minerals, amino acids, and other nutritional supplements you may require. Often, they make excellent (and tasty) additions to your normal meals. Rarely are they suitable as meal replacements.

FIGURE 7-19

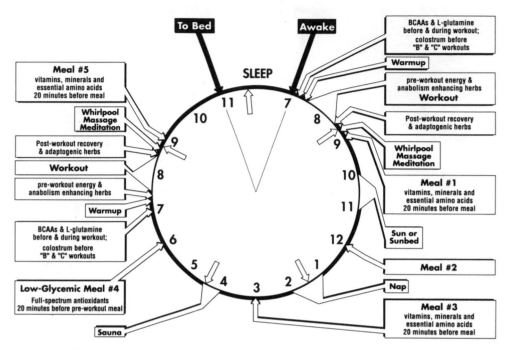

⇨ **Time of significant hGH release; meals also promote a mild hGH response.**

Warning: Food & Drug Administration laws prohibit the sale of L-tryptophan (an essential amino acid) in any form other than its naturally occurring state. Therefore, Peptide-bonded aminos are your only choice. The pure L-form of broad spectrum and essential amino acid supplements on the market today are of little use because they lack L-tryptophan.

Note: High-quality protein powders are available which contain many of the vitamins, minerals, amino acids, and other nutritional supplements you may require. Often, they make excellent (and tasty) additions to your normal meals. Rarely are they suitable as meal replacements.

Now you know exactly what to do every day, you know how to do it, how much of it to do, how often you do it over a mesocycle, even how many reps, sets, and exercises per body part to do. Most important, you are beginning to get a fairly sophisticated working knowledge of *why*.

I've even given you schedules for three or four workouts per week, as well as one-a-day workouts for novices and intermediates. But I recommend two-a-day workouts for hard-core (deadly serious)

FIGURE 7-20

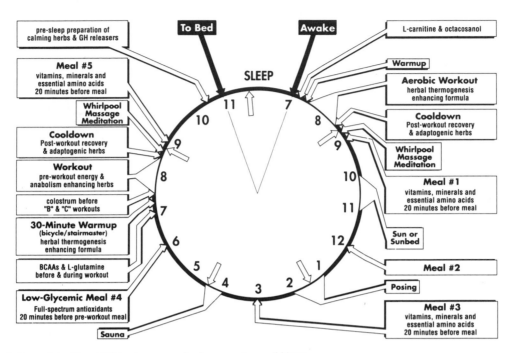

⟹ Time of significant hGH release; meals also promote a mild hGH response.

Warning: Food & Drug Administration laws prohibit the sale of L-tryptophan (an essential amino acid) in any form other than its naturally occurring state. Therefore, Peptide-bonded aminos are your only choice. The pure L-form of broad spectrum and essential amino acid supplements on the market today are of little use because they lack L-tryptophan.

Note: High-quality protein powders are available which contain many of the vitamins, minerals, amino acids, and other nutritional supplements you may require. Often, they make excellent (and tasty) additions to your normal meals. Rarely are they suitable as meal replacements.

competitive bodybuilders who have the discipline and guts to engage in maxed out, scientific training, eating, and sleeping. To them, nothing else matters!

I said this earlier, and I'll say it again: Bodybuilders *can* become champions without drugs. While your genetics may play an important part in how you ultimately fare in bodybuilding, make no mistake about the fact that discipline, self-belief, and passion far outweigh whatever hereditary advantages you may possess.

FIGURE 7-21

Variable Split Training Program for Intermediate and Beginning Bodybuilders

(Workout three days per week)

RECOVERY DAYS PER INTENSITY LEVEL

BODY PART	A	B
*Chest	2	3
Shoulders	2	3
Back	3	4
*Biceps	2	3
Triceps	2	3
Midsection	1	2
*Legs	3	4
Calves	1	2
Forearms	1	2

DAYS 1–12 OF THE MACROCYCLE

BODY PART	1	2	3	4	5	6	7	8	9	10	11	12
*Chest	—	B	—	—	—	B	—	—	—	—	A	—
Shoulders	—	A	—	B	—	—	—	—	A	—	B	—
Back	—	—	—	A	—	B	—	—	—	—	A	—
*Biceps	—	B	—	B	—	B	—	—	—	A	A	—
Triceps	—	A	—	B	—	B	—	—	A	A	B	—
Midsection	—	A	—	B	—	—	—	—	A	A	B	—
*Legs	—	B	—	—	—	B	—	—	A	B	—	—
Calves	—	A	—	B	—	B	—	—	A	B	B	—
Forearms	—	—	—	A	—	B	—	—	—	—	A	—

DAYS 13–31 OF THE MACROCYCLE

BODY PART	13	14	15	16	17	18	19	20	21	22	23	24	25	26	27	28	29	30	31
*Chest	B	—	—	B	—	—	—	A	—	—	B	—	—	—	B	—	—	A	—
Shoulders	—	—	—	A	—	B	—	—	—	—	A	—	B	—	—	—	—	A	—
Back	B	—	—	—	—	B	—	B	—	—	—	—	—	—	B	—	—	—	—
*Biceps	B	—	—	B	—	B	—	A	—	—	B	—	B	—	B	—	—	A	—
Triceps	—	—	—	A	—	B	—	—	—	—	A	—	B	—	—	—	—	A	—
Midsection	—	—	—	A	—	B	—	B	—	—	A	—	B	—	—	—	—	A	—
*Legs	B	—	—	B	—	B	—	—	—	—	B	—	B	—	B	—	—	B	—
Calves	—	—	—	A	—	B	—	—	—	—	A	—	B	—	—	—	—	A	—
Forearms	B	—	—	—	—	A	—	B	—	—	A	—	B	—	B	—	—	A	—

Notice that "C" workouts are not included for beginning bodybuilders. Only you can decide when you're ready to handle the extreme level of intensity afforded by "C" workouts. Certainly, "C" workouts should be avoided for the first 3–6 months of your bodybuilding career.

In this example chart, I have assumed that your weak body parts are chest, biceps, and legs. Notice that these three body parts are marked with an asterisk (*). You must adjust this chart to reflect your own individual strengths and weaknesses. Since you're working out only three days a week, it's almost impossible to follow the basic periodization philosophy of alternating heavy and light workouts—too many days are off days. Hence, you'll notice that for body parts that take longer to recover (i.e., legs and back), all of your workouts are of "B" intensity. These two body parts are trained twice weekly (e.g., Mondays and Fridays). The remaining body parts follow a variation of the heavy-light system.

You should notice that the prescribed number of recovery days is not always adhered to. That's because of the rest days. Rather than skipping the body part that falls on a rest day, it's moved forward or backward a day or two.

Be sure to do a gastrointestinal cleanse for three days prior to beginning this mesocycle.

FIGURE 7-22

The ABC Training Progress Log

DIRECTIONS

Keep a record of your reps and sets when doing your A, B, and C workouts for each exercise you perform. To ensure maximum progress, your intensity—body part per body part and workout per workout—should approximate the "ABC" model presented on page 53 of this book. Set up your training log in a manner similar to that presented below, or simply photocopy these charts multiple times and insert them into your training logbook.

Name _____ Date _____

Supplements _____

BODY PART AND INTENSITY (A, B, OR C INTENSITY, AND PERCENT OF MAX)	EXERCISE		1st SET	2d SET	3d SET	4th SET	5th SET	6th SET	7th SET	8th SET	9th SET	10th SET	11th SET	12th SET
Chest	bench press	reps												
		lb.												
	dumbbell bench press	reps												
		lb.												
	incline dumbbell bench press	reps												
		lb.												
	other exercise(s)	reps												
		lb.												
Shoulders	seated dumbbell presses	reps												
		lb.												
	frontal dumbbell raises	reps												
		lb.												
	lateral raises	reps												
		lb.												
	other exercise(s)	reps												
		lb.												
Back	back extensions	reps												
		lb.												
	stiff-legged deadlifts	reps												
		lb.												
	pulldowns	reps												
		lb.												
	high pulls	reps												
		lb.												
	bent rows	reps												
		lb.												
	other exercise(s)	reps												
		lb.												
Biceps	EZ curls	reps												
		lb.												
	dumbbell curls	reps												
		lb.												
	preacher curls	reps												
		lb.												
	incline dumbbell curls	reps												
		lb.												
	other exercise(s)	reps												
		lb.												
Triceps	French presses	reps												
		lb.												
	nose crushers	reps												
		lb.												
	pushdowns	reps												
		lb.												
	weighted dips	reps												
		lb.												
	other exercise(s)	reps												
		lb.												

BODY PART AND INTENSITY (A, B, OR C INTENSITY, AND PERCENT OF MAX)	EXERCISE		1st SET	2d SET	3d SET	4th SET	5th SET	6th SET	7th SET	8th SET	9th SET	10th SET	11th SET	12th SET
Legs	safety squats	reps												
		lb.												
	hack squats	reps												
		lb.												
	lunge walking with dumbbells	reps												
		lb.												
	stiff-legged deadlifts	reps												
		lb.												
	leg curls	reps												
		lb.												
	glute-ham raises	reps												
		lb.												
	other exercise(s)	reps												
		lb.												
Midsection	Russian twists	reps												
		lb.												
	crunchers	reps												
		lb.												
	sidebends left and right	reps												
		lb.												
	other exercise(s)	reps												
		lb.												
Forearms	regular wrist curls	reps												
		lb.												
	reverse wrist curls	reps												
		lb.												
	Thor's hammer	reps												
		lb.												
	grip exercise	reps												
		lb.												
	other exercise(s)	reps												
		lb.												
Calves	strength shoes (note time worn each day)	reps												
		lb.												
	standing calf machine	reps												
		lb.												
	seated calf machine	reps												
		lb.												
	other exercise(s)	reps												
		lb.												

Always note the percentage of max you're training with for each exercise you perform in order to gauge your progress and to avoid overtraining.

FIGURE 7-23

Beginning Through Advanced Bodybuilding Training Progress Log

DIRECTIONS

Set up your training log in a manner similar to that presented below, or simply photocopy these charts multiple times and insert them into your training logbook.

Name _____ Date _____

Supplements _____

BODY PART	EXERCISE		OVERLOAD SETS (WARM-UP SETS NOT INCLUDED)											
			1st	2d	3d	4th	5th	6th	7th	8th	9th	10th	11th	12th
Chest	_____	reps												
		lb.												
	_____	reps												
		lb.												
	_____	reps												
		lb.												
Shoulders	_____	reps												
		lb.												
	_____	reps												
		lb.												
	_____	reps												
		lb.												
Back	_____	reps												
		lb.												
	_____	reps												
		lb.												
	_____	reps												
		lb.												
Legs	_____	reps												
		lb.												
	_____	reps												
		lb.												
	_____	reps												
		lb.												
Arms	_____	reps												
		lb.												
	_____	reps												
		lb.												
	_____	reps												
		lb.												
Midsection	_____	reps												
		lb.												
	_____	reps												
		lb.												
	_____	reps												
		lb.												
Supplemental Exercises	_____	reps												
		lb.												
	_____	reps												
		lb.												
	_____	reps												
		lb.												

Always note the percentage of max you're training with for each exercise you perform in order to gauge your progress and to avoid overtraining.

8

TESTING THE EFFECTIVENESS OF ABC TRAINING: A RESEARCH REPORT

For years the before-and-after photo technique has been used by purveyors of fitness products. The old Charles Atlas ads (which still can be found in comic books) perfected the technique. Almost all of the current sports nutrition companies use it in one way or another or, more often than not, abuse it.

Let's get real. You cannot put on 30 pounds of muscle and at the same time lose 40 pounds of fat in six or eight weeks as some of the contemporary leaders in the sports nutrition industry claim. Not even close! Photos offered as proof for these claims of phenomenal gains—and they're as common as drug abuse in our sport—all suffer from one or more of the following maladies.

- The person depicted in the photo was secretly using anabolic steroids
- The person depicted in the photo provided his own "before" photo, which may have been taken months or years earlier than the advertised time frame
- The ad people secretly airbrushed (touched up) the "after" photo
- The company's ad people as well as the subject are in cahoots with one another, attempting to dupe consumers into believing the wild claims

I realize that I'll be accused of being less than kind by casting blame on the perpetrators of this kind of misleading advertising. I have no doubt, however, that in the face of such outrageous claims there is guilt. The simple truth, apparent to virtually everyone who is "of iron," is that no matter how good the products are, or how good the training program accompanying the products is, the human species is not capable of such rapid muscle mass increase.

But let's say for the sake of argument that the model, not the company, is the guilty party. Still, the company involved puts up with such shenanigans, turning its back knowing that it's in its best interests (marketing-wise) to do so. Company representatives will say, "We aren't guilty of deception. Our before-and-after model lied to us. What can we do?"

And then they'll give a public display of mock remorse—and vindication—and reap their ill-gained profits at your expense.

IS REALITY MARKETABLE?

I suspect that these less-than-honest marketing techniques seem necessary and justified to the purveyors. "After all," they say, "how can you sell reality?" The perception they're trying to sell is that you *can* make great gains in muscle mass or fat loss in a short time. The reality is that the time it takes is far greater than they would have us believe.

The perception under which marketeers operate is that consumers of bodybuilding products and training techniques want to believe the radical claims. The unfortunate reality is that they aren't as likely to buy the product if the gains appear minimal. Reality and perception, it seems, are worlds apart, and marketeers have long known that by manipulating the perception of their product, it sells better. Reality is either totally irrelevant or nearly so in their world, because (they believe) it doesn't often sell product.

Having been deeply involved in bodybuilding and fitness all my life, I've acquired a pretty good feel for what can be accomplished through integrated training. I have always believed that through meticulous application of science, you can successfully amplify the gains you'll make in a given time frame. Maybe not to the point of gaining 30 pounds of muscle in six or eight weeks, but certainly far beyond the morally bankrupt perceptions of the dishonest marketeers out there.

Exactly how much improvement can you expect? Enough to satisfy the marketeers? Don't bother trying—they don't care. Enough so that reality becomes the saleable perception? Well, wouldn't that be a new twist!

Enough so that it satisfies you? You bet.

THE ACID TEST

As Director of Research & Development for ICOPRO, Inc.,* I was fortunate to have the opportunity to test the effectiveness of integrated training under rigorously controlled conditions. The integrated variable split system (the "ABC" system) of bodybuilding described in detail in the preceding chapters served as my research model.

FIGURE 8-1

Subject Profile

Length of Study: Nine weeks (9/21/92 through 11/21/92)

Average Training Experience	
Men	5.89
Women	6.1
Subjects	
Men	17
Women	5
Average Age	
Men	29.1
Women	33.8
Average Height	
Men	5'10"
Women	5'6"

The ICOPRO Experiment

Thirty subjects from gyms around the Stamford, Connecticut, area participated in the experimental group. They were given a year's membership in the gym of their choice for their participation in the nine-week research period. They were also informed that there would be a $1,000 prize given to those whose results were selected for use in an advertising campaign. All trained once or twice daily, with Sundays off. All followed precise integrated training schedules and routines very similar to those covered in this book.

---

*ICOPRO, Inc., a bodybuilding and sports nutrition corporation, is a division of TitanSports, Inc., the parent company of the World Wrestling Federation and World Bodybuilding Federation. ICOPRO™ is the acronym for Integrated Conditioning Programs.

FIGURE 8-2

Means for Comparison

When reviewing the pre- and post-blood test results, compare the mean values given with the following ranges of normal.

white blood count (th/cmm) 4.5–10.0
red blood count (m/cmm) 4.10–5.51
hemoglobin (g/dl) 14.4–16.4
hematocrit (%) 42–49
glucose (mg/dl)...70–110
sodium (mmol/l) 135–151
potassium (mmol/l) 3.5–5.1
total protein (g/dl) 6.6–8.6
albumin: serum (9g/dl) 3.5–4.8
albumin/globulin ratio (ratio) 1.1–2.3
cholesterol (mg/dl) 100–200
triglycerides (mg/dl) 40–200
CHOL/HDL (mg/dl)..45–65
CHOL/LDL (mg/dl) 50–130
CHOL/HDL ratio (ratio) 4.5–6.4

All subjects were administered stringent urinalyses by an accredited drug testing laboratory before, during, and after the experiment in order to absolutely eliminate the possibility of drug (anabolic steroids) abuse. All were administered blood tests to monitor nutritional status and nitrogen balance tests to determine nutritional/training effectiveness.

Figures 8-3 through 8-6 are records of the ICOPRO subjects' anthropometric, health and fitness, and performance scores before and after the experimental period.

Note that this experimental treatment is a radical departure from the typical marketing procedure of merely presenting before and after photos with dubious authenticity or control for illegal drugs.

In a nutshell, folks, the ABC system of integrated bodybuilding just plain works better than any bodybuilding system there ever was. The support for this statement is self-evident in the raw data contained in the tables on pages 68–70.

FIGURE 8-3

Body Composition Comparisons

	Pretest	Posttest
Body weight		
Men	181.3	177.67
Women	147.8	140.3
Percent body fat		
Men	15.4	11.6
Women	25.5	22.2

Girth Measurements (in inches)

	Pretest	Posttest
Chest Girth		
Men	40.5	42.25
Women	36.8	36.1
Upper-arm girth		
Men	15.2	14.77
Women	11.5	11.7
Forearm girth		
Men	11.76	12
Women	9.75	10
Waist girth		
Men	33	31.66
Women	27.5	26.25
Hip girth		
Men	37.67	37.19
Women	37	35.8
Thigh girth		
Men	23.76	24.93
Women	23.35	22.65
Calf girth		
Men	15.18	15.4
Women	14.6	14.4

Skinfolds (in millimeters)

	Pretest	Posttest			Pretest	Posttest
Biceps				**Abdominal**		
Men	4.5	3.4		Men	17.43	13.21
Women	5	4.7		Women	12.8	11
Subscapula				**Thigh**		
Men	14.8	11.61		Men	12	8.7
Women	13.2	10.4		Women	22.2	19.3
Triceps				**Pectoral**		
Men	8.78	5.58		Men	12.5	9.14
Women	14.4	11.7		Women	(not taken)	(not taken)
Suprailiac						
Men	7.68	6.37				
Women	7.8	7.2				

FIGURE 8-4

Health and Fitness Comparisons

	Pretest	Posttest
Resting heart rate		
Men	67.82	67
Women	70.4	60.8
Blood pressure		
Men	128/73	129/71
Women	117/69	111/63
Psychological stress level		
Men	4.7/3.7	1.5/.95
Women	6.8/6.2	1.6/1.2
Nitrogen retention		
Men	929	755
Women	1290	710

FIGURE 8-5

Blood Tests

(Analyses provided by St. Joseph's Medical Center, Stamford, CT)

	Men— Pretest	Women— Pretest	Men— Posttest	Women— Posttest
WBC	7.10	6.83	6.24	6.35
RBC	5.10	5.15	5.41	5.40
Hemoglobin	15.40	15.30	15.10	15.16
Hematocrit	44.30	43.80	43.24	43.08
Glucose	84.00	87.00	91.20	89.60
Sodium	140.00	138.00	141.20	139.20
Potassium	4.30	4.40	4.42	4.44
Total protein	7.30	7.40	7.30	7.42
Albumin: serum	4.40	4.30	4.46	4.46
Albumin/globulin ratio	1.50	1.40	1.58	1.50
Cholesterol	176.00	151.00	167.40	155.20
Triglycerides	92.00	84.00	101.00	88.60
CHOL:HDL	51.00	48.00	42.60	45.60
CHOL:LDL	107.00	87.00	104.60	91.80
CHOL:HDL ratio	3.70	3.30	4.12	3.61

FIGURE 8-6

Performance Profile

	Pretest	Posttest

Explosive Strength

Vertical jump

Men	21.18	22.7
Women	16.7	15.85

Seated medicine ball throw (best attempt out of five)

Men	14.13	14
Women	9.75	9.95

Agility

Zigzag run

Men	6.19	5.31
Women	7.3	5.96

Anaerobic Strength Endurance

Medicine ball throws in 2–3-second intervals within 12″ of best throw

Men	12	9.5
Women	11.5	9.2

Limit Strength Tests (One Rep at Max)

Exercise	Pretest	Posttest
Sit-ups		
Men	41	55
Women	20.4	30
Curl		
Men	110	125
Women	65	77.6
Upright row		
Men	106	135
Women	79	83.3
Standing press		
Men	147	160
Women	72.4	88.3
Bench press		
Men	245	295
Women	112	123.3
Squat		
Men	326	370
Women	171.6	182.5
Bent over row		
Men	178	210
Women	101.4	107.5

PART THREE

BODYBUILDING EXERCISE TECHNIQUES

DEDICATED TO BARRY DE MEY

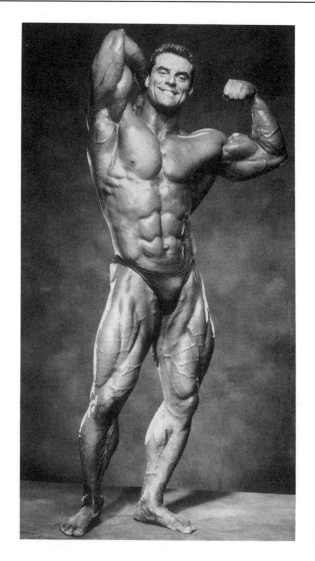

Barry De Mey

9

INTRODUCTION TO EXERCISE TECHNIQUE

All bodybuilders have their favorite exercises for each body part. Trying to pry you away from yours would be like taking your favorite teddy bear away from you. Often, however, some of the exercises I've seen bodybuilders doing in the gym are about as useful as a teddy bear—you know, movements that are comfortable and familiar or somehow perpetuate some real or imagined mystique you've ascribed to yourself and to your social station within the gym. The simple truth is, you just like certain exercises. As for the notion that your favorites are better than others, well, maybe and maybe not.

Rather than force you to give up your teddy bear, let me offer some advice that you may find very useful. Maybe you can keep your teddy bear (it's probably not hurting anything for you to do so) and, at the same time, begin doing some of the tried-and-true permutations of all of the body-part exercises in such a way that you will derive maximum benefit.

THE BEST WAY TO DO ALL EXERCISES

Every muscle in your body has an origin and insertion point. The practice of twisting and turning which way and that while doing an exercise is futile in affecting the shape a muscle will eventually assume. Your genetic predisposition will determine each muscle's shape. But you *can* make each muscle bigger.

Your muscles' origin is usually the connection closest to the midline of your body. That means it's the nonmoving end of the muscle. Your job is to force the insertion point of the muscle toward the origin point—through the "belly" of the muscle—while placing it under adaptive overload stress. Most often, that means that you should just pile on a lot of pig iron and lift the damned bar. Don't get cute!

What to Do About Poor Genetics

As I see it, there are five options open to you if you're one of the unlucky ones who, upon conception, got a swift kick in the proverbial genes. These options are discussed in detail in Part Nine. Then again, you can simply forget about the problem, and—for love of what you do—lift the damned bar!

A Word about "Cheating" Exercises

You may, during training sessions designed to emphasize your fast-twitch (white) muscle fibers, "swing" or "heave" the weight. Refer to Part Eight for a complete discussion of the usefulness and correct techniques for incorporating this advanced training method into your integrated "ABC" training regimen *before* you attempt it.

A Word about Forced Reps

Forced reps are when you're using a weight that's too heavy to do, say, 12 reps, but you do them anyway, with your partner helping you do the last 3–5 reps. The theory is that you'll receive better overload throughout the entire set.

Under certain conditions, the theory makes sense. Refer to Part Eight for a full discussion of this advanced bodybuilding technique *before* you attempt to incorporate it into your training strategy.

FIGURE 9-1

Muscles and Their Actions

Muscles of the Lower Extremities

LOCATION	ANKLE	ANKLE	KNEE	KNEE	HIP	HIP	HIP	HIP
Action	Dorsiflexion	Plantar Flexion	Flexion	Extension	Flexion	Extension	Adduction	Abduction
Tibialis anterior	X							
Gastrocnemius		X	X					
Soleus		X						
Rectus femoris				X	X			
Vastus medialis				X				
Vastus lateralis				X				
Biceps femoris			X			X	X	
Semimembranosus			X			X		
Semitendinosis			X			X		
Iliopsoas group					X			X
Adductor group					X		X	
Gluteus medius						X		X
Gluteus maximus						X		
Tensor faciae latae				X	X			X

Muscles of the Upper Extremities

LOCATION	SHOULDER	SHOULDER	SHOULDER	SHOULDER	ELBOW	ELBOW	FOREARM	FOREARM	WRIST	WRIST
Action	Flexion	Extension	Adduction	Abduction	Flexion	Extension	Supination	Pronation	Flexion	Extension
Pectoralis major	X		X							
Deltoid, anterior	X									
Deltoid, medial				X						
Deltoid, posterior		X		X						
Latissimus dorsi		X	X							
Biceps brachii	X			X	X		X			
Triceps brachii		X	X			X				
Brachioradialis					X		X	X		
Forearm flexor group								X	X	
Forearm extensor group							X			X

Muscles of the Trunk, Head, and Neck

LOCATION	TRUNK	TRUNK	TRUNK	TRUNK	SCAPULA	SCAPULA	SCAPULA	HEAD-NECK	HEAD-NECK	HEAD-NECK	HEAD-NECK
Action	Flexion	Extension	Rotation	Lateral Flex.	Elevation	Depression	Retraction	Flexion	Extension	Rotation	Lateral Flex
Rectus abdominis	X			X							
External abd. oblique	X		X	X							
Internal abd. oblique	X		X	X							
Erector spinae group		X									
Trapezius					X	X	X				
Pectoralis minor						X					
Latissimus dorsi						X					
Splenius cervicis									X	X	X
Splenius capitis									X	X	X
Sternocleidomastoid								X		X	X

10

BODYBUILDING EXERCISES

SHOULDER EXERCISES

Shoulders
Target Muscles

Deltoids (front, middle, and rear shoulders)

1. Supra-spinatus
2. Infra-spinatus
3. Teres minor
4. Subscapularis
5. Spine of scapula
6. Clavicle
7. Humerus
8. Biceps brachii—
   Long head
9. Biceps brachii—
   Short head
10. Teres major

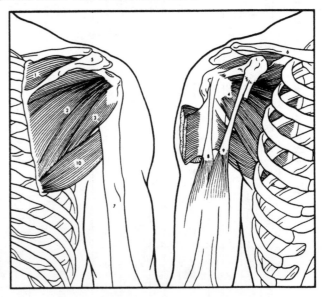

Lateral Dumbbell Raises

Your middle deltoids (three heads share a common tendon of insertion) raise your arms laterally. Using two dumbbells hanging in front of you, raise them up in a sideward direction to about head height several times. Higher isn't necessary, as the middle delts are finished contracting by the time your hands are at head height. Going higher involves the serratus anterior muscles.

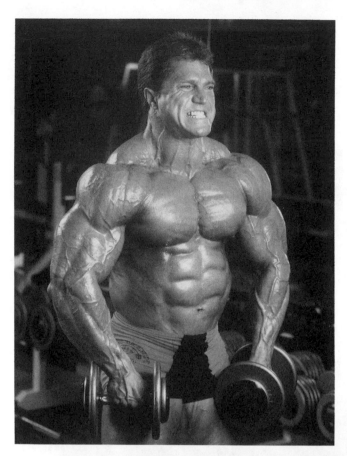

**Lateral
Dumbbell
Raises**

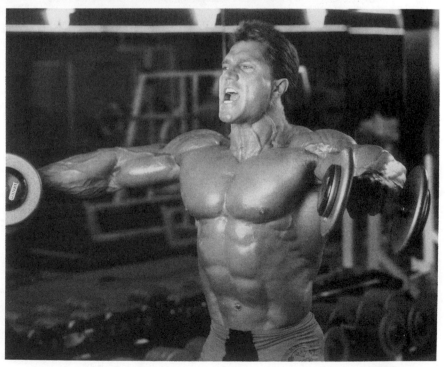

Upright Rows

This is another exercise for the middle deltoids. Holding the weighted bar in front of you with a close overhand grip, pull it upward along your torso, almost to your chin, while keeping your elbows above the bar.

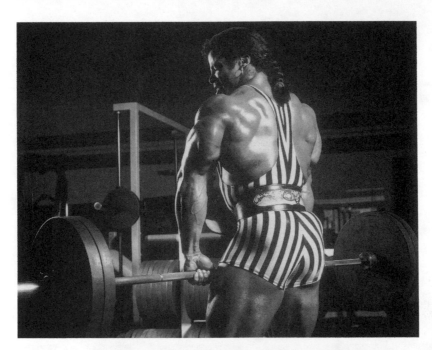

Upright Rows

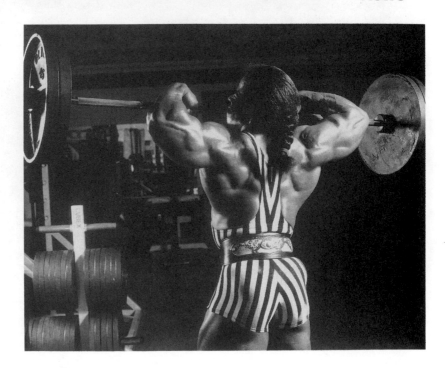

Shrugs

Your trapezius muscles (called *traps*) elevate and support your shoulder girdle (i.e., pull your shoulders toward your ears). Simply hold a bar in front of you and "shrug" your shoulders straight upward. You don't have to rotate your shoulders—just shrug.

An alternative method is to shrug with heavy dumbbells while either seated or standing. The straight bar must be held out in front of you, while seated dumbbell shrugs allow the arms to hang naturally at your sides. This makes dumbbell shrugs a bit more comfortable and definitely easier on your lower back. Holding a heavy bar in front of you requires a strong contraction of your erector spinae muscles.

Normal shrugging technique (as explained above) activates the two upper portions of your trapezius (i.e., trapezius I and II). By leaning forward (about 20–30 degrees) and then shrugging straight up—not toward your ears, but vertically toward the ceiling—you

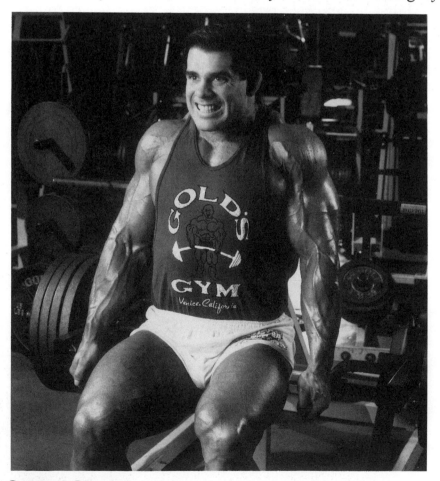

Seated Shrugs

will activate trapezius III and IV. You may wish to support your upper body against a padded surface (like a preacher curl bench) in order to alleviate unnecessary stress on your lower back while leaning forward.

Seated Press Behind the Neck

While seated on an upright back bench, remove the bar from its cradles and lower it until it touches the back of your neck. Then, press it straight back upward to arm's length. Repeat this movement for the requisite number of reps.

Despite its popularity among bodybuilders, I'm mildly opposed to this exercise for at least two reasons. First, assuming that you wish to do complete presses to lockout, seated dumbbell presses accomplish the same thing without the same interference from having to crunch your upper back muscles in order to get the bar down to your neck. Having to contract your rhomboids, your trapezius III and IV, and your posterior deltoids only serves to limit the amount of adaptive stress being delivered to your middle deltoids. Second, after the bar has passed the top of your head, your deltoids are no longer the prime movers in the movement. The deltoids are statically contracting at that point, and the serratus anterior and triceps muscles take over to finish the press to lockout.

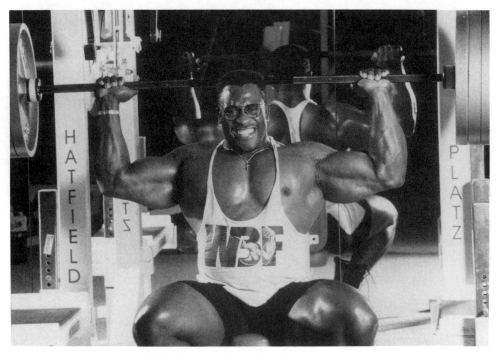

Seated Presses Behind the Neck

Actually, you can press much more weight to a head-height position than you can press completely overhead. The reason for this is your middle deltoids are much stronger than the combined strength of your triceps and serratus. Does it not, therefore, make more sense to use a heavier weight and do partial presses? I think it does, and the simple reason is it will deliver a greater adaptive stress to your middle delts.

Seated Dumbbell Press

Bring the dumbbells to your shoulders, sit down on either a padded back bench or a flat bench with no back, and follow the same directions for seated presses behind the neck.

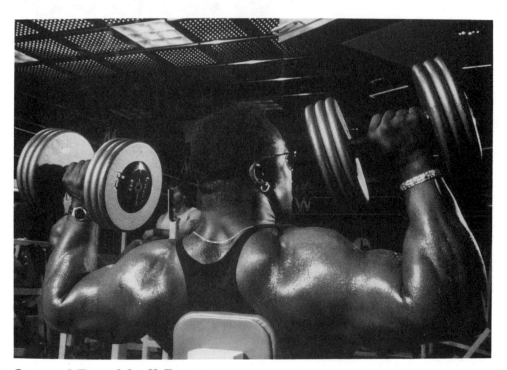

Seated Dumbbell Presses

Seated partial presses are my personal favorite middle-deltoid exercise. As I noted earlier, you will be able to use more weight with partials than you can with full-lockout presses, and that spells greater deltoid development.

Front Raises

The traditional method of exercising your frontal deltoids is to raise either dumbbells or a bar upward and to the front of your body with

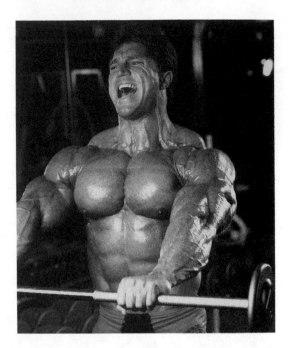

Front Barbell Raises

slightly bent elbows. If dumbbells are used, they can be raised alternately or simultaneously.

I think there's a better way. Using dumbbells, alternately raise them upward and to the front as described above, but with one significant difference. Before raising the dumbbell in your right hand, lean 20–30 degrees to the right. Before raising the left one, lean to the left in a similar fashion. The dumbbells are raised to about head height at arm's length in front of your face.

The rationale for this departure from traditional technique is that your frontal deltoids originate and insert at about that angle from the vertical plane of your body. Bending sideward while performing the dumbbell raises places the targeted frontal delt perpendicular to the floor, thereby making its contraction (force output) more efficient. Do that, and the adaptive stress is improved.

Inverted Flyes

The back part of your shoulders (posterior deltoids) usually work synergistically with several other pulling muscles of the upper back. You can come pretty close to isolating them with inverted flyes (your trapezius III and IV as well as your rhomboids are always activated to work synergistically with your posterior delts). Bend forward to a position where your torso is nearly parallel with the floor, and, grasping the dumbbells, raise them laterally (away from your sides) in a flying movement. Keep your elbows slightly bent to avoid undue elbow stress.

CHEST EXERCISES

Chest
Target Muscles

Clavicular pectoralis
(upper chest)
Sternal pectoralis
(lower chest)

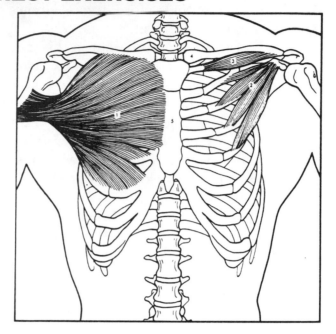

1. Pectoralis major
2. Pectoralis minor
3. Subclavius
4. Clavicle
5. Sternum

Bench Press

Your pectoral muscles (called *pecs*) are developed with bench presses. *Never* bench press alone! It's potentially dangerous, so have a spotter close by at all times. Have your spotter help you lift the bar out of the uprights and to a position directly over your chest. Lower the weight to your chest and press it back up to arm's length again. After performing the required number of reps, have the spotter assist you in placing the bar back on the uprights. You can emphasize your pecs more if your elbows are away from your sides (per-

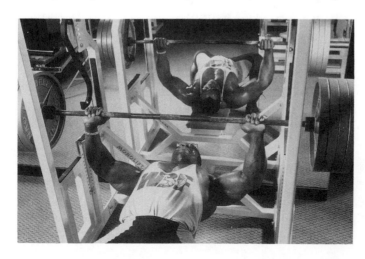

**Bench Presses
(Monolift)**

pendicular to your torso) during the movement, and you can emphasize your front deltoids more if your elbows are kept close to your sides during the movement.

Much of the danger inherent in this exercise can be eliminated by using a Monolift machine. This new device allows you to position the bar directly over your chest before you unrack the bar. While bench pressing, special spotting platforms ensure that, should the bar be dropped accidentally or should you miss the lift, the weight will not come down on you. Rather than require your training partner to help you rack the bar, he rotates the cradle hooks under the bar while it's still held over your chest.

There are two particularly troublesome techniques I see all too often among bench pressers. One is the dangerous practice of using a thumbless grip. The notion that a thumbless grip will somehow alter the angle or quality of stress you're delivering to your pecs is outrageously dumb. Keep your thumbs around the bar!

The second practice is just as outrageous. I've heard benchers say that keeping your feet off the floor—suspended over the bench or resting on the bench—somehow improves the isolation of the pecs and therefore the adaptive overload being delivered to your pecs. The truth is that while your feet are off the floor, you're always slightly off balance on the narrow bench you're lying on, and various stabilizer muscles are attempting to keep you from falling off the bench. This superfluous muscular activity detracts from the stress you can deliver to the pecs. It is certainly *not* improving it. Besides, being off balance while a heavy weight is hovering over your face and throat is downright asking for trouble!

Dumbbell Bench Press

I favor dumbbell bench presses over benching with a bar because you can achieve greater adaptive stress with dumbbells. Lowering the dumbbells will tend to force you to keep your upper arms perpendicular to your torso. Many benchers allow their elbows to drift inward toward their sides while using a straight bar. This happens because there's a natural tendency to use the anterior (frontal) deltoids to assist in moving the bar, thereby robbing the pecs of some stress.

Also, dumbbells allow you to employ a little-known technique, which I developed some years ago, that will improve the adaptive stress being delivered to your pecs. By carefully (under total control) allowing the dumbbells to drift slightly off balance toward the

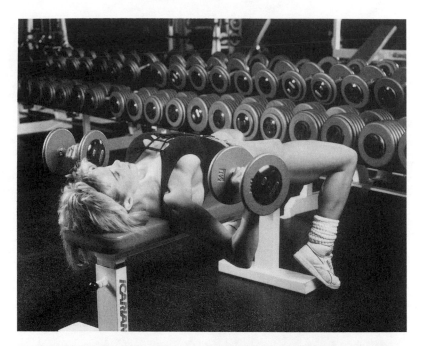

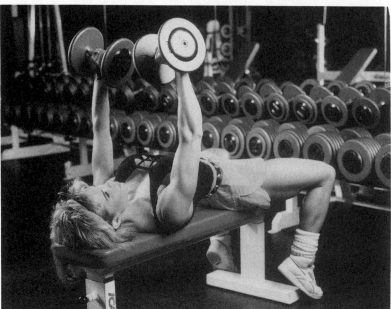

Dumbbell Bench Presses

outside, you will have to fight harder to raise them. This controlled outward drift allows you to use superior weight while getting the same benefits afforded by regular flyes. Regular flyes are done with very light weights, whereas modified dumbbell benches employ far heavier weight.

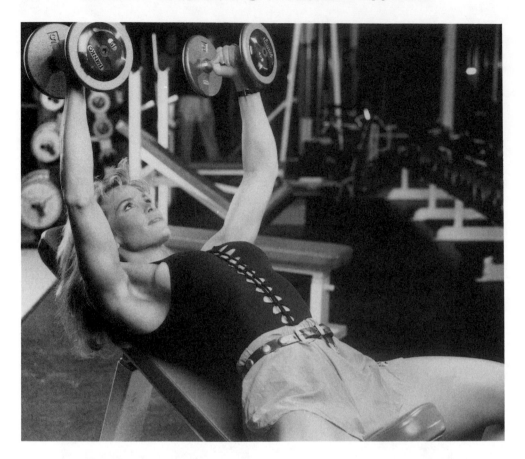

Flyes

Speaking of flyes, here's another great exercise for your pecs. Raise the dumbbells to arm's length over your chest. In a flying motion, lower the dumbbells laterally (outward from your body) until they're at the same level as the bench you're lying on. Then, raise them back up to arm's length. You'll find that the exercise is more comfortable if you bend your elbows slightly during the movement. You shouldn't keep your arms totally straight, as doing so places undue stress on your elbow joint.

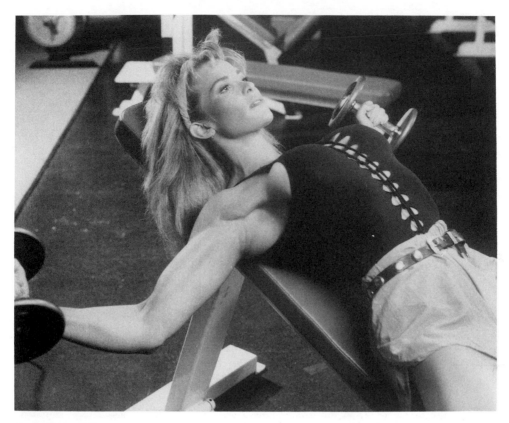

Incline Flyes

Do not perform this movement explosively, since many smaller muscles located inside your shoulder joint (i.e., your rotator cuff muscles) can easily be damaged if you do.

Incline Flyes

To target your clavicular pectorals (upper chest) as opposed to the sternal pectorals (lower chest), as regular flyes do, simply adjust your bench to somewhere between 20–30 degrees of incline. Follow the same instructions given for flyes.

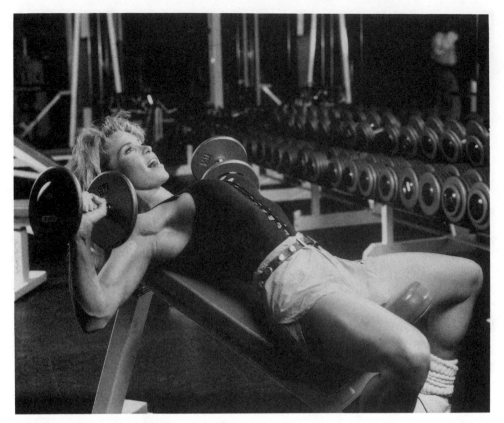

Incline Dumbbell Presses

Incline Dumbbell Presses

To target your clavicular pectorals (upper chest) as opposed to the sternal pectorals (lower chest), as regular dumbbell bench presses do, simply adjust your bench to somewhere between 20–30 degrees of incline. Follow the same instructions given for dumbbell bench presses.

Incline Bench Press

To target your clavicular pectorals (upper chest) as opposed to the sternal pectorals (lower chest), as regular (straight bar) bench presses do, simply adjust your bench to somewhere between 20–30 degrees of incline. Follow the same instructions given for regular bench presses.

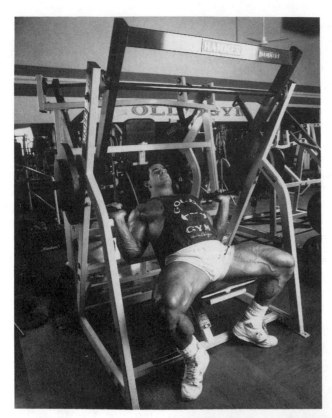

Incline Bench Presses (Machine)

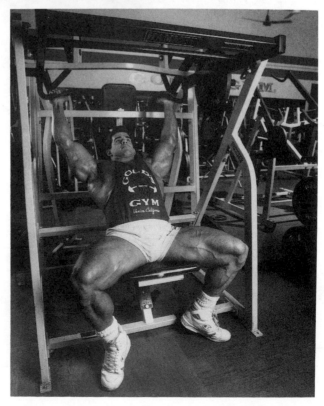

Cable Crossovers

This is a great way to achieve good isolation for your upper or lower pecs. Standing between two cable towers equipped with both upper and lower cables, grasp (for example) the upper handles and adjust your foot spacing, body position, and body lean in such a way that you're receiving maximum stress on your lower (sternal) pecs. With elbows slightly bent, pull diagonally downward across your body and continue until your hands pass one another in front of your hips. This crossing over of your hands will ensure complete contraction of your pecs. You cannot achieve the same complete pectoral contraction with dumbbells or a barbell.

The same technique applies to upper (clavicular) pec crossovers. Begin with your arms at a downward angle and, after pulling the handles diagonally upward and out in front of you, finish by crossing over upward and out in front of your face.

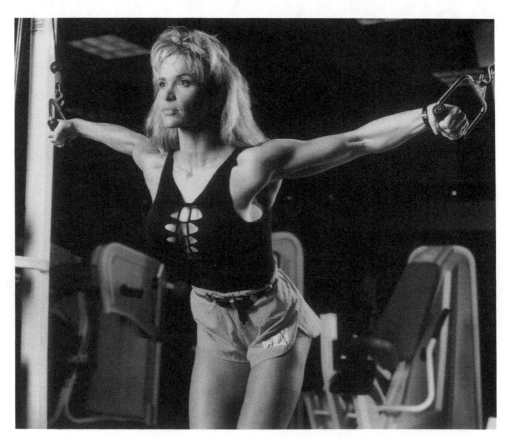

Cable Crossovers

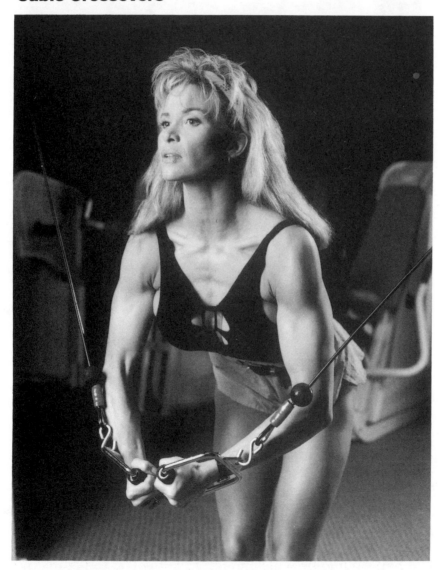

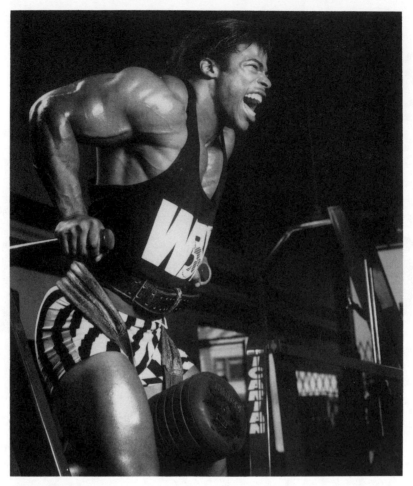

Weighted Dips

Dips

Most bodybuilders use dips for anterior deltoids or triceps. By keeping your torso upright between the two parallel bars while dipping, most of the stress is borne by these two muscles. With a slight adjustment to your body's position, however, dips become an excellent auxiliary exercise for the lower pecs.

Supporting your weight between the two bars, begin dipping. As your body descends, lean forward with your shoulders and keep your hips back. The movement then becomes very similar to decline bench presses, except that *you're* moving instead of the bar.

The bars should be wide enough to allow you to get maximum stretch while in the bottom position. As with regular dips, you can hang as much weight around your waist (with a specially designed dip belt) as you can handle, so you can do the appropriate number of reps.

Pec Deck

The pec deck exercise simulates dumbbell flyes. Because you're using a machine, the direction (angle) of movement is predetermined for you. Sometimes that's good, and sometimes that's bad. Whether it's good for you will depend on both the machine's design and your own anatomical peculiarities.

I've found very few pec decks that do not cause me to experience shoulder-joint irritation. On the other hand, you may like the exercise. It's your call.

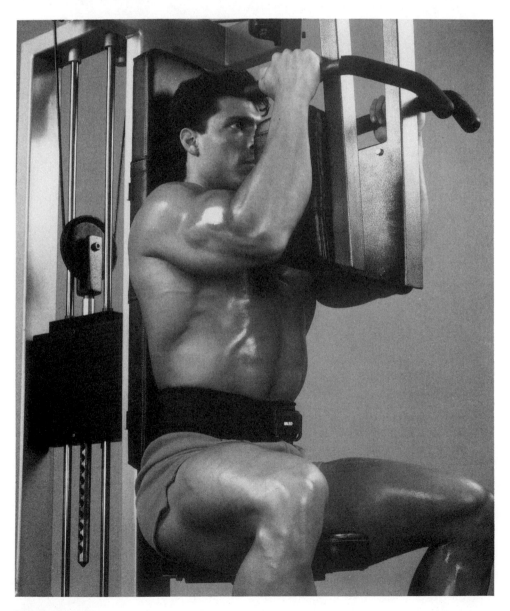

Pec Deck

BACK EXERCISES

BACK
Target Muscles

Latissimus dorsi
  (arm depressor muscles)

Rhomboids
  (downward rotators
  of the scapulae)

Trapezius
  (shoulder elevators)

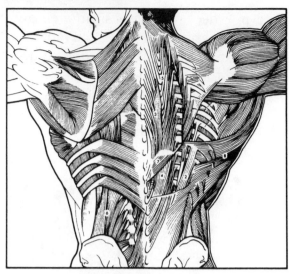

1. Internal Oblique
2. Ilio-costalis ★
3. Spinalis dorsi ★
4. Longissimus dorsi ★
5. Transversalis cervicis ★
6. Quadratus lumborum

7. Trapezius (sectioned)
8. Latissimus dorsi
9. Levator anguli scapularis
10. Rhomboideus minor
11. Rhomboideus major
12. Serratus posticus inferior

★ Muscles of the Erector Spinae

BENT OVER ROWS (AND VARIATIONS)

This exercise is exactly like inverted flyes (described as a posterior deltoid exercise), except you use a bar instead of dumbbells. Bending forward to a position where your body is nearly parallel to the floor, pull the bar to your lower chest, making sure that your elbows lead the way.

If your intent is to target your posterior delts, rhomboids, and lower trapezius muscles, you should ensure that your elbows are kept perpendicular to your torso, not close to your sides. Doing rows with your elbows closer to your sides is a variation that'll target your lats principally, not your posterior delts.

There are many variations to bent over rows, some employing dumbbells and others employing specially designed machines. *One-arm rows*, for example, are done using a very heavy dumbbell in one hand while resting your opposite hand and knee on a flat bench. This exercise variation can also be tailored to hit either the upper back (elbow facing outward) or the latissimus (elbow close to your side).

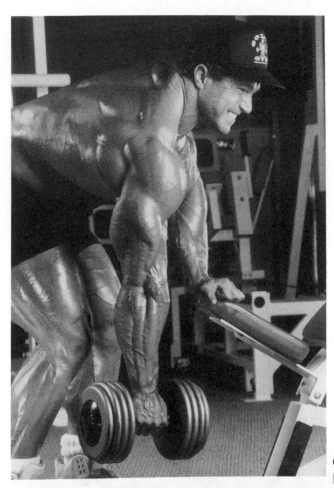

**One-Arm
Dumbbell Rows**

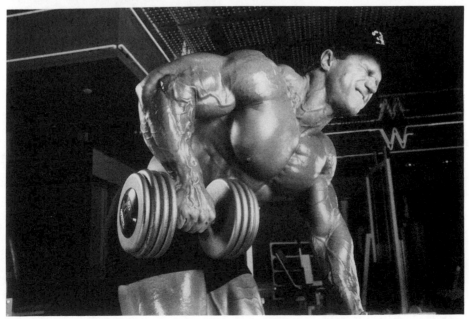

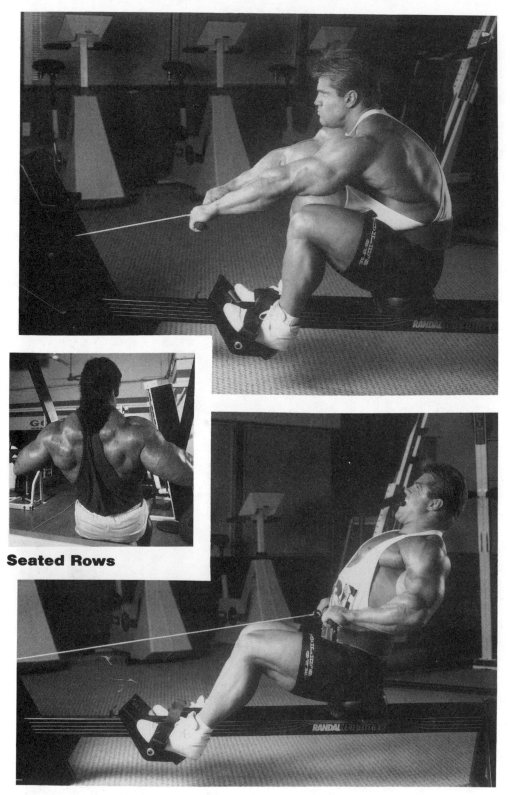

Seated Rows

Long Cable Pulls

Long cable pulls (also called *seated rows* when performed with a machine) are exactly like bent over rows, but you're seated instead of leaning over the bar while standing. Again, elbow position is key in determining which muscle(s) are targeted.

T-bar rows are also exactly like bent rows, except the weighted bar you're pulling on is attached to the floor and allowed to pivot. The many different T-bar handle designs you'll encounter all essentially make it easier to keep your elbows in (for lats) or out (for upper back).

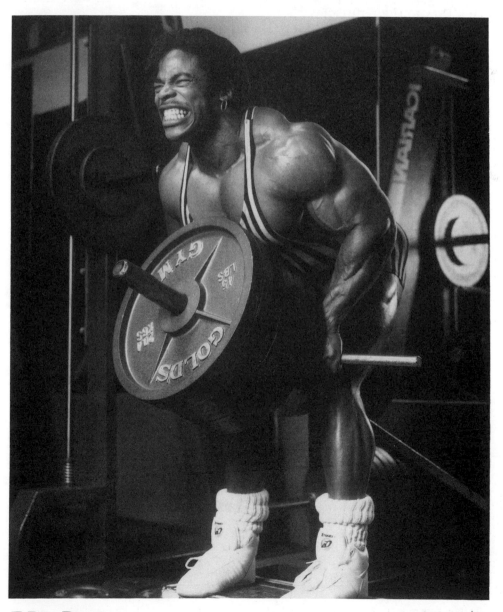

T-Bar Rows

Pulldowns

With a wide grip on the overhead pulley bar, pull the bar straight down as though you were pulling the bar straight through the middle of your head. Of course, you can't *really* do this, so simply flop your head back out of the way. Don't lean backward while doing lat pulldowns, as this will tend to involve other (nontargeted) muscles of your upper back. This exercise is done exactly like chin-ups, except the bar comes down instead of your body going up. It's great for developing your lats and not so great for developing your other back or shoulder muscles.

Some bodybuilders like to do pulldowns behind their neck. I'm not convinced that this is a wise technique. Doing so requires that you contract all of the nontargeted muscles of your upper back (i.e., all four aspects of your trapezius, your rhomboids, and your posterior deltoids) in order to get the bar down behind your head. Why do this? It tends to rob you of maximum overload for your lats (your targeted muscles). Also, pulling the bar so far down that your forearms are not perpendicular to the floor, but are instead almost parallel to the floor, involves the inward rotators of your upper arm (rotator cuff muscles). Again, this tends to rob your lats of maximum overload.

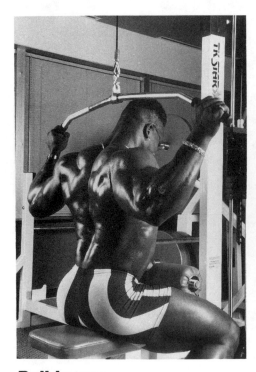 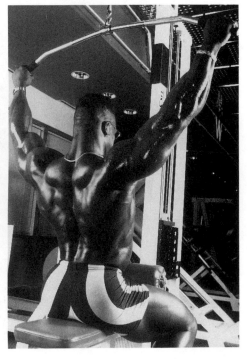

Pulldowns

One variation on lat pulldowns that I introduced a few years ago while training a few strength athletes is catching on in a big way in bodybuilding circles. It's called *lat shrug-downs*. Using more weight than you can pull down to your chin, attach your hands to the bar with lifting straps and have your partner pull you down so you can hook your legs under the thigh pads. Shrug downward with the weight by activating the lats. Do *not* pull with your arms; leave your arms totally uninvolved. I believe this variation is more effective than the traditional full-range pulldowns at developing mass and strength.

Pull-Ups

Pull-ups (or chin-ups) are great for developing your lats, the big V-shaped muscles under your arms that extend down the length of your back. If you can't do at least 8–10 regular pull-ups, try lat pulldowns with a weight that's lighter than your body's. Pulldowns and pull-ups are really identical exercises. Simply hang from a bar and pull yourself upward until your chin touches the bar.

The practice of using variable grip widths is OK, but *just* OK. I'm not convinced that any differential shape to your lats will result from employing different grips.

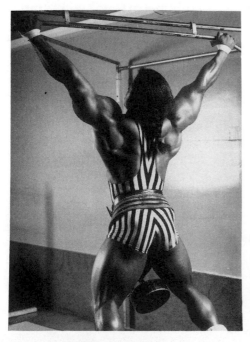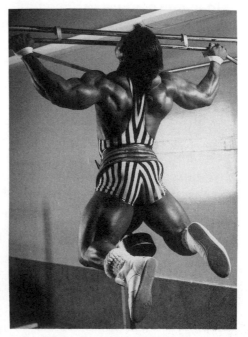

Weighted Pull-Ups

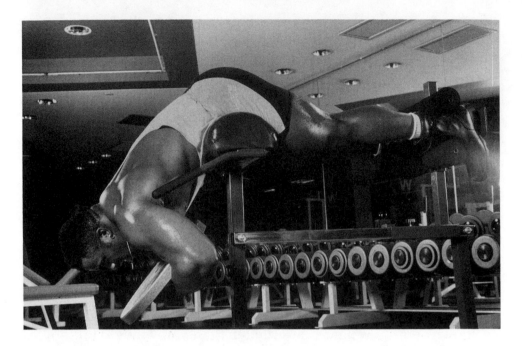

Back Extensions

By far the biggest muscles of your lower back are the erector muscles. They're also the most visible. Naturally, they're the most important lower back muscles involved in bodybuilding. Your erector spinae muscles are designed to extend (and hyperextend) your spine. They do *not* act on your hip joint, so there's no reason to engage in exercises which require hip joint movement.

The best way to target your erectors is with back extensions. This exercise requires the use of a specialized bench quite unlike the ones you're probably used to seeing around the gyms. The "hyper" benches you are used to seeing are, in my opinion, relatively worthless. The bench of choice is called a glute-ham-gastroc machine by its inventor, Dr. Mike Yessis because those muscles are the ones the Russians target with a similar exercise. Glute-ham-gastroc raises are discussed in the section dealing with leg and hip exercises.

To use the glute-ham-gastroc machine to target your erectors, your feet are secured by two foot pads backed by a metal plate that

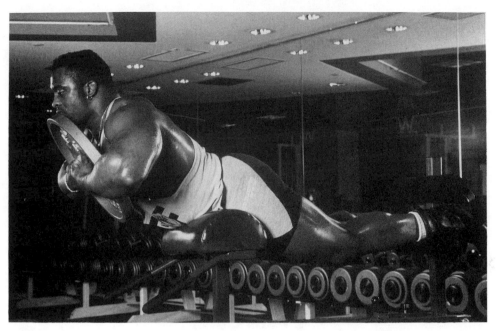

Back Extensions

prevents your feet from slipping through. Your belly button is placed in the middle of the padded support. Your knees are bent. Then, your feet push against the metal plate in order to lock your upper legs against the padded bench. All of this ensures that only your erector muscles are targeted, not your hip extensors (gluteals). Simply assume the described position and flex your spine (round your back downward). Hold as much weight behind your head as you can, and extend your spine (straighten it back out again). You should not raise way up by arching (hyperextending) your back, as doing so places too much strain on the intervertebral discs of your lumbar spine. Repeat for the desired number of reps.

This exercise is quite probably the only low back exercise you will ever have to do as a bodybuilder. It is that effective. Deadlifts, squats, glute-ham raises, and explosive high pulls all involve the lower back muscles as either stabilizers or synergists. However, none is done for the express purpose of developing your lower back.

UPPER ARM EXERCISES

Upper Arms
Target Muscles
Biceps (front of upper arm)
Triceps (back of upper arm)

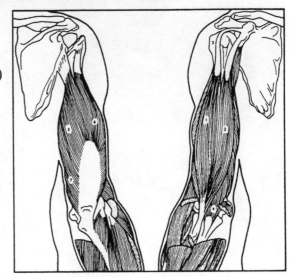

1. Biceps brachii—long head
2. Biceps brachii—short head
3. Head of humerus
4. Brachialis
5. Triceps—scapular head
6. Triceps—lateral head
7. Triceps—medial head

Biceps Curls

Your biceps brachii and brachialis are the major muscles that flex your elbow. Simply curl the weight upward by flexing your elbow. You may use dumbbells, a barbell, a cable arrangement, a machine, or an EZ curl bar. It's a myth that doing them in differing patterns to hit every angle will yield differential development. The elbow is a simple hinge joint and therefore is capable of only flexion and extension.

One note of exception is that since the biceps are comprised of two muscles (with different origins, but sharing a common tendon of insertion), you may achieve a small level of differential development between the long and short heads. Incline curls will prestretch the long head, which may *possibly* result in greater development of that head. Conversely, preacher curls (sometimes called *Scott curls* after the great Larry Scott, first Mr. Olympia winner) unload the long head somewhat, thereby theoretically placing greater overload on the short head of the biceps brachii and the underlying brachialis. Another exception is seen with hammer curls, which are performed while the forearms are pronated in order to activate the brachioradialis while curling the bar (or dumbbells).

Variations of curls abound. Here are a few noteworthy ones. Be aware that, with the exceptions noted above, all are either identical or so similar as to be functionally identical in effect.

- Preacher curls
- One-arm preacher curls
- Alternate dumbbell curls
- Concentration curls
- Barbell curls
- EZ curls
- Cable curls
- Machine curls
- Hammer curls

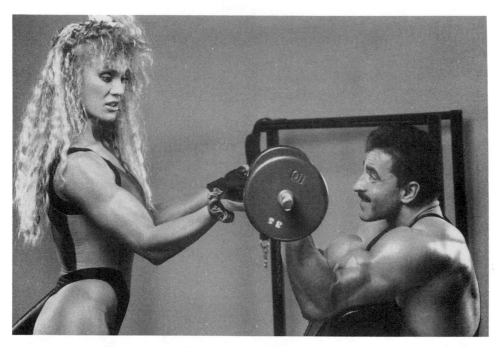

Preacher Curls (with EZ Curl Bar)

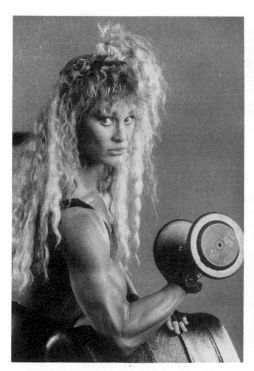

One-Arm Preacher Curls

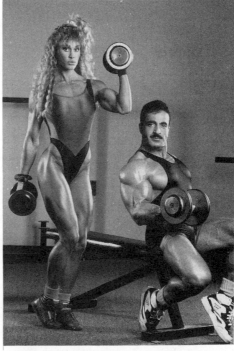

Alternate Dumbbell Curls (Seated and Standing)

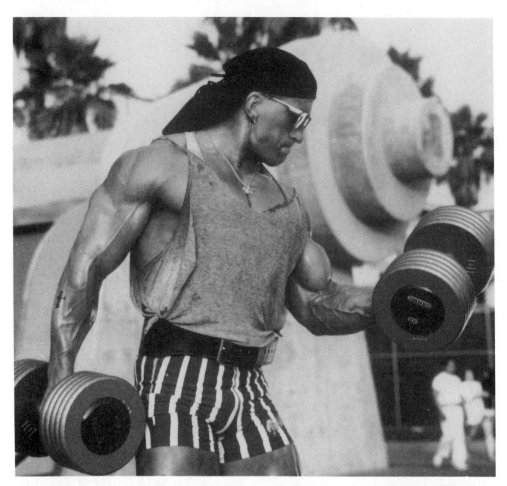

Alternate Dumbbell Curls (Using Cheating Technique)

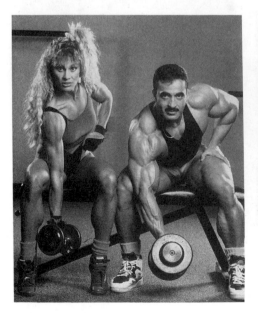

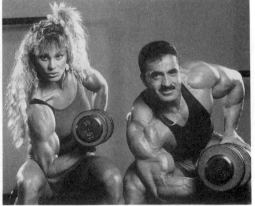

Concentration Curls

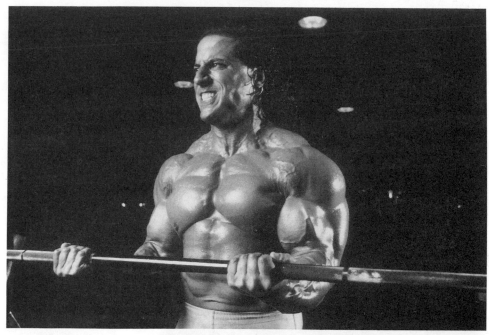

Barbell Curls

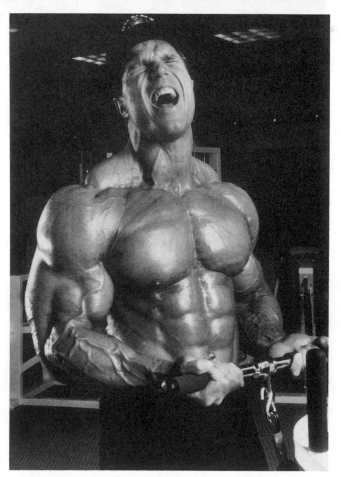

Cable Curls

Nose Crushers

If you're not careful, the weight will fall on your nose, so use a spotter when performing this exercise. Lying on a flat bench with an EZ curl bar and your elbows pointing upward, press the weight from your face to a position overhead. This exercise is for all three heads of the triceps.

As is the case with the biceps, your triceps is really three different muscles sharing a common tendon of insertion. Theoretically, it may be possible to get a slight amount of differential development in each of the heads as follows:

• Prestretch the long head (thereby providing greater overload stress on it) by doing French presses
• Unload the long head (thereby placing greater overload stress on the short head) by doing pushdowns
• All triceps exercises will stress the medial head

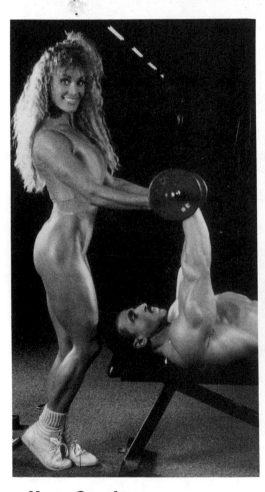 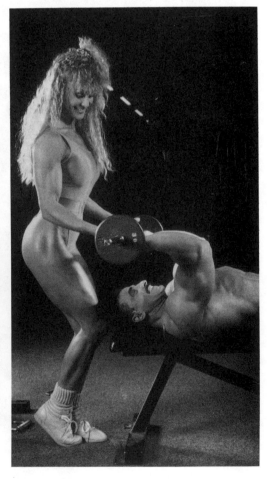

Nose Crushers

Triceps Pushdowns

Another exercise for the triceps, pushdowns require an overhead pulley machine and a special V handle. Holding your elbows against your sides, push down on the handles until your arms are straight. The practice of allowing your elbows to drift forward when lowering the weight in preparation for the next rep allows you to use a heavier weight because of the synergy afforded by your posterior deltoids during the pushdown movement. Such synergy isn't necessarily bad, but it's probably not that helpful, either.

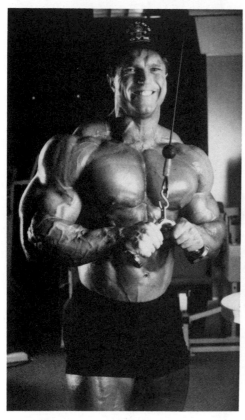 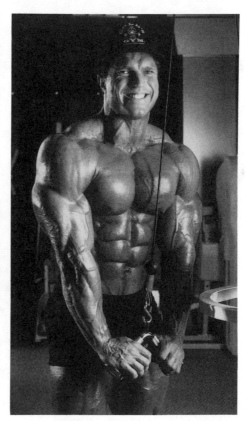

Triceps Pushdowns

As with biceps curls, variations of triceps exercises abound. Here are a few noteworthy ones. Be aware that, with the exception noted above, all are either identical or so similar as to be functionally identical in effect.

- Triceps pushdowns
- French presses
- Nose crushers

- Triceps extensions
- Cable kickbacks
- Dumbbell kickbacks

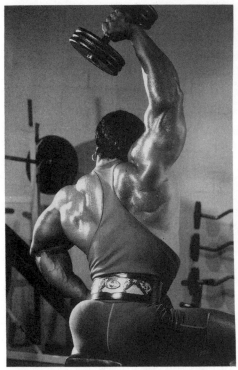

**Seated French Presses
(One-Arm)**

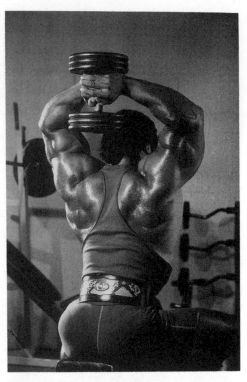

**Seated French Presses
(Two-Arm)**

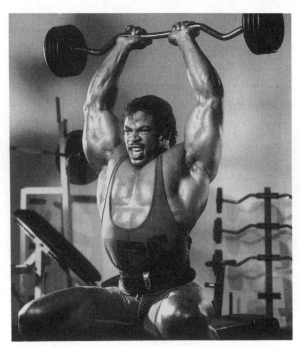

**Seated French Presses
(with EZ Curl Bar)**

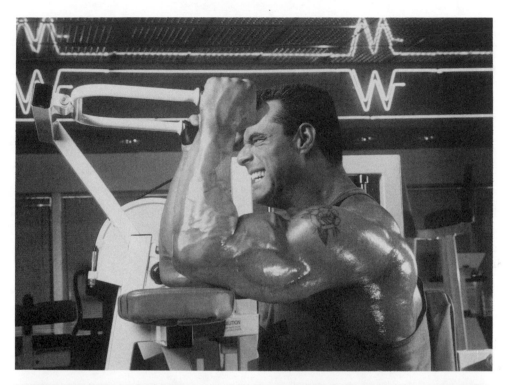

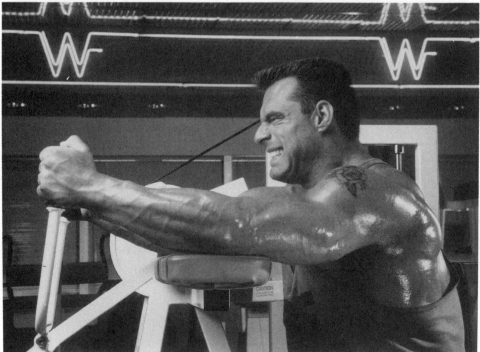

Triceps Extensions (Machine)

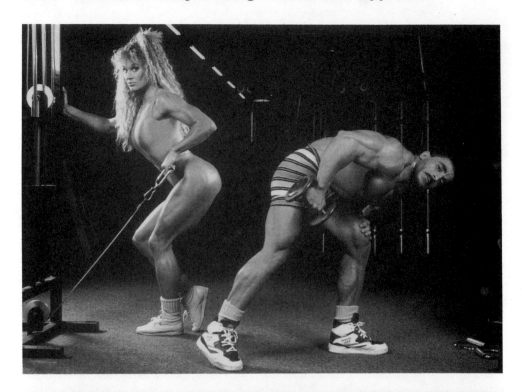

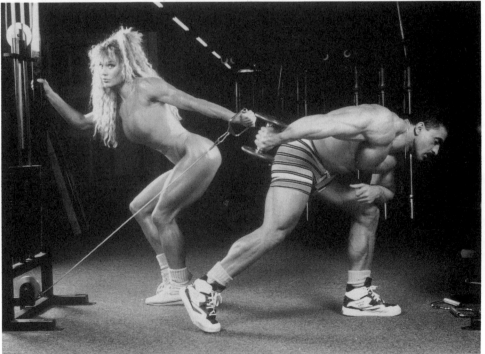

**One-Arm Cable Kickbacks and
One-Arm Dumbbell Kickbacks**

Bench Dips

Place two benches about 3–4 feet apart and get between them. Your feet are resting on one bench and your hands support your weight on the other. With a weight plate on your lap, lower yourself carefully down between the benches (your hands will tend to slip off the edge of the bench if you're not careful). Push back up to a straight-arm support position. This exercise builds your triceps as well as the anterior (front) deltoid muscles of your shoulders.

Parallel Bar Dips

This exercise was discussed under the heading of chest exercises, but it's a good one, so it bears repetition. Supporting your body weight with extra weight attached around your waist if you are able, lower yourself between the bars and press back to a straight-arm support position again. To target your triceps and anterior deltoids to a maximum degree, you must maintain a very erect torso. Leaning forward will relocate some of the stress into your lower pectorals.

FOREARM EXERCISES

Forearms
Target Muscles

Radio-ulnar pronator
   and supinator muscles

Flexors of the fingers

Wrist flexors and
   extensor muscles

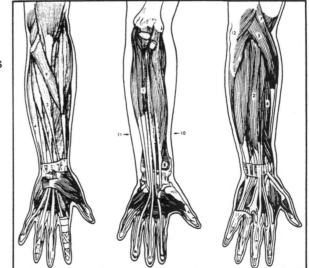

1. Flexor profundus digitorum
2. Extensor communis digitorum
3. Flexor carpi radialis
4. Flexor carpi ulnaris
5. Extensor carpi radialis longior
6. Extensor carpi radialis brevior
7. Supinator longus
8. Pronator quadratus
9. Pronator radii teres
10. Radius
11. Ulna
12. Elbow

Wrist Curls

Forearm curls develop many of the muscles of your forearms. Holding the bar in your hands, rest your forearms on your thighs while seated and allow the bar to hang over the ends of your knees. You can do them palms up or palms facing downward (reverse wrist curls). Let the bar roll to the ends of your fingers and then curl the bar all the way up to a fully flexed position (regular wrist curls) or to a fully hyperextended position (reverse wrist curls).

The finger-roll action will target the small muscles of the forearms which control finger flexion. Exercising them together with the wrist extensors and flexors, your forearms will achieve maximum size.

MIDSECTION EXERCISES

Abdominals
Target Muscles
Abdominals (stomach)

1. Pectoralis major
2. Rectus abdominis
3. External obliques
4. Internal obliques
5. Transversalis
6. Linea alba
7. Linea transversae
8. Linea similunaris
9. Psoas
10. Erector spinae
11. Quadratus lumborum
12. Serratus

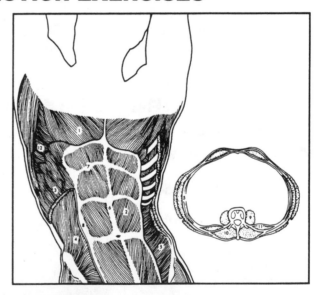

Crunchers

Most bodybuilders don't think of their abdominals (or *abs*) as important to maintaining a strong lower back, but they are exactly that! In addition to achieving that washboard effect all bodybuilders strive for, here's an exercise that is vital for maintaining a healthy, injury-free spine.

Lying on the floor with your legs draped over a bench, curl your head toward your knees so that your abs pull your trunk upward. Don't try to raise your lower back up off the floor. Instead, simply crunch your trunk by pulling your ribs toward your hips. Use a weight plate behind your head if this movement is too easy for you.

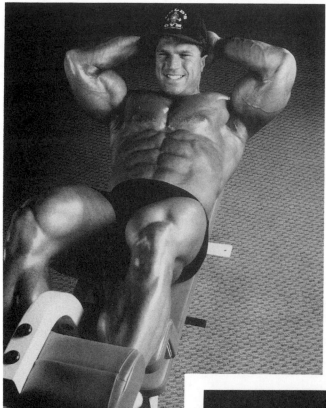

Regular Crunchers

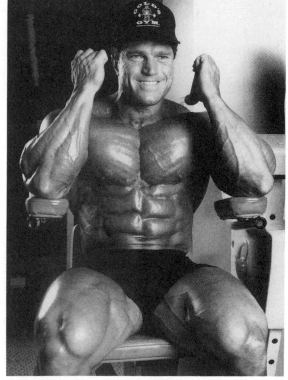

Crunchers (Machine)

The abs perform one function—they flex your spine. *Period.* That's what all abdominal exercises should do—nothing more, and nothing less. There are many variations of crunchers, and there are just as many crunch machines. All, however, have one thing in common—bringing the ribs and pelvis closer together (spinal flexion) by contracting the abdominal muscles.

Your abdominals are designed to provide you with stabilizing force for your upper and lower body. The midsection, after all, is the link between the upper and lower body. That means your primary training aim should be developing the limit strength of your abs. Thus, heavy weights should be used more often. Doing reps endlessly isn't going to give you any better washboard appearance.

Prestretch Crunchers: This variation of crunchers is by far the most effective abdominal exercise. I developed this variation during the seventies and patented the first abdominal machine ever. The patent was successfully protected when a large equipment company tried to infringe upon it—that's why you don't see this particular design element incorporated into any of the dozens of different designs of abdominal machines.

But you *can* do this variation with no specialized equipment. Simply follow the directions given for regular crunchers, but put about 6–8 inches of padding under your glutes and lower back. When lying back, your shoulders have to go all the way back until they touch the floor, thereby prestretching your abdominal muscles prior to contracting them during the crunch movement.

This prestretch offers the advantage of having to contract through roughly double the normal range of motion afforded by regular crunchers or other ab machines. That equates to roughly double the adaptive stress and double the benefits.

Reverse Crunchers: This exercise has the same basic effect as crunchers. However, your knees come toward your face instead of vice versa. Some bodybuilders believe that they can get better lower abdominal development with this exercise. I personally doubt it. It's more tenable that the entire abdominal wall benefits equally from either variation.

You can make this exercise more difficult by raising the incline board that you're lying on a bit higher. Begin with your knees and hips completely flexed. When raising your knees toward your face, you shouldn't swing them upward, as the ballistic movement will tend to remove some of the desired stress. Instead, raise them up.

For nearly double the beneficial effect, you can prestretch your abs by supporting your shoulders and upper back on a 6–8-inch-thick padding. That way, your spine hyperextends slightly so your glutes can touch the bench—and force your abdominals into a pre-stretched position—between each repetition.

Russian Twists

The Russians are famous for their great athletes. One of the exercises that all Russian athletes do for the abdominal muscles, the internal oblique muscles, and the external oblique muscles has become known as Russian twists. Every time you twist, swing a bat, or throw, you use these important muscles. As for its usefulness to bodybuilders, this exercise tightens the entire midsection in a girdle effect.

Study the accompanying photo of this exercise. Notice that your lower back remains in contact with the ground or, better yet, in contact with an SI pad for your sacroiliac, or lower back. Your feet are positioned close to your buttocks (knees bent). Holding a small weight directly over your face at arm's length, twist all the way to the right and then to the left several times. Do not allow your torso or shoulders to come in contact with the ground while twisting back and forth. This is a difficult exercise—but it has a great effect.

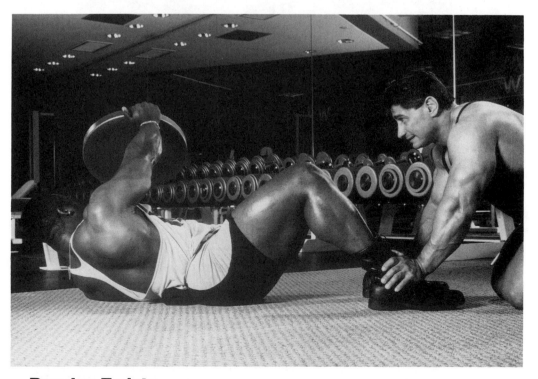

Russian Twists

Hanging Leg Raises

The myth is that hanging while raising your knees upward is going to selectively develop your lower abs. Actually, hanging leg raises is the ultimate version (the highest-stress version) of reverse crunchers. Reread the description of reverse crunchers, and then attempt to do hanging leg raises. Bet you can't! The only people I've ever seen capable of doing this exercise correctly are accomplished gymnasts.

Your best bet is to do reverse crunchers. Remember, flexing your hips during the knee raise develops your hip flexors (iliopsoas) and your grip (forearm) muscles, *not* your abs.

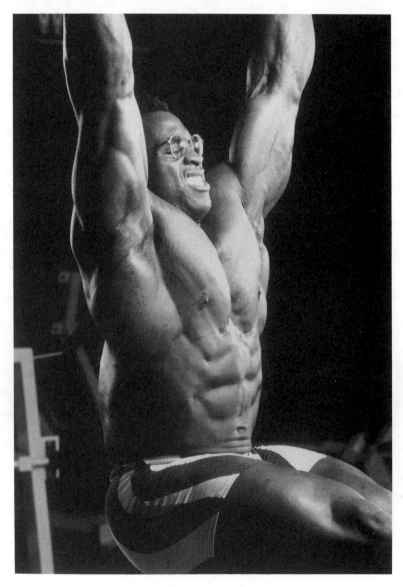

Hanging Leg Raises

Cable Crunchers

Of all the exercises I've ever seen, this is perhaps the most ill-conceived. Hanging onto a cable and then pulling downward on it may indeed involve your abs a bit, but really your body weight is pulling the cable down, not your abs. Your abs are only statically contracting in a stabilizing effect while you raise your knees off the floor slightly so your body weight can act on the weighted cable.

You'd be just as well off merely standing in front of a mirror flexing your abs.

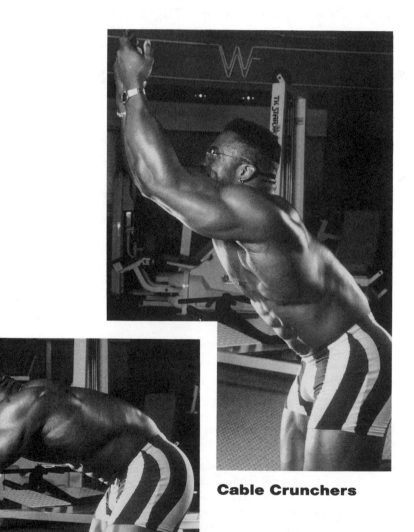

Cable Crunchers

Sidebends

Here's yet another preventive exercise for your spine. This time, you're exercising two very large muscle groups that help stabilize your lower back—your obliques and your quadratus lumborum muscles. Both are extremely important to bodybuilders and athletes alike in that they must be strong to prevent back injuries.

Of course, bodybuilders benefit from the fact that, as with Russian twists, the girdle effect comes into play. Your toned obliques will tend to trim your waist. Simply bend directly sideward toward the side holding the dumbbell. The other arm is behind your head to prestretch your targeted obliques.

HIP AND UPPER-LEG EXERCISES

Hips
Target Muscles

Gluteus maximus
  (your butt)

Gluteus minimus
  (under your hip pocket)

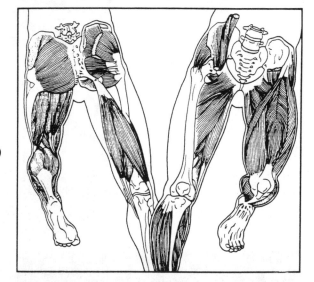

(Opposite) "Dr. Squat," a world champion powerlifter, was challenged to a squatting contest by "The Golden Eagle"—Tom Platz, a world champion bodybuilder known for his motto, "Dare to dream." The Golden Eagle got beat soundly (600 to 840) in maximum weight lifted. Both men weighed in at 198 pounds.
On the flip side, when it came time for the reps contest, Dr. Squat got his butt whipped. The Golden Eagle performed 23 reps with 525 pounds to Dr. Squat's 11 reps.
Why such a difference? Simple. Bodybuilders and powerlifters require different types of strength (see Unit One). Bodybuilders need primarily anaerobic strength endurance, while powerlifters need primarily limit strength.

Squats

Every bodybuilder should do squats, but you have to do them right. You must maintain a very erect body position when descending into the deep squat position. Leaning too far forward can be dangerous for your lower back. To do squats correctly, be prepared to have your coach help you find the proper foot spacing and bar position on your back. Over time, anyone can learn how to do them correctly.

You should also learn how to go down into the squat position low enough. The top of your thighs should be about parallel to the floor, or slightly lower, in a well-executed squat. Higher than that, and you're losing some of the benefit to your quads.

There are many variations to the squat movement. One extremely important one is the lunge squat. Lunge squats can be done to the left, right, or forward, placing the weight on the lead leg. The quad muscles of the lead leg are targeted with both front and side lunges. Side lunges also target the groin muscles (especially the adductor gracilis of the opposite leg).

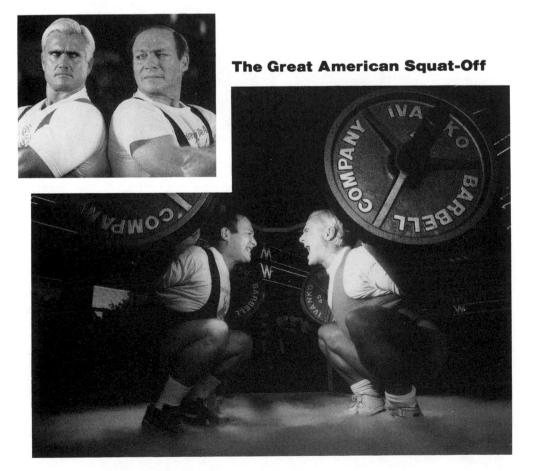

The Great American Squat-Off

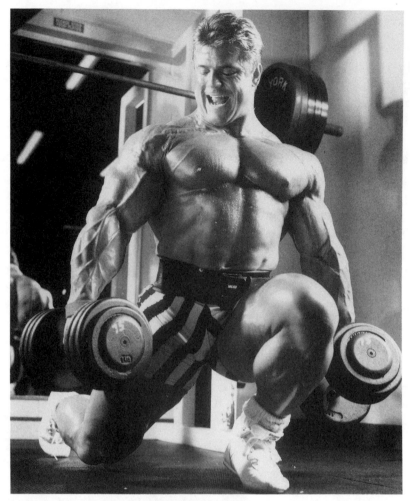

Lunge Walking with Dumbbells

From a front lunge position, you can twist to the opposite side of your lead leg while ascending from the lunge position. I had originally developed this exercise for athletes like down-linemen or shot putters who are required to explode laterally out of a lunge or squat position. Bodybuilders benefit, too, in that fuller leg development is achieved in the sartorius and adductor muscles of the upper leg. Twisting squats, as they're called, require a special harness to wear on your chest and shoulders to hold the short bar in place. Do *not* attempt to do twisting squats with a long bar or with the bar placed on your shoulders. Loss of control in this exercise can mean groin, knee, and lower back injury.

Here are the noteworthy variations to the squat movement that have been employed over the years.

- Powerlifting Squats (wide, intermediate, or narrow stance)
- Olympic squats (also called high bar squats or bodybuilding squats)
- Leg presses (angle of weight ascent ranging from 0 degrees to 90 degrees)
- Hack squats (with barbell or machine)
- Safety squats
- Twisting squats
- Lunge squats
- Side lunge squats
- Partial squats
- Box squats
- Jefferson squats
- Overhead squats
- Magic circle squats
- Sissy squats
- Front squats
- Platform squats
- Zane squats
- Bear squats
- Front Harness Squats
- True squats

All are good, all have their unique benefits, and at least one or two should always be incorporated into your leg-training regimen

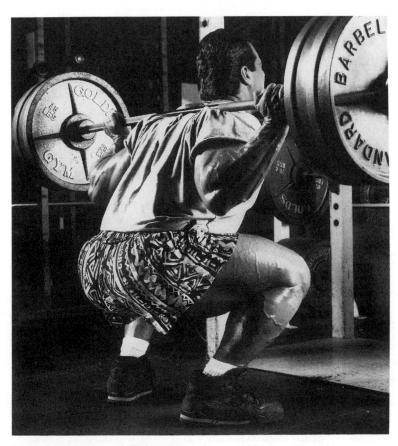

Bodybuilding Squats

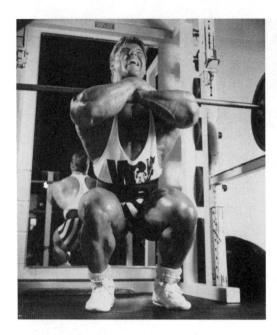

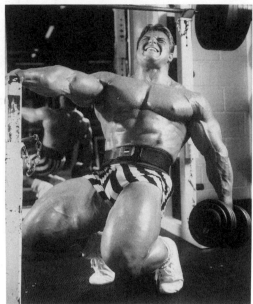

Front Squats   **Sissy Squats**

for bodybuilding excellence. A few are important enough to bear special mention.

Safety Squats: Here is a great way to do squats right! The specially designed bar makes it easier to get deep enough into the squat position and easier to keep your back straight, with far less danger of injuring your lower back or knees. Refer to Part Eight for a full discussion on squatting techniques employing both the regular straight bar and the safety squat bar.

Safety squats are also more comfortable because of the padded yoke resting on your shoulders. This special bar is called a safety squat bar although it has become widely referred to as the Hatfield bar because of my longstanding endorsement of its benefits. Notice that it allows you to use your hands to both hold yourself in a perfect, upright squatting position as well as spot yourself if the weight becomes too heavy. In my opinion, every bodybuilder should do squats this way.

Hack Squats and Leg Presses: Hack squat machines and leg press machines come in handy if you haven't learned how to do squats properly yet, you don't have a safety squat bar, you don't have a spotter to help you do squats, or your back is tired or injured and you can't do regular squats. They're good substitutes for regular or safety squats, but not a replacement for them.

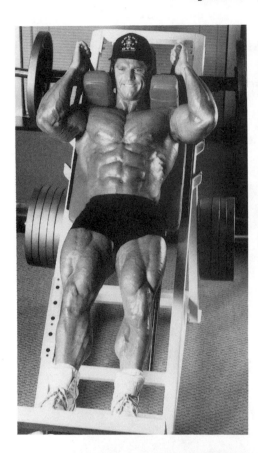
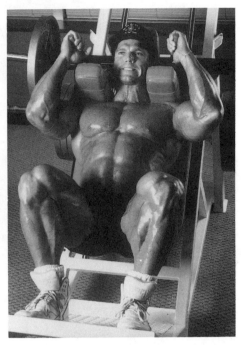

Hack Squats (Machine)

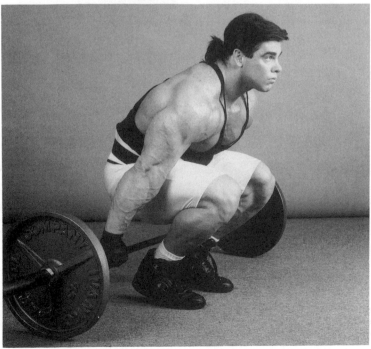

Barbell Hack Squats

Hack squat machines come outfitted with a weighted sled that rolls up and down on tracks or slides on linear bearings, and shoulder pads so you can support the weight while squatting. Leg press machines' padded shoulder supports are stationary, on the other hand, and a sled device similar to those used on hack squat machines is pressed upward at varying angles, depending upon the design of the specific leg press machine.

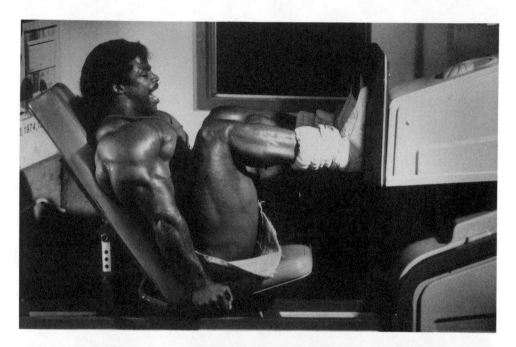

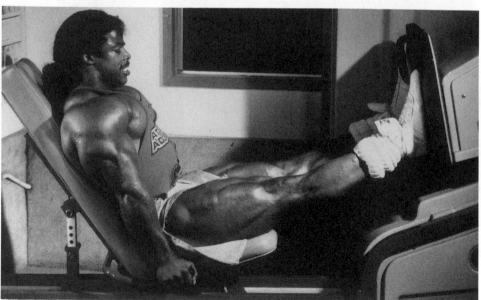

Seated Leg Presses

Stiff-Legged Deadlifts

A lot of bodybuilders use stiff-legged deadlifts to exercise their lower back. Because your lower back is more efficiently and effectively developed with back extensions, there is no need to do any other exercise for your lower back and especially not stiff-legged deadlifts!

Stiff-legged deadlifts are particularly effective for developing your hamstrings (the back of your upper legs). The traditional way

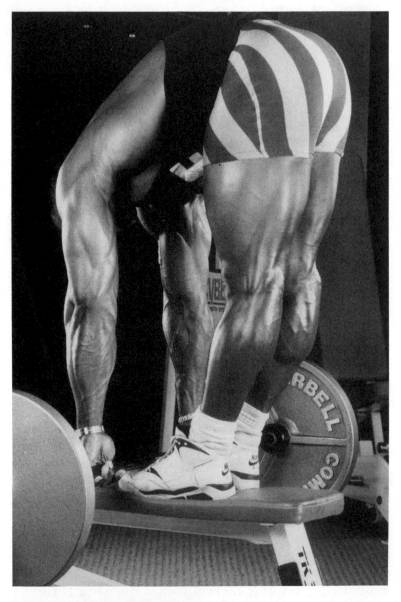

**Stiff-Legged Deadlifts
(to Insteps While Standing on Elevated Platform)**

of performing this exercise is to lower the weighted bar all the way down to your bootstraps while standing on a platform or bench with stiff legs or slightly bent knees. In this way, it's believed, you'll get maximum effect on your hams. This may be true to a degree, but you're also going to unnecessarily expose your lumbar spine to injury. Those intervertebral discs down there come loose all too easily.

I believe I've developed a better way to perform this exercise. With barbell in hand, poke both your butt and belly outward. In this position, you look kind of like one of the Keystone Kops you see in the 1920s movies. This variation of stiff-legged deadlifts has thus become known as *Keystone deadlifts*.

This seemingly strange position will prestretch your hamstrings because of the forward tilt of your pelvis. While maintaining this position, slowly lower the barbell to your knees, keeping the bar close to your legs during the descent and ascent.

You must *not* go more than an inch or two below your knees. By the time you reach your (slightly unlocked) knees, your hip joints have fully flexed. Further lowering of the bar is accomplished only through hyperflexion of your spine—a no-no!

You will feel a decided burn in your hams and glutes when Keystones are done correctly. You should feel virtually no discomfort or stress in your lower back. If you do, experiment with the movement until you feel no discomfort at all. The nice thing about doing stiff-legged deadlifts this way is that you can use a far heavier weight, thereby getting better adaptive stress applied to the target muscles, without any low back trauma at all.

One more important caution: *never* do this exercise explosively! You'll risk pulling a hamstring or blowing out a lumbar disc.

Bodybuilders are well-advised to steer clear of heavy deadlifting movements, as they are potentially dangerous to the lower spine.

Leg Curls

The back of your upper legs is comprised of three muscles called the hamstrings. Lying on your stomach, curl the padded lever upward using your hamstrings.

A lot of hamstring machines are designed with a downward angle that begins around your waist. The rationale is that it's easier for you to press your knees into the bench while curling the padded roller upward. I think this technique is somewhat counterproductive. By not pressing your knees into the bench while curling the weight up, you are more effectively targeting your hamstrings.

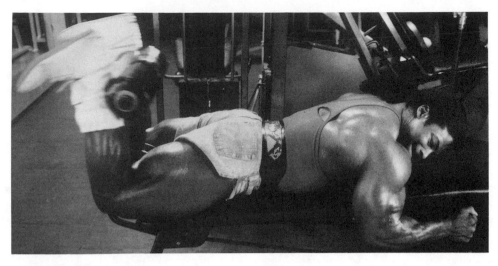

Leg Curls

Probably the best hamstring exercise for bodybuilders is standing leg curls because you're fighting directly against the force of gravity. In regular leg curls, there's a large, less-than-efficient horizontal component to the movement. Also, you're less likely to press your knees into the pad in order to make the movement easier through synergistic action of other muscles.

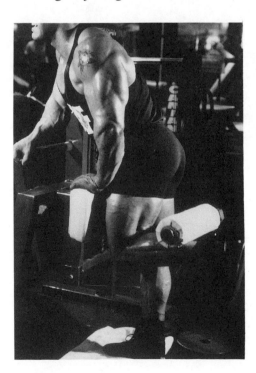

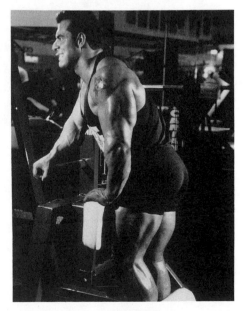

Standing Leg Curls

Leg Extensions

The front of your thighs is called the quadriceps. *Quad* means four. You have four important muscles that have different origin points, but share a common objective—to extend your knee joint. All your knee joint is capable of doing is flexion and extension anyway. That makes leg extensions an excellent quad developer.

Sitting with your feet under the padded lever, raise the weight with your quads.

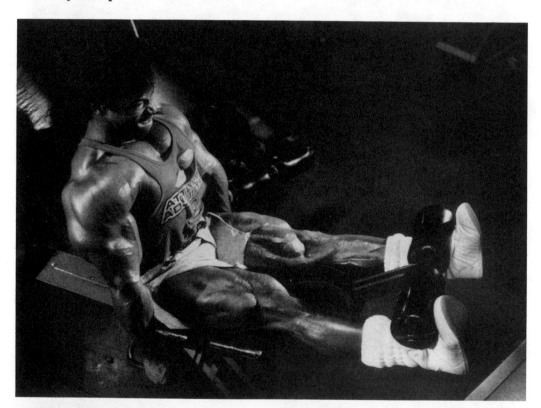

Leg Extensions

LOWER-LEG EXERCISES

Lower Legs
Target Muscles

Gastrocnemius
(calf muscles)

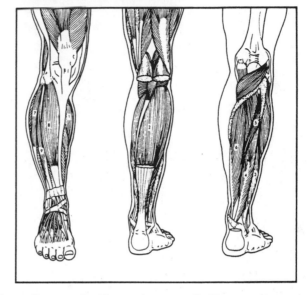

1. Gastrocnemius (sectioned)
2. Soleus
3. Peroneus brevis
4. Flexor longus hallucis
5. Tibialis posticus
6. Flexor longus digitorum
7. Peroneus longus
8. Tibialis anticus
9. Extensor longus digitorum
10. Gastrocnemius (sectioned)

Calf Raises

Seated calf raises are good. They stress your gastrocnemius muscles. Their drawback is that while you are seated, part of your gastrocs (some of the upper fibers cross the knee joint) are uninvolved.

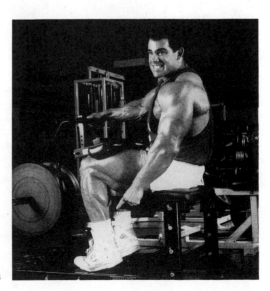

Seated Calf Raises

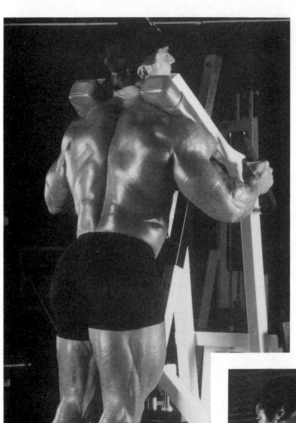

Standing Calf Raises

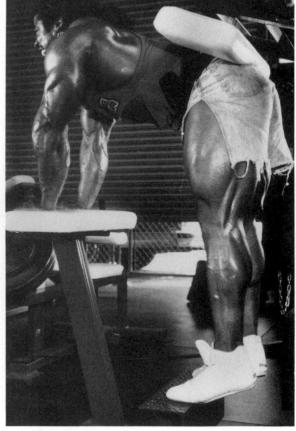

Donkey Raises

Standing calf raises and donkey raises are better because they involve the entire gastroc. In case you didn't know it, donkey raises got their name because, in the absence of a calf raise machine years ago (before modern gyms were profitable enough to be well-equipped) your training partner would have to sit on your back in donkey-and-rider fashion to provide resistance while you bent over to perform the raises.

Strength-Shoe Training

Sneakers with special platforms attached to the soles keep your heels off the ground while running, jumping, and walking. Wearing these strength shoes for an hour or so each day while you're running, jumping, and walking will make your calf muscles incredibly strong and put meat back there better than any calf exercise I've ever seen.

Be careful, though! You must gradually work up to wearing them for an hour. Begin by wearing them only five minutes a day. Add five minutes every third day or so—don't push it. You'll find that these shoes will put at least a couple inches of size and add up to five inches to your vertical jumping ability in three to four months.

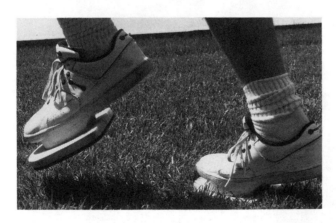

Strength Shoes

SPECIAL AND COMPOUND EXERCISES
Explosive High Pulls

This exercise is one of the best total-body exercises for athletes requiring explosiveness in their sport. Bodybuilders have traditionally avoided the movement, for reasons totally unknown to me. I think it's a great exercise for shoulders, traps, upper back, lower back, gluteal, and hamstring development.

The movement will stimulate your fast-twitch (white) fibers in these muscles. Other exercises for these muscles aren't as well suited to the kind of explosive movement necessary to get white fiber recruitment. It's a step-by-step movement done very explosively.

First, raise the weight off the floor by pulling only with your

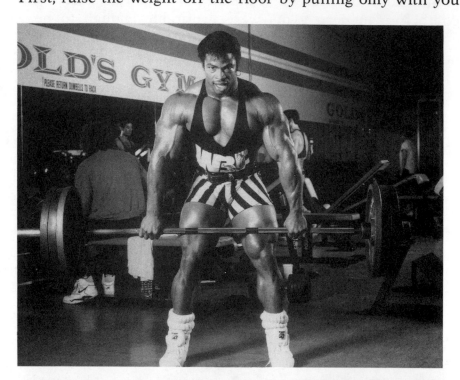

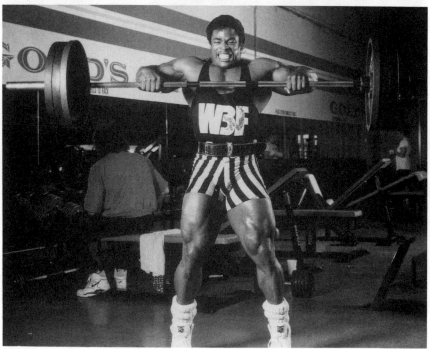

Explosive High Pulls

legs. Then, as the weight passes your knees, continue the pull upward with your back. Finally, as you approach an upright position, add to the speed of the bar by pulling with your shoulders and arms. Momentum is overcome throughout the movement by your continued attempt to accelerate the bar.

It's a difficult movement to master, so don't try to do all three steps at once. Practice the movement at a very slow speed until you learn the skill of being totally explosive.

Glute-Ham-Gastroc Raises

Your butt muscles are called the gluteus maximus, or glutes. Your hamstrings (hams) are the backs of your upper leg. Your calf muscles are called your gastrocnemius muscles (or gastrocs). A glute-ham-gastroc exercise is one that sequentially strengthens all three of these muscles in one movement.

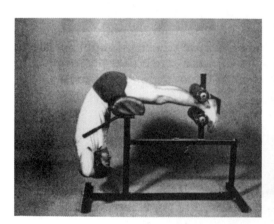 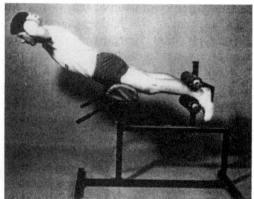

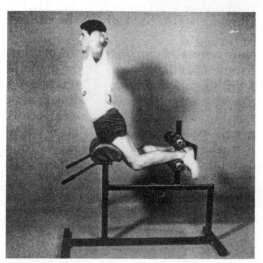

Glute-Ham-Gastroc Raises

This is an exercise developed in Russia and perfected by American sports scientist Dr. Mike Yessis. It is the single best weight-training exercise for improving speed and explosiveness in running and jumping. Bodybuilders can also benefit markedly from this exercise for the same reasons cited for explosive high pulls.

Study the photo carefully. Notice that you use your glutes to raise your body to a straight (horizontal) position. Your hams continue the movement to pull you up to a bent-knee level, and the gastrocs help the hams finish the movement.

You will need the specially-built machine shown in the photo in order to do this exercise. It's the same one you'll use to do back raises and Russian twists.

Aerobics

I'm an ironhead through and through. I've been known to poke fun at aerobic-type folk because of how skinny and undernourished they look. But, kidding aside, it's wise for you to remember that they got to look that way because of the aerobic exercises they do.

Do *you* want to look like that? No, indeed! So steer clear of doing too much aerobic training. Opt instead for a careful, integrated approach to fat control. That'll include getting bigger muscles (which burn more calories than little ones), following the five rules of sound bodybuilding nutrition (refer to Part Five), and relegating aerobic training to periods when it's really needed. That, fellow iron freaks, ranges somewhere between rarely and almost never!

But, in deference to those of you who insist on continuing to do aerobics all the time, here are the items you'll no doubt opt for:

- Exercycle (OK as a calorie burner)
- UBE (an acronym for Upper Body Exercycle; recommended for bodybuilders who are bent on using an exercycle for their lower legs. Why forget your upper body?)
- Treadmill or jogging (bad because of the pounding your knees and hips will have to endure; if you *must* jog, at least do so in soft sand or in knee-deep surf)
- Stairmaster™ (better than the exercycle or treadmill)
- Aerobics classes (good grief!)
- Versa-Climbers™ (the very best aerobic exercise there is for serious bodybuilders—*if* you have the guts!)

Some Common Forms of Aerobic Training:

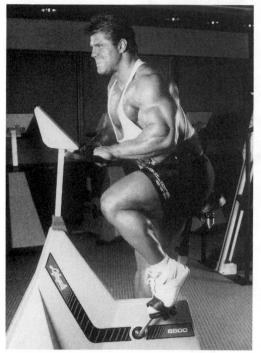

Exercycle

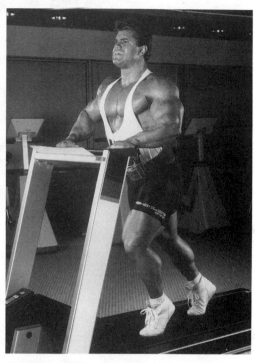

Treadmill

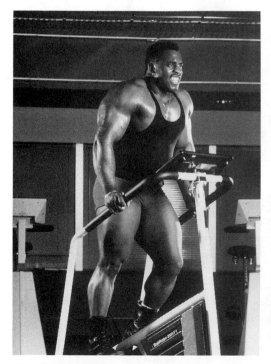

Stairmaster

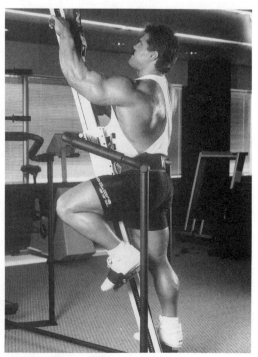

Versa-Climber

PART FOUR

SPECIAL FORMS OF STRENGTH TRAINING

DEDICATED TO DANNY PADILLA

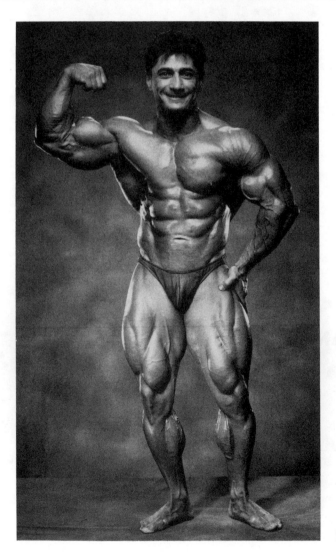

Danny Padilla

11

ANAEROBIC STRENGTH

Everyone knows what *aerobics* means. All the pencilnecks chime in, "With oxygen!" Except for a gym-hardened few, the word *anaerobics* has little meaning to people, except for a possible fleeting cognition relating to the opposite of aerobics. Yet, did you ever stop and reflect upon the fact that virtually 95 percent of everything you do in your bodybuilding life is anaerobic?

How come so much emphasis is given to aerobics? The ol' ticker, my friends—your heart—is strengthened. Whatever added lifestyle benefits accrue from the tedium of aerobic training that anaerobic training can't do much more efficiently and effectively is beyond me, but, as you know, I'm hard-core. I don't mean to debate the relative merits of anaerobic training versus aerobic conditioning. What I'd like to do instead is discuss the benefits of improving your anaerobic power in order to maximize muscle mass.

ANAEROBIC STRENGTH DEFINED

Let's get real specific for a moment and define in more exact terms what I mean by the term anaerobic strength as discussed in Part One, and how it relates to bodybuilding specifically.

During high-intensity training your energy requirements are met in large part by metabolic processes which do not require oxygen consumption. Thus, the ability of your muscles to consume adenosine triphosphate (ATP) begins to exceed that of the aerobic mechanism. In other words, your oxygen-delivery system is limited in its ability to bring oxygen to the working muscles, so other metabolic processes must take up the energy slack.

In the process of anaerobic work (work which takes place without the presence of sufficient oxygen) a tremendous oxygen debt is incurred. The phosphagens (ATP and creatine phosphate, CP for short) are the immediate sources of anaerobic energy. However, the phosphagen pool is very limited and can only sustain (at best) a brief anaerobic burst of muscle contraction. Most of your anaerobic energy must come from some other source. That's glycogen—sugar stored in your muscle cells.

So far, pretty straightforward. But to understand where most of your anaerobic energy comes from you'll have to understand lactic acid (l.a. for short) far more fully.

Glycogen breakdown (to resynthesize more CP and ATP) produces much of this caustic substance. Let's explore a few key reactions involving l.a.:

- Maximal l.a. production
- l.a. removal after exercise
- l.a. as a substrate for glycogen synthesis
- l.a. and your muscle's pH (acid/alkaline balance) in regard to your muscle's tension-producing capability

Energy During Maximum Muscle Contraction

How long does an average maximum lift take? Maybe two or three seconds, right? Well, by the time you've maximally tested your muscle's strength of contraction for one brief second, you're already into the third stage of muscle energetics—the glycolytic stage.

Within 1.26 seconds of maximum contraction, for example, 80 percent of your muscle's ATP is derived from CP degradation, and 20 percent from l.a. production. By the time your muscle has contracted for a period of 2.52 seconds, fully 50 percent of your ATP comes from l.a. production (Eric Hultman and Hans Sjoholm, 1983).

By the time you've contracted maximally for six seconds, your power output has begun to decrease despite the fact that your muscle's CP content is still at least 65 percent of its basal level. Continuing beyond six seconds, your CP content diminishes, your ATP diminishes, and acidosis—a build-up of l.a.—begins to severely hinder work.

It's pretty obvious, then, that your inability to generate maximum muscle contraction after six seconds or so stems from a multiplicity of factors rather than from a depletion of any single energy source.

ANAEROBIC STRENGTH

Anaerobic strength, then, can be defined in lay terms as your ability to continue to perform maximum muscle contractions over time (i.e., throughout a given set). Fatigue—the mortal enemy of bodybuilders not capable of withstanding severe oxygen debt and the metabolic corollaries—is very often misunderstood.

The misunderstanding resulted from the often-quoted research conducted in 1929 by Hill and Kupalov, who reported that fatigue was the result of a decrease in intracellular pH resulting from lactic acid accumulation.

In 1970, however, this view was changed as a result of new research conducted by Spande and Schottelius. Their research led them to conclude that a decrease in creatine phosphate (CP) inside the muscle was the main contributory factor in fatigue. They measured fatigue by simply monitoring the muscle's decreased force output.

By 1978, however, even that view was changed. With the aid of some incredible new technology—nuclear magnetic resonance imaging (NMR)—Dawson, Gadian, and Wilke discovered that a decrease in a muscle's tension-producing ability was directly proportional to increases in hydrogen ions and of free ADP (a metabolic by-product of ATP degradation) rather than resulting from either l.a. concentrations or CP content.

Eric Hultman and Hans Sjoholm, reporting their research at the International Symposium on Human Muscle Power (McMaster University, Hamilton, Ontario, 1984), concluded that anaerobic power—the ability to continue maximal work—stems from several factors, including decreased ratio between ATP and ADP, decreased muscle pH, and depletion of ATP (by as much as 60 percent).

The biochemical processes that bring about fatigue, according to Hultman and Sjoholm, are the formation and the breakdown of the muscles' actin-myosin cross-bridges. The cross-bridges are activated by the breakdown of ATP molecules. ATP breaks down into ADP and P, giving off energy in the process. That released energy ultimately causes the cross-bridges on the actin-myosin myofibrils to contract. Muscle contraction, then, is a result of thousands of microscopic cross-bridges grabbing, releasing, and regrabbing their way across one another, causing the actin and myosin to slide across one another.

What stops this cross-bridging is a lowering of your intramuscular pH—your cellular environment becomes too acidic from the buildup of lactic acid. Lactic acid activates other enzymes within the cell that are supposed to assist in the energy transfer system of the cell. Also, the regeneration of ATP is slowed below a critical threshold necessary to maintain contraction. You're using up your ATP too quickly during intense muscle contraction for resynthesized ATP to be effective in maintaining contraction.

How Can You Improve Your Anaerobic Strength?

Mind you, all of these enzymatic reactions take place in seconds. Pushing heavy weights for 8–10 reps and 10–12 sets, for example, reduces your intracellular environment to a junkpile of metabolic wastes and enzymatic poisons.

The critical question for all anaerobic athletes (which includes bodybuilders) is whether there is a way of improving anaerobic power. There is. You can delay the processes involved in fatigue, you can amplify your limit strength level (providing the net effect of making whatever work you're doing less taxing), and you can speed the recovery process markedly. It's best to do all three.

Here are some pointers.

- Pay attention to your mineral balances, especially your calcium/magnesium and sodium/potassium ratios
- Ensure that you've adopted a long-term commitment to sound nutrition, as it is only over time that you can achieve efficiency in intramuscular energetics
- Use branched-chain amino acids to assist in maintenance of an adequate amino acid pool (blood-borne aminos) for protein turnover during and following training
- Inosine is known to activate enzyme activity (specifically, pyruvic acid), allowing cellular activity to progress until more ATP can be biosynthesized
- By far the most important way to improve anaerobic strength, however, is to engage in high-intensity training of the white (fast-twitch) muscle fibers. That's where most of the enzymatic activity takes place and where your anaerobic powers are the greatest
- Highly trained bodybuilders are capable of tolerating lactate levels as much as 30 percent higher than untrained individuals. The mechanism presumed to contribute to this improved tolerance is motivation. However, it's just as certain that improved ability to improve ATP/ADP ratios, resynthesize ATP, and reduce lactate buildup will also contribute to improved

anaerobic power. That takes high-intensity training supported by sound nutritional practices.

- The use of buffers (alkaline substances) to reduce your blood acidity can assist in improving anaerobic power, especially in untrained or out-of-shape athletes. The longstanding buffer of choice is sodium bicarbonate—baking soda

- Substances which scavenge ammonia (a toxic by-product of amino-acid breakdown) appear to assist in rapid recovery both during and following intense training/competition

- Kinotherapy (active rest during the recovery phase following intense training) causes a compensatory effect in the fatigue centers of the central nervous system. Exercise antagonistic muscles mildly during rest periods (e.g., electrical stimulation on triceps following a biceps workout)

- Massage therapy, performed properly, can facilitate recovery in several ways, such as reactivation of peripheral circulation, resorption, decreased muscle tension, and elimination of toxins

- Techniques such as oxygen therapy, chemotherapy, psychological therapy, acupressure, ultrasound, and a host of other potentially rejuvenating techniques can be used to great advantage

It seems to me that if you're serious about bodybuilding you'll begin to get acquainted with your most important attribute—your anaerobic strength. This attribute will give you the edge you need in gaining strength. You will then discover that the true secret to improving your training efficiency is your ability to recover.

12

STRENGTH WITH MASS
FOR SPORTS

In Part One, you learned that strength can take many different forms. The precise form(s) for you will depend upon the requirements of your sport. Indeed, your selection of strength forms to train for will totally shape the kind of training you will perform. The different forms of strength are both acquired and displayed by forcing your body to apply maximum or near-maximum force within the bounds of your sport's metabolic requirements.

Although some overlap exists, acquiring one kind of strength will not necessarily improve the others. Your training has to be targeted to the specific requirements of your sport. If you need more than one kind of strength, you have to train for more than one.

You can get massive, of course. Many sports require that the participants be as big and muscular as possible. But, if you choose not to put on added muscle mass, you can achieve precisely the kind(s) of strength you require in your sport without gaining an ounce of body weight. Or, if you train and eat properly for your sport, you can gain as much body weight as you need, ensuring that the added weight is muscle, not fat.

If sheer muscle mass is your objective, Figure 12-1 gives you a fairly clear idea as to the kind of strength you'll have to work on in addition to those required in your sport. It gives you a breakdown of which kinds of strength different classes of athletes require. Also, if you look back in Part One, you'll be able to understand the exact factors which contribute most to improved muscle mass.

All bodybuilders want bigger muscles. That's part of that sport's requirements, and training like a bodybuilder will give you your

ENERGY SOURCES

ATP/CP · GLYCOLYTIC · OXIDATIVE

FIGURE 12-1

Energy and Strength Requirements for Various Sports

SPORT	TYPE OF FORCE DELIVERY	TYPES OF STRENGTH REQUIRED
High jumping Javelin Pitching Batting	Ballistic (non-weight-bearing) burst of maximum force	Speed-strength (especially starting strength)
Weightlifting Shot put	Instantaneous burst of maximum force	Speed-strength and limit strength
Powerlifting	Briefly sustained maximum force output	Limit strength and speed strength
100m Run	Instantaneous bursts of maximum force time after time	Linear anaerobic strength endurance (ATP/CP) and starting strength
200m Run	Instantaneous bursts of maximum force time after time	Linear anaerobic strength endurance (ATP/CP and glycolytic), and starting strength
Football Boxing Karate Judo Gymnastics	Maximum force output time after time (both ballistic and weight-bearing)	Nonlinear anaerobic strength endurance (ATP/CP and glycolytic), speed-strength, and limit strength
400m Run	Instantaneous bursts of maximum force time after time	Linear anaerobic strength endurance (glycolytic)
Tennis Wrestling Basketball Soccer	Intermittent bursts of force over a long period of play	Nonlinear anaerobic strength endurance (ATP/CP and glycolytic), nonlinear aerobic strength endurance, and speed-strength (especially starting strength)
Crew Mid-distance races (800m run) (Mile/1500m run)	Near-maximum force output repetitively performed over time	Linear anaerobic strength endurance (glycolytic) and linear aerobic strength endurance
Long distance races (Marathon) (Biathlon) (Triathlon) (Nordic skiing)	Submaximum force output repetitively performed over time	Linear aerobic strength endurance and linear anaerobic strength endurance (glycolytic)

greatest returns in mass. However, if you compete in a sport other than bodybuilding, you should not make the mistake of training like a bodybuilder all the time. Concentrating only on getting big muscles will not necessarily aid you in becoming a better athlete in your sport.

The sport of bodybuilding was purposely omitted from Figure 12-1 because it doesn't make sense to put it there at all levels of force output and strength categories. Just remember that the key to successful bodybuilding training—success beyond your greatest expectations—is to inject variation in your training.

Athletes in sports other than bodybuilding can and often should get massive muscles, but never at the expense of performance capabilities and only rarely to the same extreme as a bodybuilder. The all-important strength-to-weight ratio must be preserved. That's why you never see a 300-pound heavyweight boxer or gymnast. Even among the behemoths occupying down-lineman spots in professional football the strength-to-weight factor reigns supreme.

The bigger and stronger your muscles get, the faster and more agile you will be, or, if you're an endurance athlete, the more stamina you will get. However, there is a point for all athletes in every sport where, if you begin getting too big, your efficiency as an athlete begins to go down. You may gain greater absolute strength by getting bigger muscles, but you will lose some of the other important types of strength in the process. For example, factors like quickness (starting strength plus reaction time) and aerobic strength are typically reduced as you grow to a bodybuilder's proportions.

GUIDELINES FOR TRAINING

Some very important guidelines can easily be incorporated into your training methods. The single most important guideline for all athletes—not just bodybuilders—is to "cycle" your training. Cycling your training can help isolate the conditioning objectives of most immediate concern, allowing you to direct your best efforts to those particular aspects important to you at any specific stage of your training.

The theory behind cycle training (or *periodized* training, as the former Soviet sports scientists like to call it) is basically this: by breaking conditioning routines into discreet time periods, you can more efficiently establish the types of strength and speed you need first, in order to prepare you for the more intense training techniques that will come later in your precompetition training. For instance, you must first develop a basic foundation of limit strength before you can move on to train for any of the other types of strength. Using another example, you don't try to sprint at full speed before conditioning your leg muscles to withstand that kind of punishment.

Cycle training must be planned carefully and undertaken only with a complete commitment. It's a program in which each mesocycle of your training must be completed in its proper sequence for the overall effort to have the effect you desire. If you let up in one phase of your cycle, you won't reach the level you're shooting for in the next phase, and so on.

13

AEROBIC OR ANAEROBIC?

As you learned in Part One, aerobic simply means with oxygen and anaerobic means, just as simply, without oxygen. Remember, though, that within the anaerobic category, you have to account for the differences between ATP/CP (explosive) sports and glycolytic (mid-distance) sports. Neither of these two anaerobic categories of sports require that oxygen be supplied to the working muscles until *after* the skill is completed. Then, you pay back to your muscles the debt of oxygen you owe them so you can explode again.

You need to be aware of these three terms to understand what's happening in your body under the stresses of different kinds of exercise routines or in your sport. Most importantly, you have to understand that anaerobic conditions result when you participate in all-out sports such as sprinting, jumping, weightlifting, football, and baseball. In these sports, the contraction time demanded of your muscles is very low. But, if you have to repetitively contract your muscles explosively, as you might down after down in football, you begin getting fatigued. Your force output begins to diminish, and when this happens, your muscles continue to function as long as they can. They're using stored sugar—glycogen—to keep them going. When there is no more available glycogen, the level of lactic acid in your muscles builds and you experience muscle fatigue. Oxygen is then required in order for you to continue. You might be able to pay back the oxygen your muscles require to remove the lactic acid in between downs, plays, or reps. If you cannot, or if you don't have enough time to recover, you will not be able to play as explosively as when you were fresh.

FIGURE 13-1

Pathways of Muscular Energetics

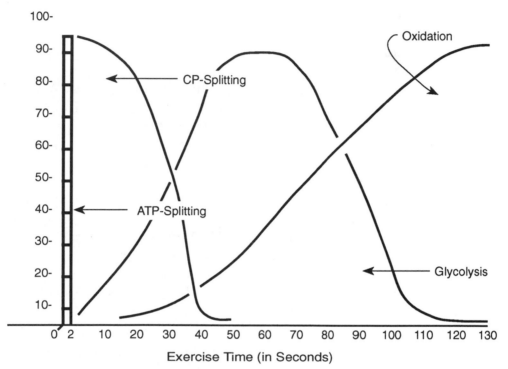

Percentage of the Energy-Delivering Processes

Exercise Time (in Seconds)

If you are an explosive athlete, and in the beginning phase of cycle training, your greatest outputs come in the categories of (1) amount of work done (or a high total number of pounds lifted per workout), (2) moderate oxidative and glycolytic strength endurance, (3) limit strength, and (4) general fitness. These areas are where you should attempt the most, push your body to the max.

Your lowest output, at the start, should come in (5) intensity of effort (no limit attempts with the weights), (6) maximum anaerobic strength endurance (glycolytic), (7) skill/body control, and (8) speed-strength (starting strength and explosive strength). These are the areas where you should attempt the least, while concentrating on the other four factors.

The key to the cycle training program is to reverse this order of output gradually, so that factors 1 through 4 begin to decrease, while factors 5 through 8 begin to increase. At the end of the cycle, you should see a complete turnaround, and your greatest efforts should come from factors 5 through 8, while the least of your work occurs in factors 1 through 4.

Glycolytic athletes require almost the same approach to their initial training cycle as do the ATP/CP athletes. The difference is that glycolytic athletes have to really hit the anaerobic endurance aspect hard—without neglecting their skills, their explosiveness, and their limit strength—as they approach their competition. However, if you're an endurance athlete just beginning a training cycle, limit strength training and general fitness are still the most important elements of your initial training. Then, you get into speed work and hill work and finally into high-level cardiovascular (oxidative) work.

The basic philosophy of cycle training is that simple. Of course, each sport has its peculiarities, as does each athlete. These peculiarities notwithstanding, there are some very tried-and-true methods of training for these three classes of sports that apply to all athletes within each category.

Now let me throw you a curve ball. Separating all sports into three categories is very simplistic. Actually, all sports require some oxygen. Without oxygen you would die. There is considerable overlap between these areas, as you can see from Figure 13-1, which shows the different muscle energy sources.

You'd be wise to keep in mind the different levels of oxygen required for different sports. The different levels were summarized in Figure 12-1, which lists the different sports and the types of strength required in each. You will see that they're arranged beginning with the ATP/CP sports, on to the glycolytic sports, and through the aerobic sports.

In the midrange of oxygen consumption—the glycolytic sports—are wrestling, basketball, and soccer, tennis and racquet sports. Cross-country skiing and marathon running are almost 100 percent aerobic, however. Most pure strength events—the ATP/CP sports—such as shot putting and weightlifting are almost totally anaerobic, meaning no oxygen other than that needed to sustain life is necessary.

HOW TO TRAIN FOR AEROBIC OR ANAEROBIC STRENGTH

Anaerobic and aerobic athletes train very similarly. The principal difference is that aerobic athletes train while in severe need of oxygen for very long periods of time. Anaerobic athletes in explosive

ATP/CP sports don't. Anaerobic athletes from glycolytic sports train while in severe oxygen debt, too, but only for short, intermittent periods. In Chapter Fourteen, you will note the strikingly similar schedules for anaerobic versus aerobic athletes. But don't overlook the important differences, either!

14

AN EXAMPLE OF AN INTEGRATED TRAINING REGIMEN FOR AEROBIC AND ANAEROBIC SPORTS

GENERAL OBJECTIVES

- Organize all aspects of training so that each element of your training is in harmony with all the others, or integrated
- Reverse the effects of disuse from not training; in other words, add muscle mass and strength to long-unused muscles (establish foundation)
- Eliminate weaknesses or rehabilitate from injuries
- Remain injury-free

SPECIFIC OBJECTIVES

- Your weaknesses must always be tended to *first* in any training program
- It is understood that differences in training objectives exist between different sports; however, the similarities that exist far outweigh the differences
- Preparation will entail one macrocycle of about twelve weeks' duration
- The twelve-week macrocycle is broken down into four mesocycles of three weeks' duration each

Mesocyclic Objectives

Mesocycle One:
- Maximize muscle mass
- Minimize fat

- Improve general strength and fitness foundation (especially weaknesses), including *moderate* aerobic threshold training for anaerobic and aerobic athletes alike
- Work on specific skills (weaknesses)
- Begin pushing anaerobic threshold by doing 3–6 two-minute drills
- Begin introducing checkmark training (light plyometrics)

Mesocycle Two:
- Maximize limit strength of muscles/movements used in your specific sport (emphasis on legs)
- Push back the anaerobic threshold (maximum force output time after time—anaerobic strength endurance—by performing the two-minute drills while in both ATP/CP and glycolytic pathways)
- Aerobic-event athletes begin aerobic threshold training in earnest
- Begin training specific skills (weaknesses) in earnest
- Concentrate on between-workout recovery
- Introduce explosive strength and starting strength to anaerobic athletes by doing moderate plyometrics (aerobic athletes stay on light plyometric training)

Mesocycle Three:
- Maximize explosive strength through "compensatory acceleration" training with weights (see the discussion on this advanced form of weight training in Part Eight)
- Specific event skills must predominate all skills-training sessions
- Push back anaerobic threshold to the limits of your capabilities—high intensity for up to ten three-minute drills (includes both anaerobic and aerobic athletes)
- Aerobic athletes push back the aerobic threshold in earnest
- Maximize between-workout recovery
- Weighted plyometrics and hill/stairs-running incorporated into three-minute drills or done in addition to three-minute drills
- Aerobic athletes: attempt to conduct some of your training at altitude

Mesocycle Four:
- Maximize ballistic strength (starting strength) by doing shock plyometrics

- Heavy emphasis on anaerobic threshold (anaerobic athletes) or aerobic threshold (aerobic athletes—altitude training should be incorporated when possible)
- Maximize between-workout recovery ability
- Heavy emphasis on skills
- Emphasize speed, agility, ballistic movements
- "Overspeed" drills in final preparatory period (anaerobic athletes only)
- Weight training dropped in favor of complexes

TRAINING TECHNIQUES AND SEQUENCES

For every coach, there's a different system of training and a different level of understanding of the technologies available to enhance athletic performance capabilities. This is as true for bodybuilding coaches as for coaches in any other sport.

Your personal skill-training regimen is coach's domain. I've described some common training techniques that I've found extremely effective. With variations of each, depending upon your background and level of understanding of the end uses of these techniques, you will find them effective as well. Some, perhaps, will be revolutionary to you.

Figure 14-1 is an example of how you should incorporate all of the forms of sports training with your bodybuilding efforts.

UBE/LBE (Cybex Upper Body Exerciser)

The UBE/LBE develops anaerobic strength endurance through pushing back the anaerobic threshold of the upper extremities. UBE looks like a bicycle for your arms; LBE is the legs' bicycle ergometer and is ridden as per instructions. Neither should be done for long, slow distances during anaerobic threshold drills. However, both UBE and LBE training can be aerobic in nature simply by engaging in long, slow pedaling.

UBE/LBE Drills:
1. Set UBE/LBE at fastest speed. Go maxed out for 20 seconds ("bury" the needle), rest one minute, and repeat—then again.
2. Set UBE/LBE at medium speed. Go maxed out for one minute, rest one minute, and repeat—then again.
3. Set UBE/LBE at slow speed. Go maxed out for three minutes, rest one minute, and repeat—then again.

FIGURE 14-1

An Example of How to Integrate Variable Split Bodybuilding into an Athlete's Overall Training

WEEK	DAY	CHEST	SHOULDERS	BACK	ARMS	LEGS	ABS	PLYOS	DRILLS	AEROBIC OR ANAEROBIC	SKILLS
1	M				B		C	A		C	A
	T	A		A		B			A		B
	W		C		A		B	B		B	C
	T	A		B					B		A
	F				A	B	B	C		C	B
	S	B	C	B					C		C
2	M				B	A	A	A		C	A
	T	B	B	C					A		B
	W					A	A	B		B	C
	T		B		B				B		A
	F	C				B	B	C		C	B
	S		A	C					C		C
3	M				C	B		A		C	A
	T	C	A				B		A		B
	W			B				B		B	C
	T		B			C			B		A
	F				C		C	C		C	B
	S	B		B					C		C
4	M		B	A	B	C		A		C	A
	T	B					C		A		B
	W		C	A				B		B	C
	T				B	B			B		A
	F	A					B	C		C	B
	S		C	B					C		C
5	M	A	C		A	B		A		C	A
	T			B			B		A		B
	W	B			A			B		B	C
	T		B			A			B		A
	F			C			A	C		C	B
	S	B	B		B	A			C		C

Plyo Ball

The Plyo Ball, marketed by ISSA (International Sports Sciences Association), is a more comfortable variation of the old medicine ball. It teaches explosive and starting strength in all arm/hand/body movements and requires total body coordination at generating speed-strength. Make sure your wrists and hands are protected.

Plyo Ball Drills:
- Right and left jab positions
- Between legs (for back)
- Overhead (for midsection)
- Chest Pass
- Left and right twisting throws

Go two minutes nonstop, alternating the above-listed positions, and then rest for one minute. Repeat for 3–6 "rounds."

Sports Chute

The Sports Chute marketed by ISSA is a modified "pilot" parachute ranging in sizes from two to five feet. It is strapped to your waist and trails behind you while you are doing sprints or other running drills. The obvious objective is to provide resistance in such a way while running that speed and anaerobic threshold are improved without any disruption in your running form or skill, as often occurs with hill training or tow-training.

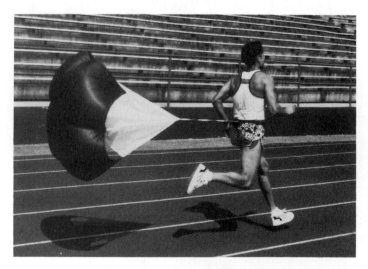

**The ISSA
Sports Chute**

Weight Training

Initially a foundation-strengthening program using a variable split format, weight training is described in greater detail in Part Two, so review Part Two carefully. Remember, the "ABC" format is a scheme accounting for the periodicity of each individual body part's ability to recover.

2-3-Minute Drill

Use two- to three-minute combinations of forward and backward sprints, skipping, hopping, jumping, and "carioca" (football-type) drills for both upper and lower body. Start out with only three two-minute drills with one minute's rest between each. Gradually (over the first mesocycle) work up to six two-minute drills with one minute's rest between, and progress to three-minute drills after the first mesocycle. Take your pulse after each drill (target: 180 beats per minute) and again one minute later (target: 120 beats per minute).

Bear in mind that this drill is nonstop—push to the absolute limits of your anaerobic tolerances.

Drill Sequence: Jog or do stepups to get warmed up. Follow these coaching commands.

- 10-yard circle sprints (two left and two right)
- Sprint 40 yards
- Stop and sprint backward
- Jump in place high ten times
- 10-yard square sprints (two left and two right)
- Get in a pushup position and give me your legs
- Run forward on your hands
- Run backward on your hands
- Run left
- Run right
- Jump up and down on your hands ten times
- Stop, get up, and carioca left 40 yards
- Carioca right back to me
- Skip 40 yards
- Skip backward back to me
- Crab-drill forward—backward—left—right
- Three-point stance starts (six or eight)

Go for a solid 2–3 minutes at a heart rate of 180 beats per minute (approximate). After a one-minute rest (getting your heart rate back to 120) you do it again, and again.

There are many variations to the 2–3 minute drill. You will find you'll do well creating your own sport-specific drills, basing the component movements on your sport's requirements and, especially, your weaknesses.

Plyometrics

This is a way of converting strength to speed through totally concentrated, instantaneous force output in every move you make.

On days where only plyos are done in the midday workout, they should be relaxed, with much rest between bouts. Each bout should last only 10–20 seconds, but (beginning with the second mesocycle) with *total* focus on starting strength.

Plyometric Drill Sequence:

Mesocycle one: go easy and slow

Mesocycle two: begin exploding

Mesocycle three: add weights and/or go uphill and stress
       explosive movements

Mesocycle four: anaerobic athletes add "shock" plyos,
       overspeed plyos, and overspeed running drills

Here's an example of how a coach calls out a plyo drill sequence:

1. Jog or do stepups to warm up
2. Easy (not "all-out") jumps, hops, skips
3. Concentrate—"laser" focus—and then do 20 yards of skips
4. Again!
5. Hop like a kangaroo
6. Again!
7. Repeat steps 3, 4, 5, and 6 backward
8. One-legged hops 30 yards (both feet)
9. Hop on your hands 10 yards
10. Repeat step 9 backward
11. Repeat step 9 left and right
12. After two weeks, incorporate between-bench hop-down— hop back up—10 reps
13. Twisting skips 40 yards
14. Twist the other way back 40 yards

Watch out for potholes in grass—always take a minute to check this out first! Tape your wrists and wear gloves for grass drills.

Complex Training

Complex training is a system which combines weight training (limit strength), shock plyometrics (starting strength), bounding-type plyometrics (starting strength with explosive strength), and the actual skill of your event (e.g., running, throwing, jumping). These four elements are done sequentially without resting between each and can be done for both upper and lower body.

The principal objective of complex training is to make the neural transfer between raw limit strength and speed-strength to skilled execution of your sport. It is a highly taxing system, so no more than three complexes should be performed for upper and lower body, respectively. It's an excellent in-season system of strength maintenance training, especially when little time is available, and it's suitable for anaerobic and aerobic athletes alike.

Lower Body Example
- Five explosive reps with 85% in the Squat (no rest)
- Five depth jumps from about 30 inches (no rest)
- Bounding like a kangaroo 30 yards (no rest)
- Five sprints from a dead stop (5 yards) (rest and repeat)

Upper Body Example
- Five explosive reps with 85% in the bench press (no rest)
- Five depth jumps from 16 inches (e.g., between two benches) (no rest)
- Bounding in a wheelbarrow position (partner-assisted) for about 10 yards (no rest)
- Five throws with a VersaBall (no rest)
- Five actual throws or swings (rest and repeat)

PERIODIZING YOUR TRAINING

Arranging the above-listed techniques of training into a cogent periodized system wherein each successive mesocycle builds on the previous one is one of the toughest operations to perform in all the world of sport.

Let me offer the following suggestion. These sequences are designed to be addressed as a triple variable split—that is, three shorter, high-intensity training bouts per day instead of one long one, with all three varied in intensity depending upon your recuperative requirements. However, as your schedule permits (school, work, etc.), you can perform these sequences quite successfully as one or two workouts.

The reasoning behind keeping them separate—especially your skills workouts—is to provide ample rest between each session in order to recover fully. If you can't separate them because of scheduling problems, then at least take a half hour or so between each. You'll find it helpful to have a nutritious snack (such as a high-energy drink or a protein candy bar) between sessions.

FIGURE 14-2

Scheduling Your Training Days for Each Mesocycle

MESOCYCLE ONE (THREE WEEKS' DURATION):

MONDAY	TUESDAY	WEDNESDAY	THURSDAY	FRIDAY	SATURDAY

Morning Training Objectives

MONDAY	TUESDAY	WEDNESDAY	THURSDAY	FRIDAY	SATURDAY
Skills	Skills	Skills	Skills	Skills	Skills
UBE	LBE	UBE	LBE	UBE	LBE
Plyo ball		Plyo ball		Plyo ball	

Midday Training Objectives

MONDAY	TUESDAY	WEDNESDAY	THURSDAY	FRIDAY	SATURDAY
2-minute drill	Plyos	2-minute drill	Plyos	2-minute drill	Plyos
(3 reps)		(4 reps)		(5 reps)	
(4 reps)		(5 reps)		(6 reps)	
(5 reps)		(6 reps)		(7 reps)	

Note: Do 3, 4, and 5 "repetitions" of two-minute drills during week one; 4, 5, and 6 during week two; 5, 6, and 7 during the third week. Rest one minute between each "repetition" of the two-minute drill.

Note: Sports Chute training follows all midday workouts for anaerobic athletes and aerobic jogging/cycling for aerobic athletes.

Evening Workout

MONDAY	TUESDAY	WEDNESDAY	THURSDAY	FRIDAY	SATURDAY
weights	weights	weights	weights	weights	weights

MESOCYCLE TWO (THREE WEEKS' DURATION):

MONDAY	TUESDAY	WEDNESDAY	THURSDAY	FRIDAY	SATURDAY

Morning Training Objectives

MONDAY	TUESDAY	WEDNESDAY	THURSDAY	FRIDAY	SATURDAY
Skills	Skills	Skills	Skills	Skills	Skills
UBE	LBE	UBE	LBE	UBE	LBE
Plyo ball		Plyo ball		Plyo ball	

Recommended: Aerobic training done at altitude.

Midday Training Objectives

MONDAY	TUESDAY	WEDNESDAY	THURSDAY	FRIDAY	SATURDAY
2-minute drill	Plyos	2-minute drill	Plyos	2-minute drill	Plyos
(4 reps)		(5 reps)		(6 reps)	
(5 reps)		(6 reps)		(7 reps)	
(6 reps)		(7 reps)		(8 reps)	

Note: Do 4, 5, and 6 "repetitions" of two-minute drills during week four; 5, 6, and 7 during week five; 6, 7, and 8 during the sixth week. Rest one minute between each "repetition" of the two-minute drill.

Note: Sports Chute training follows all midday workouts for anaerobic athletes and aerobic jogging/cycling for aerobic athletes.

Evening Workout

MONDAY	TUESDAY	WEDNESDAY	THURSDAY	FRIDAY	SATURDAY
weights	weights	weights	weights	weights	weights

MESOCYCLE THREE (THREE WEEKS' DURATION):

MONDAY	TUESDAY	WEDNESDAY	THURSDAY	FRIDAY	SATURDAY

Morning Training Objectives

Skills	Skills	Skills	Skills	Skills	Skills
UBE	LBE	UBE	LBE	UBE	LBE
Plyo ball		Plyo ball		Plyo ball	

Recommended: Aerobic training done at altitude.

Midday Training Objectives

3-minute drills	Weighted	3-minute drills	Weighted	3-minute drills	Weighted
(Hill)	plyos	(Hill)	plyos	(Hill)	plyos
(5 reps)		(6 reps)		(7 reps)	
(5 reps)		(6 reps)		(7 reps)	
(5 reps)		(6 reps)		(7 reps)	

Note: Do 5, 6, and 7 three-minute drills during weeks 7, 8, and 9. Rest one minute between each "repetition" of the three-minute drill. All three-minute drills are performed while going uphill. An uphill grade of 15%–30% works best.

Note: Sports Chute training follows all midday workouts for anaerobic athletes and aerobic jogging/cycling for aerobic athletes.

Recommended: Aerobic training done at altitude.

Evening Workout

weights	weights	weights	weights	weights	weights

Note: All weight training sessions during Mesocycle Three should emphasize "compensatory acceleration," an advanced weight training technique discussed in Part Eight.

MESOCYCLE FOUR (THREE WEEKS' DURATION):

MONDAY	TUESDAY	WEDNESDAY	THURSDAY	FRIDAY	SATURDAY

Morning Training Objectives

Skills	Skills	Skills	Skills	Skills	Skills
UBE	LBE	UBE	LBE	UBE	LBE
Plyo ball		Plyo ball		Plyo ball	

Recommended: Aerobic training done at altitude.

Midday Training Objectives

3-minute drills	Shock	3-minute drills	Shock	3-minute drills	Shock
(8 reps)	plyos	(9 reps)	plyos	(10 reps)	plyos
(8 reps)		(9 reps)		(10 reps)	
(8 reps)		(9 reps)		(10 reps)	

Note: Do 8, 9, and 10 "repetitions" of the three-minute drills during weeks 10, 11, and 12, which are the final (pre-competition) mesocycle. Rest one minute between each "repetition" of the three-minute drill.

Note: Sports Chute training follows all midday workouts for anaerobic athletes and aerobic jogging/cycling for aerobic athletes.

Recommended: Aerobic training done at altitude.

Evening Workout

Complex training		Complex training		Complex training	

PART FIVE

INTEGRATED NUTRITION FOR BODYBUILDING

DEDICATED TO MIKE QUINN

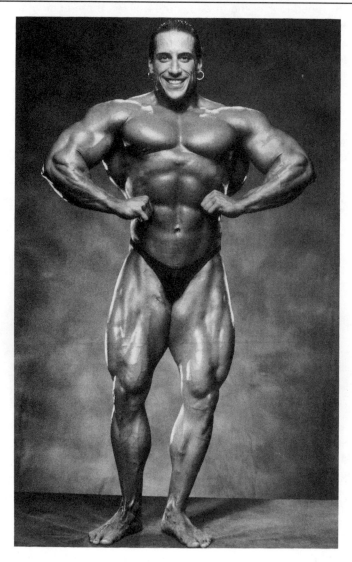

Mike Quinn

15

MAXIMUM NUTRITION FOR MAXIMUM BODYBUILDING RESULTS

In every issue of every muscle magazine, you're bombarded with an endless stream of articles and ads on dieting and supplementing. Some offer good, scientifically based information that can indeed support your training efforts. Others are, well, garbage, but you know that already. You may even be in tune enough to know the difference between the good and the bad. That's good, but it's not enough.

For example, the survival mechanisms driving you to eat are of an exceedingly primitive nature. Almost anything you put into your mouth will keep you alive. Almost anything you eat—if you eat enough of it—will make you gain weight. But bodybuilders interested in achieving their maximum muscle mass potential need more. Much more.

The chief task of society is to produce survival fare for millions of people. Historically, that task has taken precedence over performance fare for the few elite athletes out there. For the most part, athletes have been left to forage for themselves, with little or no help from those who do nutritional research. More often than not, this was due to the lack of both adequate funding for such research and a sports performance perspective.

However, because of the latest research as well as the spate of popular books on the subject of sports nutrition, this situation is slowly being rectified. This information, albeit sparse, can help you pick and choose the right diet, the right nutritional supplements, and the right training methods you need to truly reach—or at least approach—your mass potential.

Bodybuilding is an integrative science embracing knowledge from many disciplines. The hallmark of bodybuilders, of course, is their incredible musculature. They got to be that big by training with weights, but it never would have happened had they not been getting enough of the proper nutrients and calories, and not in any haphazard schedule. There are some simple rules for bodybuilders to follow when it comes to eating and supplementing.

NUTRITIONAL RULES TO FOLLOW

Rule One

Always eat at least five meals a day. Two or three meals often simply isn't enough. If your muscles don't get the calories they need, how are they going to keep going? By cannibalizing muscle tissue! That's the same muscle tissue you spent hours and much sweat to get.

Rule Two

Remember the 1-2-3 rule. In each of your five meals, one part of the calories should come from fats, two parts from protein, and three parts from carbohydrates.

Here's an example. Let's say you eat 600 calories five times a day. That's 3,000 calories. If you're following the 1-2-3 rule, each meal is broken down like this: 100 calories from fat, 200 calories from protein, and 300 calories from carbs. That's how you get massive and lean.

Rule Three

You can get even more sophisticated than the 1-2-3 rule. In fact, you *must* if you want to win. For example, when you sit down to eat, ask yourself, "What am I going to be doing for the next three hours of my life?" Then, if you're taking a nap, eat less; if you're planning on a training session, eat more. And so forth.

By carefully manipulating your caloric intake meal after meal, day after day, week after week, and month after month, pretty soon you'll look in the mirror and see something you've been waiting to see for a long, long time—cuts. What's more, you'll see *muscle*.

Rule Four

Another rule of thumb for bodybuilders trying to put on muscle mass without also putting on fat is to zigzag your caloric intake. For example, if you want to go to 240 pounds (and under 10 percent body fat) and presently weigh only 190 pounds (with 20 percent body fat), you should "amp" your calories for about four to five days, then back off for one or two. That way, you gain a pound of muscle and fat, then lose the fat. You are left with muscle. Continue like this over months of time and you will grow harder, bigger, and healthier.

Rule Five

The final rule of thumb for serious bodybuilders is that no matter how hard you try, no matter how good a cook your mama is, or where you buy your food:

- You can't always eat perfectly balanced meals
- You can't always eat five or six times daily
- There are many instances where your body requires certain nutrients in greater amounts than can be derived from diet alone
- A perfectly balanced diet cannot be maintained during periods of contest preparation or periods where a purposeful caloric restriction is imposed
- Periods of high-stress training require supernormal intake of many nutrients without a commensurate increase in caloric need
- Periods of high-stress training create a situation in which various benefits can be derived from nutritional substances not normally found in food or biosynthesized in the body in sufficient or significant quantities but which are either man-made or derived from botanical sources
- Soil depletion, toxins in the food chain, overprocessing, overcooking, free radical formation in the body, and a host of other (sometimes medically related) factors all interact to make food less than totally nutritious
- Because man has been able to improve on Mother Nature's original work in many of life's arenas, there are some superfoods available which are plainly and simply better than normal food for serious bodybuilders

While there are some truly effective and nutritious sports supplements available, there is no magic bullet in the world of sports or bodybuilding nutritional supplementation. There is no single supplement that will suddenly catapult you from an obscure beginner's level into the realm of elite sports or bodybuilding accomplishment.

Only an integrated conditioning program can truly make a significant difference in your training and sports or bodybuilding performance.

FITTING YOUR NUTRITION TO YOUR TRAINING

To be the best bodybuilder you can be is to know how to train properly, recuperate adequately, and choose the right foods, as well as how and when to eat them and when supplements are needed.

One basic concern is to estimate how many calories you need on a meal-to-meal basis. By simply adding and subtracting, you can estimate the number of calories you should be consuming per meal in order to ensure that your added weight will not become fat but will instead be converted to lean muscle. For example, let's assume that your daily caloric intake is 2,500 calories (an average of 500 calories for each of five meals). You want to put on muscle mass, so you add 500 calories to your daily intake (3,000 calories per day). Then, by adding and subtracting:

Calories in meal preceding strenuous workouts: _____
(add 300 calories to average meal)
Calories in meal preceding moderate workouts: _____
(add 200 calories to average meal)
Calories in meal preceding vigorous activity: _____
(add 100 calories to average meal)
Calories in meal preceding moderate activity: _____
(average meal)
Calories in meal preceding light activity: _____
(subtract 100 calories from average meal)
Calories in meal preceding relaxing periods: _____
(subtract 200 calories from average meal)
Calories in meal preceding a nap: _____
(subtract 300 calories from average meal)

Once you have estimated your caloric needs on a meal-to-meal basis, proper scheduling of meals is important. Five meals a day will sustain your blood sugar levels, leave you with energy for what you are going to do, and provide nutrients for use in your body throughout the day.

You can determine how many calories you should consume at the beginning of the next three-hour period by asking yourself, "What am I going to do for the next three hours?" This should take place five times a day, at three-hour intervals which will occupy the hours you are awake each day. By following an eating schedule like this, you will be capable of storing less fat while providing carbohydrates, proteins, vitamins, and minerals to your body tissues as they need them.

In order to follow scientific nutritional practices you will also need to determine how much and what kind of protein you need to consume. As you already know, small amounts of protein, depending in part on your training intensity and your lean body weight, should be available to your muscle tissue throughout the day for maximal utilization for recovery (repair and growth). By referring to the Protein Requirements table (Figure 19-1), you will be able to estimate your daily protein requirements.

Be scientific about your nutrition and you will find that you will have more energy, bigger muscles, less fat, and more productive training. Keep records of your nutritional habits, and before each meal consult a good calorie counter which lists each food's level of fat, protein, and carbohydrates. In just a couple of weeks or so, you will begin to develop an instinctive or intuitive knowledge of what kinds of food to eat, how much food to eat, and when to eat. The Food Consumption Log (Figure 15-1) should assist you in your integrative planning.

FIGURE 15-1

Daily Food Consumption Log

Instructions: Photocopy this page multiple times and insert the copies into your training log.

TYPE FOOD	SIZE PORTION	1 PART FAT	2 PARTS CARBOHYDRATES	3 PARTS PROTEIN	TOTAL CALORIES
Meal 1					
Supplements					
Meal 2					
Supplements					
Meal 3					
Supplements					
Meal 4					
Supplements					
Meal 5					
Supplements					
TOTALS		Fat	Carbohydrates	Protein	Calories

Important: For maximum results, your nutritional supplement schedule should approximate the guidelines presented in the "daily clock" of your activities (refer back to Part Two).

16

ZIGZAG YOUR WAY TO MUSCULAR WEIGHT GAIN

"I eat like a horse, and I still can't gain weight!"

"No matter what I do, I get fat if I gain weight!"

Anyone who has been around the gym world for any length of time has heard these complaints. Even off-season bodybuilders working for mass often have trouble gaining those last couple of pounds that make the difference between that horrid third-place-rendering malady known as pencilneckitis and ascendance to the winner's circle.

Scientists have long known that eating more food than your body needs—even while exercising with weights—can cause deposition of those extra calories in the form of adipose tissue. They have come up with some intriguing findings that can definitely benefit you, whether you are a bodybuilder or a fatso.

A study* completed at the University of Pennsylvania involved 18 women weighing an average of 216 pounds at the beginning of the research period. Half received a 1,200-calorie per day diet, and the other half received 16 weeks of a common meal-replacement liquid followed by a conventional weight-reducing diet. All of the fat women walked to increase their caloric burn.

While the BMRs (basal metabolic rates, the rate at which you burn calories over a 24-hour period while at complete waking rest) of both groups fell after 5 weeks, it fell significantly more for the subjects taking the meal-replacement supplement (the more strin-

---

*Wadden, T. A., et. al. "Long-term effects of dieting on resting metabolic rate in obese outpatients." *JAMA* 264, 6 (Aug. 8, 1990): 707–11.

gent of the two experimental treatments). Their BMRs quickly returned to a level considered normal for their new (lower) body weight. After 48 weeks, the BMRs of both groups had dipped an average of 9 percent, and their percentages of body fat had dropped an average of 16–19 percent.

What's interesting about this study's findings, other than the relatively predictable outcome that the crash dieters weren't any better off than the moderate dieters after 48 weeks, is that scientists had previously assumed that any drop in weight triggered a permanent, corresponding drop in BMR. A permanently lowered BMR would mean that a dieter would not burn calories as rapidly and might therefore regain the lost pounds or have real problems shedding more pounds.

This is precisely what happens during most bodybuilders' last contest peaking cycle. In the off-season prior to another contest cycle, most bodybuilders are trying to put on some muscle, but the weight invariably comes on in fat as well as muscle. Even if you're not a competitive bodybuilder, you may have the same problem of not being able to put on muscle mass without also putting on fat. Your weight training isn't forcing an anabolic response that is capable of fully exploiting your caloric intake. Calories are left over, and they are going to get stored.

Scientists are finally beginning to support what we of irondom have known for a long, long time. The "zigzag" method of muscle-mass gain works better than any other weight-gain method. Better, that is, if you continue to lead a bodybuilding lifestyle.

Several good and bad weight-gain scenarios are presented in Figure 16-1. You'll notice that as you increase your caloric intake, both your body-fat percentage and your muscle mass increase correspondingly. Then, to force your percent body fat back to a lower level without giving up hard-won gains in muscle mass, you begin eating fewer calories per meal for a brief period.

Your total body weight begins to dip, but not as low as it was at the beginning. Your percent body fat, on the other hand, is as low as it was at the beginning, meaning that the weight you've gained is only muscle. When you raise your caloric intake again, up goes your body weight—both muscle and fat. Eat less again, and down the body weight goes—again, not as low as it was before except for your percent body fat, which has come back down to its previous low level. This process continues until your body-fat percentage is at contest levels and your muscle mass is beyond any you've ever experienced at contest time.

By zigzagging your caloric intake, you ultimately allow periodic BMR adjustments to take place, bringing your BMR to a level corresponding to your new body weight. It's easy to begin losing fat again—and again—without giving up hard-won muscle mass. If you simply try going up, up, up in body weight, your BMR never has a chance to adjust, and your muscle-gaining and fat-loss efforts become harder and harder until, in thorough frustration, you begin stringent dieting again and lose all that wonderful mass that's hidden under a blanket of ugly fat.

The most important element in the entire process of zigzagging is heavy weight training. Without the heavy training, your increased weight will be primarily fat, not muscle. Don't try to gain too quickly! Even with the best-conceived weight-training program, excessive calories always add up to increased fat. Mild exercise of any kind is OK for the pencilnecks, I guess—especially those considered chronically skinny or fat—but even for such people, weight training is the single best method for ensuring that gradually increased weight will be mostly muscle.

Further, when you couple the zigzag method of eating with weight training and a careful supplement program, you will be amazed at how easy it is to put on muscle mass and how utterly enjoyable it is to keep it forever. Your new lifestyle will ensure that!

Finally, for you bodybuilders who insist on getting massive between contests—massively *fat*, that is—I have only a couple of things to say.

1. Change your slovenly ways—bigger is only better if it's only muscle!
2. If you don't change your ways, you'll never break into the winners' circle at Mount Olympus.

FIGURE 16-1

Good and Bad Weight-Gain Scenarios

EXAMPLE 1
How *Not* to Do It

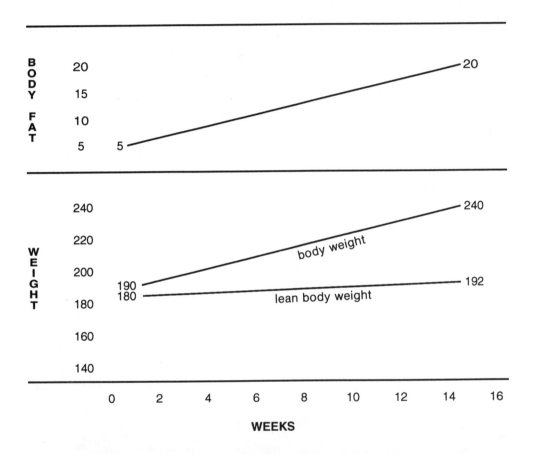

You're an athlete and in great shape. Trouble is, you're too small, and you want to put on some mass. You train harder, eat more, and get bigger—much bigger. But your lean body weight—your muscle mass—only goes up 12 pounds. Your body fat skyrockets. This is the most common scenario you'll notice among athletes wishing to put on some mass. Tch! Tch! You don't make the cut.

EXAMPLE 1
How *Best* to Do It

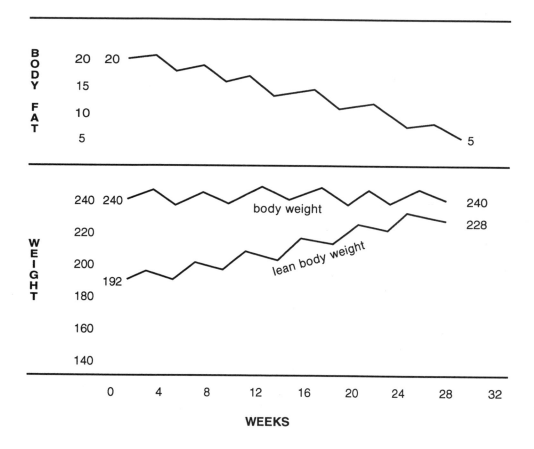

You're an athlete and in great shape. Trouble is, you're too small, and you want to put on some mass. You begin eating, supplementing, and training more scientifically, periodically adjusting your caloric intake so that your metabolism gradually adjusts to your new level of body weight and lean mass. You're not in a hurry. You have entered a level of elite sports performance that few dare dream of!

Note: The "down-zag" in caloric intake should last 3–5 days, while the "up-zig" should last a day or two.

EXAMPLE 2
How *Not* to Do It

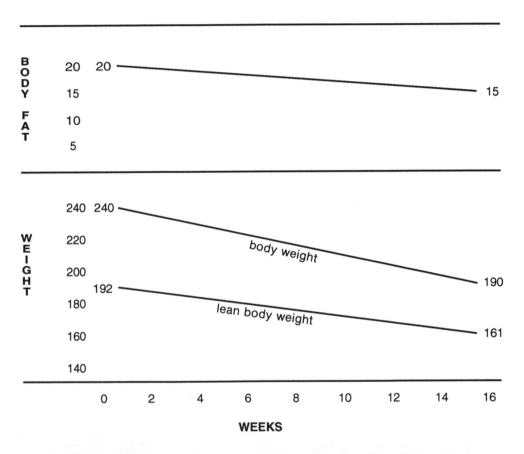

You're a fat slob. You're overweight and inactive. Your doctor tells you to lose that ugly fat, and common sense tells you the best way to do it is to go on a low-calorie diet and do some running or weight training. You lose fat, all right, but you end up losing a lot of muscle, too. Your percentage of body fat comes down five points as you lose a total of 50 pounds. Not bad, but the horror of it all is that most of the weight you lost came from precious muscle. You end up sick, weaker, and thoroughly unhealthy.

EXAMPLE 2
How *Best* to Do It

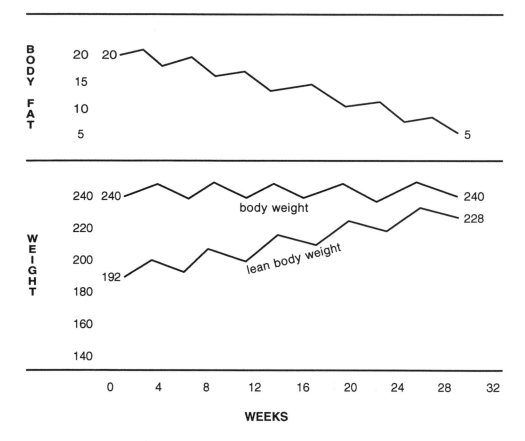

You're a fat slob. You're overweight and inactive. Doc tells you to lose that ugly fat, and scientific studies tell you that the best way to do it is to train with weights and control your caloric intake so your metabolism has a chance to continually adjust. You learn not to be in a hurry. Your body fat comes down to an excellent level over 7–8 months, and your muscle mass actually increases.

Note: The "down-zag" in caloric intake should last 3–5 days, while the "up-zig" should last a day or two.

EXAMPLE 3
How *Not* to Do It

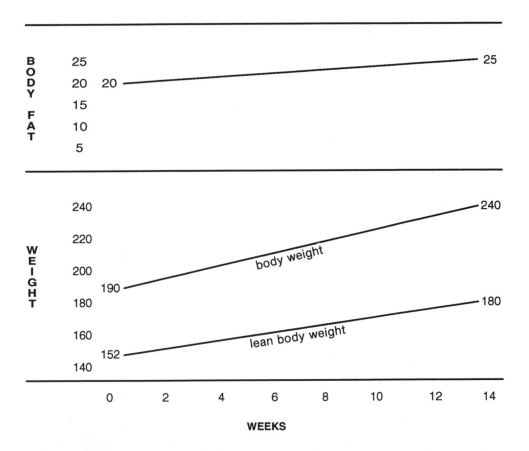

You're too small, you're overly inactive, and—even though you don't look it with your clothes on—you're soft and fat. You dream about getting big and muscular and entering a bodybuilding contest. You eat like a horse and gain weight rapidly. "Great!" you say. Guess again, fella! Sure, you put on a full 50 pounds, but you gained only 22 pounds of muscle and a full 28 pounds of ugly adipose baggage. You used to be a 190-pound person with a normal body-fat percent, but now you're a big fat slob who can't get out of his own way.

EXAMPLE 3
How *Best* to Do It

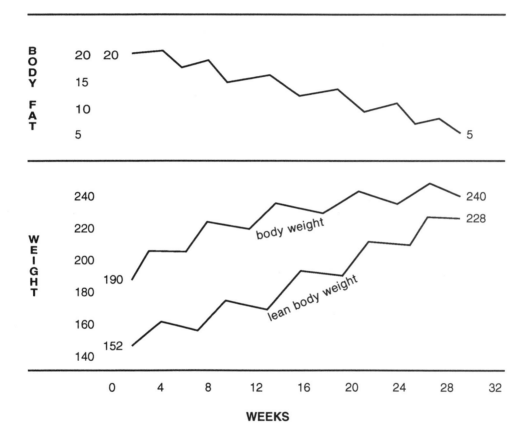

You're too small, you're overly inactive, and—even though you don't look it with your clothes on—you're soft and fat. You dream about getting big and muscular and entering a bodybuilding contest. Science guides you on your quest. You eat, train, and supplement in a zigzag pattern, allowing adjustments in your BMR to compensate for your changing muscle mass and activity level. Down comes your body-fat percentage, up goes your body weight, and you're left with a physique that any bodybuilder would be proud of.

Note: The "down-zag" in caloric intake should last 3–5 days, while the "up-zig" should last a day or two.

FIGURE 16-2

Recommended Foods for
Muscle Mass/Fat Loss Diets

BREADS AND CEREALS
Instructions: Eat 6-8 small servings
of these foods daily (spread over five meals)

Whole-wheat breads
Whole-grain cereals
Whole-grain pasta
Brown or wild rice
Plain popcorn
Lentils
Sweet potatoes or yams
Beans

Avoid
Refined or fiber-free breads, cereals, grains, and pastas

FATS
Instructions: Eat no more than two small servings
of these foods daily (e.g., during meal 1, 3, or 5)

Margarine
Butter
Mayonnaise
Vegetable oil (unsaturated) (preferably canola oil or virgin olive oil)

Avoid
Nuts
Gravy
Avocados
All rich sauces
Fried food

FRUITS
Instructions: Eat three or four
of these fruits daily (spread over 3-4 meals)

Northern hemisphere fruits preferred, with southern hemisphere fruits (e.g., bananas, mangoes, etc.) not eaten in preworkout or precompetition meals

Avoid
All dried or canned fruits

MEATS
Instructions: Eat five small servings
of these foods daily (spread over 3-5 meals)

Any lean meats (broiled)
Lean fish (broiled)
Egg whites
Lean poultry (broiled)
Lean shellfish

Avoid
Oil-packed fish, mackerel, salmon
Luncheon meats
Processed meats
Smoked fish and meats, egg yolks

DAIRY PRODUCTS
Instructions: Have 3-5 small servings
of these foods daily (spread over 3-5 meals)

Skim milk
Yogurt (nonfat or low fat)
Buttermilk (nonfat)
Frozen lowfat yogurt (in moderation)
Cottage cheese (nonfat)
Ricotta (nonfat)
Mozzarella (nonfat)

Avoid
All others, including cheeses not listed

VEGETABLES
Instructions: Eat 3-5 servings
of these foods daily (spread over 3-5 meals)

All vegetables (preferably fresh), emphasizing the vegetables with the highest glycemic indexes
All vegetable juices (preferably fresh)

MISCELLANEOUS
Instructions: Enjoy the following foods to taste

Nonfat homemade soups
Diet cola
Water (6–8 cups daily)
Tea or coffee (decaffeinated preferred;
2-3 cups maximum)
Nutritional supplements (as directed)

Avoid
Alcohol
nondiet colas

FIGURE 16-3

An Example of a Muscle-Gaining Diet*

(APPROXIMATE TOTAL CALORIES = 5,268)

MEAL	SERVINGS	FOOD	GRAMS		
			Fat	Pro	Carb
1 (8:00 A.M.)	8	Egg whites	0.0	27	3
	2	Whole-grain pancakes	6.0	7	18
	4 sli.	Whole-grain toast w/butter	14.0	10	44
	4	Apples	2.0	1	84
	16 oz.	Mass-building shake	8.4	46	100
(Approximate total calories = 1,635)					
2 (11:00 A.M.)	16 oz.	Mass-building shake	8.4	46	100
	2 sli.	Whole-grain bread	1.4	5	22
(Approximate total calories = 780)					
3 (2:00 P.M.)	1 lg.	Grapefruit	1.2	1	10
(1–2 hours before training)	3 sm.	Apples	1.5	1	63
	3 c.	Whole-wheat spaghetti	1.8	14	97
	2 c.	Kidney beans	1.8	15	15
	16 oz.	Skim milk	0.8	17	23
	16 oz.	Low-glycemic-index carbohydrate drink	0.0	1	42
	3	Broiled chicken breasts	9.0	80	0
(Approximate total calories = 1, 662)					
4 (5:00 P.M.)	16 oz.	Mass-building shake	8.4	46	100
	1 c.	Baked beans	1.0	15	40
(Approximate total calories = 890)					
5 (8:00 P.M.)	6–8	Hard-boiled egg whites	0.0	20	2
	1 sm.	Vegetable salad	0.3	2	6
	3 sli.	Whole-grain bread	2.0	8	33
(Approximate total calories = 301)					

---

*Avg. nutrient ratios: Fats 11.6%, Protein 27.5%, Carbs 60.9%

FIGURE 16-4

How Long Can I Expect to Wait to Put on Muscle?

NUMBER OF WEEKS IT'LL TAKE

		5	10	15	20	25	30
		100	10	20	30	40	50	60

	L	120	9	19	28	38	47	57
Y	E A N	140	9	18	27	36	45	54
O U R	B	160	8	16	24	32	40	48
R	O D	180	8	16	24	32	40	48
P R E	Y	200	7	15	22	30	37	45
S E	W E	220	7	14	21	28	35	42
N T	I G	240	6	13	19	26	32	39
	H T	260	6	12	18	24	30	36
		280	5	11	16	22	27	33
		300	5	10	15	20	25	30

	5	**10**	**15**	**20**	**25**	**30**

Pounds of Added Muscle Desired

17

LOSING FAT
AND KEEPING IT OFF

Convention has it that there are three ways to lose *weight*: dehydration, fat loss, and lean muscle weight loss. Regardless of your level of bodybuilding development, fat loss is the *only* acceptable route for you. Dehydration is never healthy or acceptable, and losing lean muscle mass totally counters everything the bodybuilding lifestyle stands for. Let's establish the objective of any serious bodybuilder right off the bat—to lose fat without sacrificing—and, in fact, increasing—your muscle tissue.

Diets that produce a loss in lean body weight are those most often lacking carbohydrates. Without carbohydrates in your diet, energy for training will come from fats and proteins. Your performance will decrease, you'll feel fatigued, tired, weak, and irritable; your brain will find it more difficult to operate effectively, and you will be less able to concentrate.

A loss in lean weight can also result from too little protein intake. Because training breaks down your muscle proteins, an adequate protein intake is necessary for repair and rebuilding. When protein is not available for these anabolic processes, your training will continually break down your muscle and you will actually lose valuable tissue.

According to conventional theory, *fat* loss can only be accomplished three ways: with exercise, through reduced caloric intake, or through a combination of the two. That's good, but good is never good enough for serious bodybuilders. The *best* approach to getting rid of excess fat is through integrated training. There are many, many ways that fat can be shed or avoided without committing the common mistake of sacrificing muscle tissue.

SOME FAT-LOSS POINTS TO REMEMBER

1. *Thermogenesis* is the production of body heat through oxidation of foods, physical means, and biochemical means. There are several ways to induce a calorie-burning thermogenic response in your body so that your fat-loss efforts will be far more effective: sauna, cold, certain herbs, exercise, and frequent meals are but a few.

2. Exercise maintains or increases your lean body weight. As you increase your lean weight your metabolism also increases, both during training and at rest. This is why dieting alone is not an effective means to losing fat.

3. Research shows that dieting does not reduce the number of fat cells you have, but it can reduce the *size* of these cells. It is believed that your number of fat cells is somewhat genetic and can be increased during early childhood.

4. A problem many bodybuilders face is their willingness to starve themselves in order to lose fat. By starving yourself, your fat cells learn to conserve energy (fat) more efficiently. Therefore, it gets more difficult to lose fat each time you diet.

5. The adage "you must eat to lose fat" is very true. If you lower your calorie intake too much, your metabolism will slow down and you will defeat your sole purpose of dieting—it will become more difficult to lose fat. This occurs even if you are training.

Of course, your training will then suffer. You will experience decreases in coordination and physical work capacity. Handling heavy weights becomes impossible, and you become more irritable and unable to relax. You must remember that you need to eat not only to supply your working muscles with energy and to replace nutrients lost during training, but also to lose fat.

6. Although how much you eat is important, it is just as important to know what to eat and when to eat it. This is where an integrated approach to fat-loss and bodybuilding comes in. Indeed, that's what this entire book is about.

ZIGZAG YOUR WAY TO FAT LOSS

"I eat like a bird, and I still gain weight!"

"Not matter what I do, I get fatter and fatter!"

"All I have to do is smell food and I put on weight!"

Anyone who has been around the fitness world for any length of time has heard these complaints, too. Even athletes and bodybuilders preparing for competition often have trouble shedding those last couple of pounds of third-place–rendering, muscle-masking ugliness called adipose.

Whether you're losing fat, gaining muscle, or doing both at the same time, the same nutritional science applies. The scientists cited in the preceding chapter on zigzag dieting for increasing muscle mass are gathering hard data supporting what we of irondom have known for a long, long time—that is, there's a way to lose fat and still maintain a reasonably high BMR so your fat-loss process can continue smoothly. It's called the zigzag method of fat loss, and it works better than any other fat-loss method. Why? It's permanent. Permanent, that is, if you continue to eat four or five small meals per day and exercise regularly. It allows you to maintain or improve your lean muscle mass.

Several weight-loss scenarios, both good and bad, are presented in Figure 17-1. You'll notice that as you reduce your caloric intake and increase your caloric burn, your body-fat percentage drops correspondingly, but so does your BMR. To force your BMR back to a normal level, you begin eating normally again for a brief period (never more than 36 hours).

During this brief pig-out period your body-fat level again begins to climb, but not as high as it was at the beginning. You lower your caloric intake again; down goes your body-fat. Eat normal again, and up the body fat goes—again, not as high as it was before. This process continues until your body-fat percentage is at healthful levels.

By zigzagging your caloric intake, you ultimately allow periodic BMR adjustments to take place, bringing your BMR back to a level corresponding to your new (lower) body weight. It's easy to begin losing fat again—and again. If you simply try going down, down, down in body fat, your BMR never has a chance to adjust, and your fat-loss efforts become harder and harder until, in thorough frustration, you binge out and get fat again—forever.

As with gaining muscle mass and increasing total body weight, the most important element in permanent fat loss is weight training. Remember, big muscles burn more calories than little muscles, and the more muscle you have, the higher your BMR will tend to be. Without the weight training, your fat-loss efforts will result in loss of lean tissue primarily, not fat. Don't try to lose fat too quickly! Even with weight training starvation diets will result in lost muscle rather than fat.

Walking is OK for those considered chronically fat. For those of you who are only slightly overweight, mild but regular aerobic exercise is excellent for maintaining an efficient BMR. But weight training stands out as the single best method for ensuring that gradually lost weight will come from fat stores.

Further, when you couple the zigzag method of eating with weight training, moderate aerobic exercise, and a careful diet and supplement program, you will be amazed at how easy it is to lose fat and how utterly enjoyable it is to keep it off forever.

The same admonishment on gaining muscle mass applies to those of you who need to shed body fat. For you diehards out there who insist on getting fat between contests or during the winter months of inactivity, I have only a couple of things to say:

1. Change your slovenly ways.
2. If you don't change your ways, be prepared to suffer the indignities associated with being overweight, always on a diet, and in a rut wherein you never quite realize your true potential as a bodybuilder.

FIGURE 17-1

How to Lose Fat and Still Stay Muscular and Strong

EXAMPLE 1
How *Not* to Do It

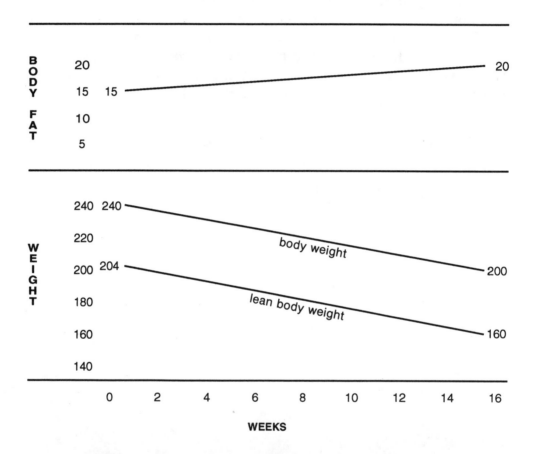

You're an athlete competing out of your optimal body weight, and your coach says to lose weight. You comply. Down goes your weight—down 40 pounds! "Great!" coach praises. But is it? No. You've lost 44 pounds of muscle and put on 4 pounds of fat. Your body-fat percentage climbed a staggering five points. You've made your weight division, all right, but now you're going to lose even more matches than you were losing at the higher body weight.

EXAMPLE 1
How *Best* to Do It

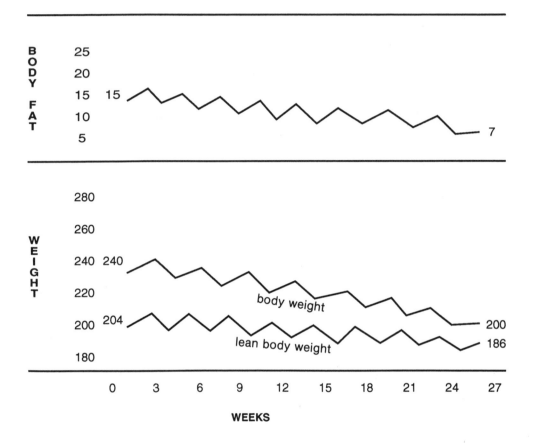

You're an athlete, and you're not winning in your body-weight division. Your coach determines that you are out of your optimal weight division and need to lose 40 pounds. Carefully planned training coupled with a programmatic fat-loss program allows you to drop to 200 pounds and bring your body fat down from a previous 15 percent to a far more competitive 7 percent—where it should be!

Note: The "down-zag" in caloric intake should last 3–5 days, while the "up-zig" should last a day or two.

EXAMPLE 2
How *Not* to Do It

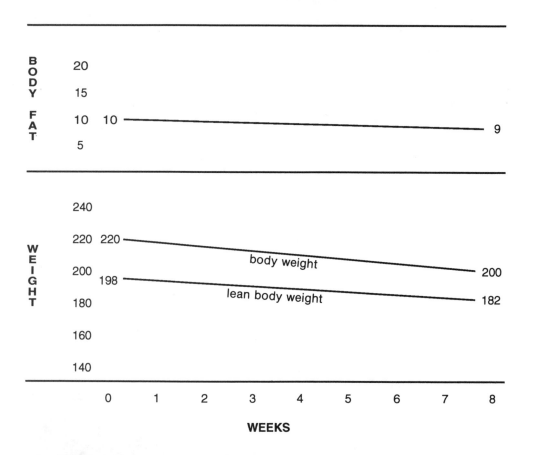

You're a competitive bodybuilder, and you have a contest in two months. You go through the traditional chicken-only diet to get cut up. You lose a full 20 pounds, and your body-fat percentage drops a point. But wait! Of the 20 pounds you lost, only 4 pounds were fat. You actually lost a full 16 pounds of the muscle you worked diligently to put on over months of grueling training.

EXAMPLE 2
How *Best* to Do It

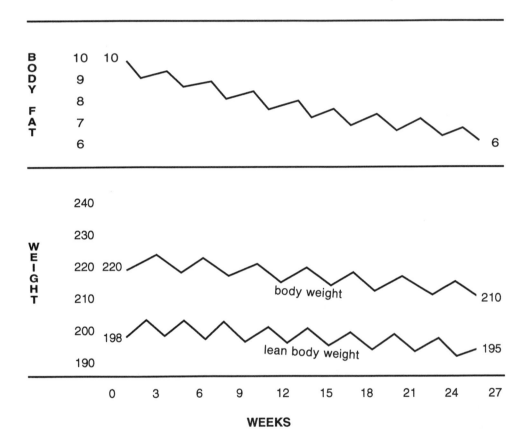

You're a competitive bodybuilder, and there's a contest coming up that you feel is critical for your career. Six months out, you begin to carefully pare away fat with an eye toward preserving that precious muscle you worked so diligently to put on over months of grueling, back-breaking work. In the off-season, you never let your body weight or body fat get out of control. Slowly, the fat melts away. A full seven pounds of it goes, and only three pounds of muscle was sacrificed. However, you end up at contest time a full 4 percent lower in body fat, and that's enough to expose the tremendous muscular achievement your hard work has produced.

Note: The "down-zag" in caloric intake should last 3–5 days, while the "up-zig" should last a day or two.

EXAMPLE 3
How *Not* to Do It

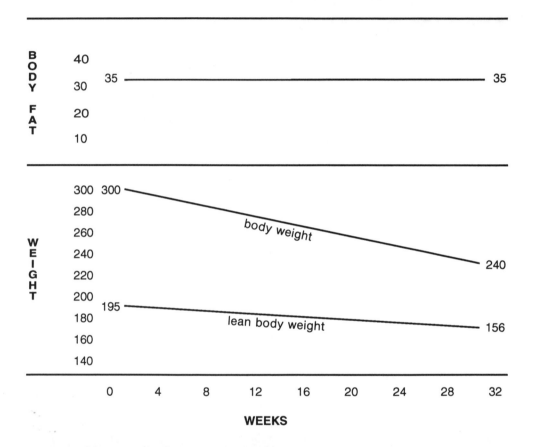

You're fat, and your doctor informs you that unless you lose 60 pounds, your health will be in jeopardy. You comply. You go on a crash diet and lose 60 pounds in six months. You lose 21 pounds of fat, but you also lost 39 pounds of precious muscle. What's worse, your total body-fat percentage didn't drop a bit. Before, you were a large fat person; now, you're a smaller fat person.

EXAMPLE 3
How *Best* to Do It

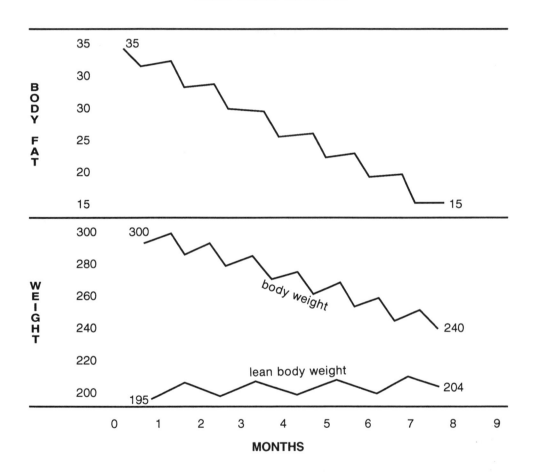

You're fat, and you know it. So do your doctor, your friends, and your coworkers. Your self-image is at an all-time low and your health is in jeopardy. You go on a carefully constructed long-term diet, combining spurts of low caloric intake with integrated training and light aerobics. The fat begins to disappear—slowly at first, but surely. In nine short months, you've lost a full 60 pounds and succeeded in bringing your total body-fat percentage from a whopping 35 percent to a normal and healthy 15 percent. Predictably, you begin seriously thinking about entering a bodybuilding contest.

Note: The "down-zag" in caloric intake should last 3–5 days, while the "up-zig" should last a day or two.

EXAMPLE 4
How *Not* to Do It

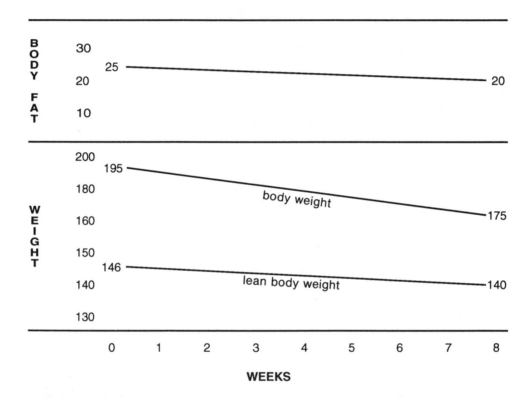

WEEKS

You're of average activity level, body build, and weight, except as you get older you notice a bit of fat appearing around your waistline. You go on a diet and lose 20 pounds in two months. Your body-fat level came down from 25 percent to a more normal 20 percent. You look better in your clothes, sure, but when you look closely, you'll see that you lost 14 pounds of fat and sacrificed a full 6 pounds of muscle in the process.

EXAMPLE 4
How *Best* to Do It

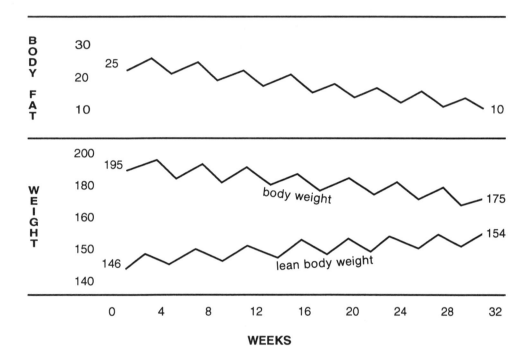

You're of average activity level, body build, and weight, except as you get older you notice a bit of fat appearing around your waistline. You go on a carefully planned diet, integrating it with just as careful exercise and nutritional supplementation. Unlike the average well-meaning dieter, you're in no hurry to lose the weight. You lose 20 pounds in 8 months, and your body-fat level came down from 25 percent to an extremely healthy 10 percent. You look better in your clothes, sure, but you look even better in a bathing suit! When you look closely, you'll see that you actually lost 28 pounds of fat and gained a full 8 pounds of muscle in the process. Predictably, you begin seriously thinking about entering a bodybuilding contest.

Note: The "down-zag" in caloric intake should last 3–5 days, while the "up-zig" should last a day or two.

PLANNING YOUR FAT-LOSS STRATEGY

When you plan a fat-loss program, certain measures can make it easier for you to achieve your goal of getting hard and lean without giving up muscle in the process.

1. Gustation (Taste). If you like certain foods, you will be more inclined to eat them. You should learn how to prepare foods that are good for you and in a way that they taste good.

2. Satiety. Foods that satisfy your hunger and blood-sugar levels will leave you less likely to snack. These foods should have a glycemic index (the rate at which they are converted to blood sugar) of under 50. (A chart showing the glycemic indexes of many popular carbohydrate foods is presented in Chapter Twenty-Two.) Eating five meals each day keeps your blood-sugar levels elevated and does not allow you to get hungry.

3. Health. Getting the most from your integrated training efforts is the primary immediate objective. Accomplish this through applying a balanced diet and nutritional supplementation as part of your integrated training program. This lifestyle commitment will promote health and, if you're healthy, your muscle-building and fat-loss efforts are far more effective.

4. Meal-to-Meal Calorie Control. To be the best bodybuilder you can be, you must know how to train properly, recuperate adequately, and choose the right foods and how and when to eat them, and which nutritional supplements are needed.

5. Follow the five rules of sound bodybuilding nutrition presented earlier in this Part.

6. Pay special attention to the calorie-control formula presented earlier, as this formula will ensure that your calories are all being accounted for during each three-hour period of your day.

FIGURE 17-2

An Example of a Fat-Loss Diet*

Note: To achieve your prescribed caloric intake, adjust each meal's food portions up or down. Do *not* eliminate foods!

			APPROX. GRAMS		
MEAL	**SERVINGS**	**FOOD**	**Fat**	**Pro**	**Carb**
1 (8:00 A.M.)	3	Egg whites	0.0	10.0	1.2
	1 med.	Whole-grain pancake	6.4	6.8	17.6
	1 slice	Whole-grain toast	.7	2.4	11.0
	1 pc.	Fresh fruit	.5	.3	21.0
	8 oz.	Skim milk	.4	8.4	11.8
(Approximate total calories = 434)					
2 (11:00 A.M.)	1 pc.	Fresh fruit	.2	1.2	15.4
	2 slice	Whole-grain bread	1.4	4.8	22.0
	1 sm.	Chicken breast	3.1	26.7	0.0
	6 oz.	Skim milk	.3	6.3	8.9
(Approximate total calories = 385)					
3 (2:00 P.M.)	½	Grapefruit	.1	.8	9.7
(1½ hours before training)	1 sm.	Broiled chicken breast	3.1	26.7	0.0
	1 sm.	Apple	.5	.3	21.0
	1 c.	Kidney beans	.9	7.7	7.5
	8 oz.	Skim milk	.4	8.4	11.8
(Approximate total calories = 418)					
4 (5:00 P.M.)	8 oz.	Fruit juice	.5	1.7	25.8
	1 sm.	Chicken breast	3.1	26.7	0.0
	1 med.	Vegetable salad	.3	2.0	6.0
	6 oz.	Skim milk	.3	6.3	8.9
(Approximate total calories = 347)					
5 (8:00 P.M.)	3	Egg whites	0.0	10.0	1.2
	1 sm.	Vegetable salad	.3	2.0	6.0
	1 slice	Whole-grain bread	.7	2.4	11.0
(Approximate total calories = 140)					

*Calorie Totals: Fat 209, Protein 647, Carbs 869, Calories 1,724
Avg. Nutrient Ratios: Fats 12%, Protein 38%, Carbs 50%

FIGURE 17-3

Factors Contributing to Obesity and
What to Do about Them

POSSIBLE CAUSES

Excessive stimulation of appetite
  center

Adipose cell hyperplasia

Hyperlipidogenesis
  Increased lipoprotein
  lipase activity

Lesions

Decreased lipid metabolism
  Decreased lipolytic hormones
  Defective adipose cell lipolysis
  Abnormality in autoimmune
    innervation

Decreased lipid utilization
  Aging
  Defective oxidation of fats
  Defective thermogenesis
  Inactivity
  Underexercising

Genetic predisposition

Endocrine and metabolic
    disturbances
  Cushing's syndrome
  Gallbladder disease
  Diabetes mellitus
  Hypertension
  Thyroid disorders
  Thrombosis
  Kidney disorders
  Frohlich's syndrome

Sociocultural environment
  Stress
  Poverty (poor diet)
  Emotional disturbances
  Childbirth

WHAT TO DO ABOUT THEM

Consult your physician to either treat or
rule out all medical causes

Consult a competent person experienced
in either medical weight loss (if indicated)
or exercise and nutrition

If appropriate, join a self-help group to
effect long-term behavior modification
(e.g., OA or TOPS)

Seek support from both your family and
friends in sticking to prescribed program

Eat sensibly five times daily

Exercise sensibly every day

Use high-quality, proven nutritional
supplements to your diet and exercise
program, especially during periods of
calorie restriction or during periods of
higher-than-usual exercise intensity

Avoid fad diets and crash diets of all kinds

When approved, consider using a high-
quality meal-replacement drink

Your weight-loss regimen should never be
so Spartan that you lose interest or quit
because it's too hard to stick to

FIGURE 17-4

Weeks Required to Lose Fat
Using the Zigzag Method of Dieting and a
Well-Planned Exercise Program

STARTING BODY-FAT PERCENTAGE

POUNDS OF FAT TO LOSE (without losing muscle)	5*	10*	15	20	25	30	35	40
5	20	15	10	5	5	5	6	7
10		25	20	10	10	10	12	14
15			30	15	15	15	18	21
20			40	20	20	20	24	28
25				25	25	25	30	35
30				30	30	30	36	42
35				35	35	35	42	49
40					40	40	48	56
45					45	45	54	63
50					50	50	60	70
55						55	66	77
60						60	72	84

(number of weeks needed to bring you down to a 10–15 percent body-fat level)

---

*Going below 10 percent recommended for athletes only.

When you're close to an ideal body-fat level (around 10–15 percent for average athletes, but well under 10 percent for competing bodybuilders who sometimes compete as low as 3 or 4 percent body fat), you take a bit longer to lose fat because you have very little fat left to lose. Only care over weeks of time will ensure that only fat, not muscle, is lost. Chronically obese people also take longer to lose fat, because of their very low metabolic rates and their inability to engage in strenuous (calorie-burning) exercise. By zigzagging your caloric intake and engaging in muscle-building (or muscle-preserving) exercise, metabolic-rate adjustments take place and the fat-loss process continues uninterrupted.

18

EASY METHODS OF DETERMINING YOUR BODY-FAT PERCENTAGE

A lot of different ways of determining your body-fat percentage share one common problem—they're only accurate to within plus or minus four percentage points under the best of administrative conditions. In other words, if you calculate your body-fat percentage at 20 percent, it could actually be anywhere between 16–24 percent. Practice and fastidious care will ensure that your estimates are reasonably accurate, regardless of which procedure or technology you employ.

In most cases, bodybuilders will find that the methods presented in this book tend toward the conservative. More often than not, if you measure out at, say, 10 percent body fat, you're probably closer to 6 or 7 percent, because the density of your muscles is far greater than the norm. Remember, most methods of estimating body fat are based on population norms, and bodybuilders are anything but normal people! If you're an accomplished bodybuilder (heavily muscled from years of weight training), subtract two or three percentage points from your final calculation.

Underwater weighing is the accepted standard by which the validity and reliability of all other methods are judged. Even bodybuilders will get a relatively accurate reading from underwater weighing. Underwater weighing is based on Archimedes's principle of specific gravity. If your body weighs less than an equivalent volume of water, you'll float; if it weighs more, you'll sink.

Other methods of estimating your body-fat percentage include electrical impedance, ultrasound, skinfold measurements, and anthropometric measurements. The easiest anthropometric method requires only a scale, a tape measure, and some regression equations based on population norms. The techniques for both men and women are outlined in Figure 18-1 (for men) and Figure 18-2 (for women).

One note of caution, however. Why do you even need to know your body-fat percentage in the first place? There really isn't any good reason other than merely knowing or monitoring progress. If you're fat, you know it without being measured; if you're rock-hard, you know that, too. From our perspective, it's probably more important for you to look in the mirror while naked. Too fat? Lose some fat! Too skinny? Gain some muscle!

ESTIMATING YOUR BODY-FAT PERCENTAGE

The two methods of determing your body weight presented in Figures 18-1 and 18-2 use an equation that includes several numbers which remain constant. These constants are based on such factors as the average density of your bones and the average amount of air in your lungs. As I pointed out above, the principal advantage of these estimation procedures is that all they require is a scale and a tape measure.

FIGURE 18-1

Estimating Body-Fat Percentage—Men

Step One: Multiply your body weight (nude) by 1.082.
Step Two: Add this number to 94.42.
Step Three: Multiply your waist girth (measured at the umbilicus) by 4.15.
Step Four: Subtract this number from the number obtained in Step Two to obtain your "fat-free" body weight.
Step Five: Subtract your fat-free body weight (obtained in Step Four) from your total body weight.
Step Six: Multiply that number by 100.
Step Seven: Divide that number by your total body weight to obtain your body-fat percentage.

Example: Let's say you weigh 205 pounds, and your waist measures 35 inches.

Step One: $1.082 \times 205 = 221.81$
Step Two: $221.81 + 94.42 = 316.23$
Step Three: $35 \times 4.15 = 145.25$
Step Four: $316.23 - 145.25 = 170.98$ (fat-free body weight)
Step Five: $205 - 170.98 = 34.02$
Step Six: $34.02 \times 100 = 3,402$
Step Seven: 3,402 divided by 205 = 16.59, which is your body-fat percentage

FIGURE 18-2

Estimating Body-Fat Percentage—Women

Step One: Multiply your body weight (nude) by 0.732.

Step Two: Add this number to 8.987 (save this number).

Step Three: Measure the circumference of your wrist at its widest point, and divide the circumference by 3.14 (pi) to determine your wrist's diameter (save this number).

Step Four: Multiply your abdominal circumference (measured at the umbilicus) by 0.157 (save this number).

Step Five: Multiply your hip circumference (measured at its widest point) by 0.249 (save this number).

Step Six: Multiply your forearm circumference (measured at its widest point) by 0.434 (save this number).

Step Seven: Add the numbers obtained in Steps Two and Three (save this number).

Step Eight: Subtract the number obtained in Step Four from that obtained in Step Seven (save this number).

Step Nine: Subtract the number obtained in Step Five from that obtained in Step Eight (save this number).

Step Ten: Add the number obtained in Step Six to that obtained in Step Nine. This number is your fatfree weight (your "lean" body weight).

Step Eleven: To obtain your body-fat percentage, subtract your lean body weight from your total body weight. Multiply that number by 100, and then divide the product by your total body weight.

Example: You weigh 130 pounds, and your vital measurements are as follows: wrist, 6.25 inches; abdominal, 27 inches; hip, 38 inches; and forearm, 10 inches.

Step One: $130 \times 0.732 = 95.160$

Step Two: $95.16 + 8.987 = 104.147$

Step Three: $6.25 \div 3.14 = 1.990$

Step Four: $27.0 \times 0.157 = 4.239$

Step Five: $38 \times 0.249 = 9.462$

Step Six: $10 \times 0.434 = 4.340$

Step Seven: $104.147 + 1.990 = 106.137$

Step Eight: $106.137 - 4.239 = 101.898$

Step Nine: $101.898 - 9.462 = 92.436$

Step Ten: $92.436 + 4.340 = 96.776$ (your lean body weight)

Step Eleven: $(130 - 96.639) \times 100 = 3,336.10$; and $3,336.10 \div 130 = 25.556$

Your body-fat percentage is 25.556.

ALTERNATIVE BODY-FAT ESTIMATION PROCEDURES

Two alternative methods of estimating body-fat percentage require the use of skinfold calipers to measure the folds of fat at four different sites on your body. These calipers measure the thickness of the outer layer of fat on your body, the measurements of which are automatically plugged into regression equations. Several numbers included in the regression equations remain constant. These constants are based on such factors as the average density of your bones and other tissues, and the average amount of air you have in your lungs.

Once you have measured the skinfolds at the sites indicated, you can easily compute your body-fat percentage through the use of a nomogram (Figure 18-3) or tables of norms (Figure 18-4). These techniques require no math.

How to Use Skinfold Calipers

Measuring body fat with calipers takes a bit of practice. In measuring most of the body sites used in the equations, the calipers should be held vertically or, as is the case with subscapular and suprailiac measurements, at a slight angle to conform to the natural fold of the skin.

Firmly pinch the skinfold with your thumb and forefinger, being sure to grasp only the skin and fat directly beneath the skin. While holding the fold of fat away from the underlying muscle, place the calipers over the fatfold in such a way that a representative fatfold thickness is within the jaws of the calipers, and read the measurement. Perform the measurement a few times before you trust your judgment.

11 Thigh
16 chest
12 waist
8 Bicep

47

FIGURE 18-3

Two Skinfold-Site Methods of Calculating Body-Fat Percentages for Men and Women

PERCENT BODY FAT/MEN

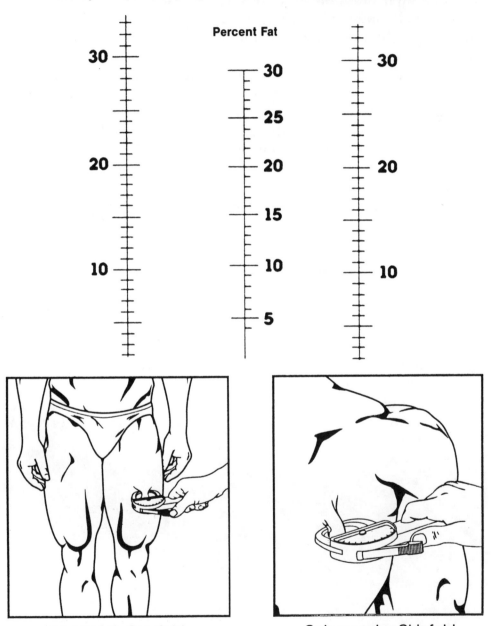

Mid-Thigh Skinfold

Subscapular Skinfold

Directions: Locate your thigh and subscapular skinfold values in the corresponding columns. Draw a straight line from one value to the other, crossing over the middle scale of values. The point on the middle scale where the line intersects is your percentage of body fat.

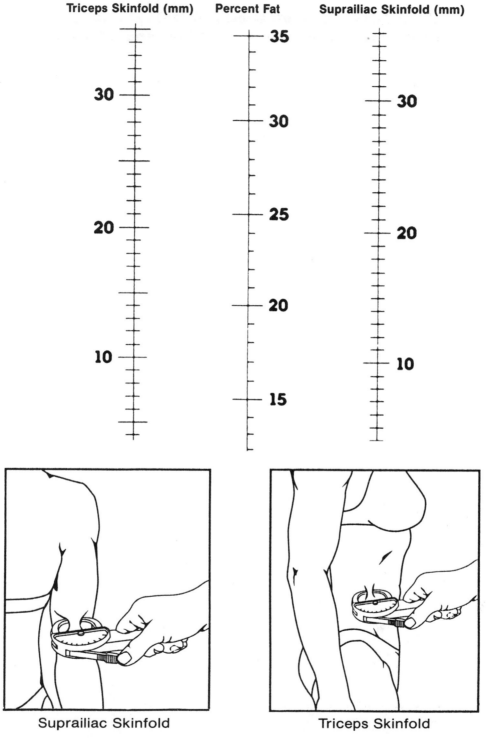

Suprailiac Skinfold   Triceps Skinfold

Directions: Locate your triceps and suprailiac skinfold values in the corresponding columns. Draw a straight line from one value to the other, crossing over the middle scale of values. The point on the middle scale where the line intersects is your percentage of body fat.

FIGURE 18-4

Skinfold-Site Methods of Determining Body-Fat Percentages for Men and Women

The equivalent fat content, as a precentage of body weight, for a range of values for the sum of four skinfolds (biceps, triceps, subscapular, and suprailiac) of men and women of different ages.

TABLE A: MEN

Skinfolds (mm)	Ages 17–29	30–39	40–49	50+
15	4.8	—	—	—
20	8.1	12.2	12.2	12.6
25	10.5	14.2	15.0	15.6
30	12.9	16.2	17.7	18.6
35	14.7	17.7	19.6	20.8
40	16.4	19.2	21.4	22.9
45	17.7	20.4	23.0	24.7
50	19.0	21.5	24.6	26.5
55	20.1	22.5	25.9	27.9
60	21.2	23.5	27.1	29.2
65	22.2	24.3	28.2	30.4
70	23.1	25.1	29.3	31.6
75	24.0	25.9	30.3	32.7
80	24.8	26.6	31.2	33.8
85	25.5	27.2	32.1	34.8
90	26.2	27.8	33.0	35.8
95	26.9	28.4	33.7	36.6
100	27.6	29.0	34.4	37.4
105	28.2	29.6	35.1	38.2
110	28.8	30.1	35.8	39.0
115	29.4	30.6	36.4	39.7
120	30.0	31.1	37.0	40.4
125	30.5	31.5	37.6	41.1
130	31.0	31.9	38.2	41.8
135	31.5	32.3	38.7	42.4
140	32.0	32.7	39.2	43.0
145	32.5	33.1	39.7	43.6
150	32.9	33.5	40.2	44.1
155	33.3	33.9	40.7	44.6
160	33.7	34.3	41.2	45.1
165	34.1	34.6	41.6	45.6
170	34.5	34.8	42.0	46.1
175	34.9	—	—	—
180	35.3	—	—	—
185	35.6	—	—	—
190	35.9	—	—	—
195	—	—	—	—
200	—	—	—	—
205	—	—	—	—
210	—	—	—	—

TABLE B: WOMEN

Skinfolds (mm)	Ages 16–29	30–39	40–49	50+
15	10.5	—	—	—
20	14.1	17.0	19.8	21.4
25	16.8	19.4	22.2	24.0
30	19.5	21.8	24.5	26.6
35	21.5	23.7	26.4	28.5
40	23.4	25.5	28.2	30.3
45	25.0	26.9	29.6	31.9
50	26.5	28.2	31.0	33.4
55	27.8	29.4	32.1	34.6
60	29.1	30.6	33.2	35.7
65	30.2	31.6	34.1	36.7
70	31.2	32.5	35.0	37.7
75	32.2	33.4	35.9	38.7
80	33.1	34.3	36.7	39.6
85	34.0	35.1	37.5	40.4
90	34.8	35.8	38.3	41.2
95	35.6	36.5	39.0	41.9
100	36.4	37.2	39.7	42.6
105	37.1	37.9	40.4	43.3
110	37.8	38.6	41.0	43.9
115	38.4	39.1	41.5	44.5
120	39.0	39.6	42.0	45.1
125	39.6	40.1	42.5	45.7
130	40.2	40.6	43.0	46.2
135	40.8	41.1	43.5	46.7
140	41.3	41.6	44.0	47.2
145	41.8	42.1	44.5	47.7
150	42.3	42.6	45.0	48.2
155	42.8	43.1	45.4	48.7
160	43.3	43.6	45.8	49.2
165	43.7	44.0	46.2	49.6
170	44.1	44.4	46.6	50.0
175	—	44.8	47.0	50.4
180	—	45.2	47.4	50.8
185	—	45.6	47.8	51.2
190	—	45.9	48.2	51.6
195	—	46.2	48.5	52.0
200	—	46.5	48.8	52.4
205	—	—	49.1	52.7
210	—	—	49.4	53.0

Directions: Measure the skinfolds at your biceps, triceps, subscapular, and suprailiac sites (all measurements are in millimeters). Add these values. In the column corresponding to your age and sex, you'll find your percentage of body fat.

FIGURE 18-5

Desirable Body-Fat Levels for Different Sports

SPORT	MEN	WOMEN	SPORT	MEN	WOMEN
Basketball	7–12%	14–20%	Tennis	8–13%	15–21%
Football			Distance running	5–10%	10–12%
Linemen	10–15%	—	Track and field		
Backs	7–12%	—	Jumpers	7–10%	10–13%
Gymnastics	4–8%	10–12%	Throwers	8–12%	10–15%
Soccer	7–10%	—	Sprinters	4–8%	10–13%
Swimming	5–8%	10–15%	*Wrestling	4–8%	—
*Weightlifting	5–10%	10–15%	*Powerlifting	5–10%	10–15%
**Physique	4–8%	9–12%			

*Athletes in the heavier weight divisions typically exceed these guidelines by 3–4 percentage points. To exceed them by more than this margin is pure and simple slovenliness.
**Elite male bodybuilders are usually closer to the 8-percent level as opposed to the 4-percent level because they've put on extra mass via fat deposits in the muscles themselves. Their subcutaneous fat levels, however, remain extremely low in order to show cuts (muscular definition).

19

YOU ARE WHAT YOU EAT

A solid foundation for integrated training begins with a solid nutritional program. For your body to perform on an optimal level, you must feed it the right combinations of nutrients. A well-planned diet is just as important to your overall training program as the exercises you do; indeed, these two elements should never be regarded as separate. They are both a part of integrated training.

Many people, including athletes, are still ignorant about the amounts of protein, carbohydrates, vitamins and minerals, and other forms of supplements they need on a daily basis. This situation must be remedied. You have to pay strict attention to what you eat, and when, and also why. Just as with training exercises, there are reasons behind scientific eating. Once you establish those reasons for eating the way you do, you're on your way to becoming a serious athlete.

Athletes eat for many reasons beyond mere indulgence or survival. These reasons include

- To gain muscle mass
- To lose fat
- To acquire greater strength (all forms)
- To improve mental focus and concentration powers
- To improve energy for explosive sports
- To improve energy for mid-distance types of sports
- To improve cardiovascular (endurance) sports energy
- To promote tissue repair
- To increase between-workout or between-game recovery

- To reduce pain stemming from fatigue
- For general (overall body) health

Let's get one thing clear. The *macro*nutrients (protein, carbohydrates, fats, and water) and the *micro*nutrients (vitamins, minerals, and trace elements) are by far more important in achieving a solid nutritional foundation than any other supplements you can take. That being the case, let's discuss them.

MACRONUTRIENTS

Protein

Contrary to what some nutritionists think, bodybuilders *do* need more protein when they are training. It is estimated that bodybuilders require anywhere from .925 grams to 2.0 grams of protein per kilogram of body weight per day (c. Meredith, 1988). This is far and above that required by sedentary individuals.

Protein makes up nearly half of your body's dry weight. All proteins are constantly being replaced. Within six months, every protein molecule in your body is broken down and replaced. Although some proteins aid in the repair and growth of your hair, skin, nails, muscles, and brain, some is lost through excretion. When you sweat some proteins are lost. During heavy exercise blood cells are destroyed, and protein is used to rebuild these cells.

It is vital to know that additional protein is needed in proportion to your muscles' demand for it. The more intensely you train, the more protein is required for repair and growth. Protein deficiencies can result in growth abnormalities and hinder tissue development. Adult bodybuilders can expect such conditions as tiredness, reduced energy, weakness, mental depression, a lowered resistance to infections and disease, slowed healing of injuries, and prolonged recovery from exercise.

More Is Not Better: Consuming more protein than your body can utilize can result in an increase in fat storage. Your liver virtually converts the excess protein into fat. Overconsumption of protein for a prolonged period of time can also increase the formation of a highly toxic ammonia called urea. Since the urea in your body must be excreted, an overabundance of urea places a strain on your liver and kidneys and is oftentimes responsible for a form of arthritis known as gout.

Protein molecules are broken down into the "building blocks of protein" commonly referred to as amino acids. There are twenty-two amino acids constructed in a certain pattern to make human protein, and of these twenty-two, twelve are easily biosynthesized in your body as needed. The other ten building blocks are essential—that is, they must be obtained through your diet because your body can't biosynthesize them. When any of these essential amino acids is deficient, the rebuilding processes become less effective.

Although you may obtain sufficient quantities of protein in your diet, the structure of the amino acids may not be optimal. This will mean less than optimal assimilation in your body and thus less protein effectiveness. For this reason, protein is rated by means of the protein efficiency ratio (PER) that reflects its quality. While some foods are classified as incomplete proteins (e.g., fruits and most vegetables), others include all the essential amino acids and are regarded as complete proteins (e.g., eggs and milk). Eggs contain all the essential amino acids in proper proportions and have the highest PER available. Therefore, egg protein has the highest assimilation of all types of protein. It is possible but sometimes quite difficult to combine foods in a way that all essential amino acids are provided.

Because of protein's delicate and complex structure, it is most times critical to peak performance that you complement your diet with protein supplements comprised of the essential amino acids.

Timing Is Critical: Timing your protein consumption is just as important as the quality. When you exercise, your body actually decreases its protein production. This can last for hours following your training, at which time a rebuilding phase begins. This is an important time to consume high-quality protein, especially the three branched-chain amino acids (BCAAs) leucine, isoleucine, and valine. Since these structural proteins are those metabolized in your muscles rather than in your liver, the time period just before and following exercise are the recommended times for BCAA intake.

As your training increases in volume, duration, or intensity, your protein requirements increase accordingly. With the increased need for quality protein, you should consume foods that have a high protein efficiency ratio. Such foods are eggs, milk, meat, and fish. Figure 19-1 gives you a means for determining your daily protein requirements.

FIGURE 19-1

Determining Approximate Daily Protein Requirements

FORMULA

Lean body weight (in pounds) × requirement factor = daily protein requirement (in grams)

Requirement Factors

.5—Sedentary, no sports or training
.6—Jogger or light fitness training
.7—Sports participation or moderate training 3 times a week
.8—Moderate daily weight training or aerobic training
.9—Heavy weight training daily
1.0—Heavy weight training daily plus sports training, or "two-a-day" training

LBW* (lb.)	.5	.6	.7	.8	.9	1.0
			Grams of Protein			
90	45	54	63	72	81	90
100	50	60	70	80	90	100
110	55	66	77	88	99	110
120	60	72	84	96	108	120
130	65	78	91	104	117	130
140	70	84	98	112	126	140
150	75	90	105	120	135	150
160	80	96	112	128	144	160
170	85	102	119	136	153	170
180	90	108	126	144	162	180
190	95	114	133	152	171	190
200	100	120	140	160	180	200
210	105	126	147	168	189	210
220	110	132	154	176	198	220
230	115	138	161	184	207	230
240	120	144	168	192	216	240

*LBW—Your fat cells require insignificant protein, so it doesn't make any sense to compute your protein requirements from total body weight. Your LBW (lean body weight, or fatfree weight) can be estimated using any one of several anthropometric, ultrasound, electrical impedance, or underwater weighing techniques.

Carbohydrates

Everyone needs energy, and the best source of energy comes from carbohydrates. Ultimately, your bodybuilding nutrition program should contain anywhere from 50 percent to 60 percent of your caloric intake in the form of carbohydrates.

Carbohydrates can be classified three ways: monosaccharides, disaccharides, and polysaccharides. Simple sugars found in honey and fruits, like glucose and fructose, fall into the monosaccharide category. Disaccharides include table sugar (sucrose) and lactose, a sugar found in milk. Polysaccharides are those sugars often referred to as complex carbohydrates, such as starches (dextrins, cellulose, pectin, and glycogen) that can be found in whole grains, vegetables, nuts, some fruits, and legumes.

When you consume carbohydrates, your digestive system converts them to blood sugar (glucose). This glucose is stored in your muscle cells and in your liver. Your brain operates with the help of glucose in your blood as energy. When your training is intense, glycogen stored within your muscles provides most of the energy for contractions. When your intensity is low to moderate, your blood-borne sugar acts as an energy source. When there is leftover glucose in your blood following a refill of carbohydrate stores, the remaining carbohydrates are stored as fat.

The glycemic index is a handy rating system that tells you what carbohydrates provide the best energy for prolonged training periods. By consuming foods with low glycemic ratings, you will experience a more stabilized blood-sugar level.

Fats

As a bodybuilder, you should realize the importance of fat in your diet. Fat is not always the villain responsible for clogging your arteries and packing on your waistline. Rather, fat acts as a secondary source of energy during training or competition. Fat-based energy becomes available soon after carbohydrate stores in your muscles deplete.

Often referred to as *lipids*, fats can be found in solid or liquid form. Even though carbohydrates are your body's major source of energy, fats are the most highly concentrated source of energy over carbohydrates and proteins. Fats have nine calories per gram, while carbohydrates and proteins contain only four, so it's easy to see why foods high in fat are also high in calories.

There are a host of reasons why our bodies need fat. Fats act as the storage substance for excess calories that you consume, and this applies not only to fats but also the excess carbohydrates and proteins. Fat is an essential ingredient in maintaining healthy skin and hair and acts as a carrying agent in the transportation of the fat-soluble vitamins A, D, E, and K. Fats in our diet provide us with essential fatty acids the body does not manufacture (linoleic acid, linolenic acid, and arachadonic acid); these essential fatty acids aid in the responsibility of many bodily functions, including the regulation of blood pressure. Fats help regulate levels of cholesterol in your blood and provide satiety because they increase the time needed to empty food from your stomach.

An important question that you must be able to answer is what kinds and how much fat should be in your daily diet. All fats are found as various combinations of saturated and unsaturated fatty acids. Fats that are saturated usually come from animal sources like meat, milk, and butter. However, coconut and palm oils are also highly saturated. With the exception of the two oils mentioned, saturated fats usually remain solid at room temperature.

Unsaturated fats are often classified as either monounsaturated fats (olive, peanut, and avocado oils) or polyunsaturated fats (corn, sesame, and safflower oils). The major criterion for choosing unsaturated fats is that they are of plant and fish origin. These fats usually remain liquid at room temperature and have a short life.

A process called hydrogenation makes unsaturated fats more saturated. This is done to preserve the shelf life of unsaturated fats. No better for you than saturated fats, hydrogenated unsaturated fats become hard at room temperature. Such is the case with margarines and shortenings. Another common term for hydrogenated fat is rancid fat.

One Fat That's Desirable: Consumed fat requires a long, complicated process to become usable energy. If we can find a fat that we could eat, absorb quickly, and use as an efficient energy source, the consumption of the fat would be helpful. State-of-the-art research tells us that medium-chain triglycerides (MCTs) might fit this bill. MCTs are fatty acids produced from coconut oil and palm kernels, among others.

MCTs are quickly absorbed, protein-sparing (anticatabolic), and provide greater energy for longer periods. MCTs deliver *twice* the energy of carbohydrates, reduce cholesterol, enhance the absorption of amino acids, induce thermogenesis, diminish your food efficiency ratio (it takes more food than normal to gain weight), and cannot contribute to stored body fat because they're used exclusively in the mitochondria of your muscle cells where they're converted to ketones. Ketones are either used for energy or excreted—never stored.

Excess intake of MCTs can lead to diarrhea and possibly complicate liver problems in some people with liver disease. MCT oil can be used on salads and in baking but not for frying and does not provide any of the essential fatty acids. However, MCTs provide a more healthful alternative to saturated fat intake by providing high-calorie intake for energy without many of the dangerous side effects of dietary saturated fat.

Cholesterol: A major concern to anyone interested in health, fitness, and performance is cholesterol. Cholesterol is another cousin to the fatty-acid family that has a link with fats in your diet. Cholesterol is found in foods that come from animals, like meats and dairy products. Both of these food types are high in saturated fats. Although cholesterol is manufactured by your body, it is a useful agent in cell-membrane and nerve-fiber construction and acts in the building of some hormones.

When the cholesterol circulating in your blood sticks to the walls of your arteries, this closes off blood flow and can lead to a heart attack or stroke. Known as the "silent killer," atherosclerosis or plaque buildup in the arteries results from a high concentration of cholesterol in your blood.

Your liver usually processes the cholesterol found in your body. This process is in part the result of cholesterol taken in through your diet, but heredity has a great influence on how much cholesterol your body actually manufactures for itself.

Through the processing of cholesterol comes two main classes of cholesterol. Low-density cholesterol, often referred to as LDL (low-density lipoproteins) because of its combination of fats with proteins, carries the cholesterol through the bloodstream to deposit it for cell building. Excess LDL that gets attached to the artery walls closes the arterial opening. High-density lipoproteins (HDL) attach to these excess cholesterol deposits and take them to your liver for remanufacturing or excretion. For this reason, LDL is labeled as "bad" cholesterol and HDL as "good" cholesterol.

Since saturated fats usually stimulate the production of LDL, a high consumption of saturated fats will raise your overall cholesterol levels and increase your risk of heart disease. But what you must know is that polyunsaturated fats can lower your levels of LDL. Recent research shows us that some polyunsaturated fats found in fish oil might provide additional benefits. This oil reduces the chances of blood clotting, thus lowering your chances of blocked arteries. In addition, monounsaturated oils like olive oil have recently been discovered to have LDL-lowering properties, a plus in lowering high cholesterol, but since fat contains a high number of calories, a high consumption of fat can easily lead to obesity. This only increases your chances of heart disease and reduces your chances of success in sports.

Fats should make up 10–15 percent of your total daily caloric intake. The (very conservative) FDA advocates limiting your fat intake to about 30 percent of your daily calories. This is too much fat! The FDA recommendation probably stems from the fact that (as usual) they're thinking of feeding the masses as opposed to the fitness-conscious few.

MICRONUTRIENTS

Vitamins

Everyone needs vitamins, and bodybuilders need more vitamins than most other people. If you want to be a successful bodybuilder, you must provide your body with everything it needs. Vitamins are undoubtedly essential to physical performance and muscle growth beyond the norm.

Each vitamin has specific responsibilities in your body. The most important vitamins essential to successful physical performance include:

Vitamin A: Maintains your skin and mucous membranes and contributes to the function of night vision. Excess vitamin A intake can be toxic, since this vitamin is fat-soluble. Vitamin A can be found in carrots and leafy yellow vegetables.

Vitamin B_1 (Thiamin): Responsible for carbohydrate metabolism along with the function of your nervous system. Intake of more than 1,000 milligrams might cause increased urination and possible dehydration. Because this vitamin is water-soluble, daily replacement is necessary. Whole grains are the best source of B_1.

Vitamin B_2 (Riboflavin): An active agent in the metabolism of energy and cell maintenance. It also is an essential ingredient in the repair of all cells following injury. Milk and eggs are excellent sources of vitamin B_2.

Vitamin B_3 (Niacin): Has numerous responsibilities in various bodily functions and is present in every cell in your body. Too much B_3 can cause hot flashes, but you can build a tolerance to this vitamin and find it helpful in the reduction of high cholesterol. Peanuts and poultry prove to be fine sources of B_3.

Vitamin B_5 (Pantothenic Acid): Essential in the formation of the chemical acetylcholine, which is crucial to nerve transmission involving memory and in the metabolism of energy. Poultry, fish, and whole grains provide you with ample levels of this vitamin.

Vitamin B_6 (Pyridoxine): Involved in the metabolism of sugar, fat, and protein. It can be found in foods like wheat germ, fish, and walnuts.

Vitamin B_{12} (Cobalamin): Refers to substances containing the mineral cobalt which is important in the metabolism of protein and fat and an aid in producing red blood cells. Sources include liver, oysters, and clams.

Vitamin B_{15} (Pangamate or Pangamic Acid): A coenzyme involved in respiration, protein synthesis, and regulation of steroid hormones. Its principal effect is to increase blood and oxygen supplies to tissue. Deficiency states produce no apparent negative effects, which leads some conservative nutritionists to the conclusion that it is not a true vitamin. B_{15} is found principally in brewer's yeast, organ meats, and whole grains.

Folic Acid (Folacin): Helper substance of the B-complex group, especially in red blood cell formation.

Biotin: Helps metabolize carbohydrates and fats. Best sources are brown rice and soybeans.

Choline: An agent helpful in the use of the B-complex vitamins. It is crucial in normal brain function (notably memory) and acts as a factor in metabolizing fat and cholesterol. The best food sources are eggs and lecithin.

Inositol: Helpful in the use of B-complex vitamins. It acts with choline in metabolizing fat and cholesterol. In addition, it plays an important role in the transmission of nerve impulses. Lecithin and wheat germ are good sources of inositol.

Para-Amino-Benzoic Acid (PABA): Essential for normal skin and hair growth. Sources include whole grains and wheat germ. It is at least partially synthesized in the intestinal flora, a fact which has led conservative nutritionists to deny a need for it in the diet.

Vitamin C (Ascorbic Acid): A water-soluble vitamin similar to the B-complex vitamins. It is involved in various bodily functions, particularly the development of connective tissue. Drugs of any kind radically increase your need for vitamin C. Citrus fruits provide a good source.

Bioflavinoids: Chemicals that contribute to the strength of your capillaries and help protect vitamin C stores in your body. These vitamins can be found in fresh raw vegetables and fruits.

Vitamin D (Calciferol): A fat-soluble vitamin that regulates calcium and phosphate metabolism in your body. This vitamin is actually formed on your skin via ultraviolet rays from light when it reacts with cholesterol in your skin. Sunlight serves as the best source, but this vitamin is also typically added to milk.

Vitamin E (Tocopherol): Another fat-soluble vitamin that has numerous responsibilities in your body. Food sources available are wheat germ, green leafy vegetables, whole grains, and vegetable oils. Look for the natural form (d-alpha tocopherol succinate) as opposed to the synthetic form (dl-alpha tocopherol acetate). Some sports-nutrition manufacturers would have you believe that the synthetic form is better than the natural. This claim is largely unfounded and is probably made because the synthetic form is far cheaper than the natural.

Vitamin K: This vitamin is implicated in proper blood clotting. It is synthesized in the intestinal flora. Because it is fat-soluble, it has the potential for toxicity if taken in large doses. There is no established RDA.

It is well established that athletes need an abundance of vitamins for optimal performance. The physical demands of training use up these substances and make replenishment critical. It is quite possible that eating five or so carefully balanced meals (and the increased caloric intake that may normally accompany such an eating schedule) every day will make supplementation with vitamins unnecessary. However—and this is a very important *however*—who does that? Almost no one I've ever met! In the interest of insurance, it's probably wise to take a low- to moderate-dosage multivitamin/mineral supplement three times daily. Use caution, however, when fat-soluble vitamins (A, D, E, and K) are consumed in large quantities because of the possibility of toxicity stemming from bodily storage of these fat-soluble vitamins.

FIGURE 19-2

Summary of Vitamins, Minerals, and Other Nutrients*

The basic Optimum Daily Allowance (ODA) is for general health and disease prevention. Some individuals may wish to use higher levels, depending upon risk factors such as pollution, stress, and personal and family history.

Please note that for some nutrients—boron, for example—RDAs and ODAs have not yet been determined. For these nutrients, I have indicated a recommended range (in the case of boron, 3–6 milligrams), followed by an asterisk (*) to indicate that this dosage is not an ODA.

QUICK-REFERENCE TABLE

Nutrient	Major Uses	Food Sources	RDA	ODA
Vitamin A: beta-carotene	Prevents night blindness and other eye problems; May be useful for acne and other skin disorders; Enhances immunity; Cancer prevention; May heal gastrointestinal ulcers; Protects against pollution; Needed for epithelial tissue maintenance and repair	Fish liver oils, animal livers, green and yellow fruits and vegetables	4,000–5,000 IU	10,000–75,000 IU (in a mixture of A and beta-carotene)
Vitamin D	Required for calcium and phosphorus absorption and utilization; Prevention and treatment of osteoporosis; Enhances immunity	Fish liver oils, fatty saltwater fish. Vitamin D-fortified dairy products, eggs	400 IU	400–600 IU
Vitamin E	Antioxidant; Cancer prevention; Cardiovascular disease prevention; Improves circulation; Tissue repair; May prevent age spots; Useful in treating fibrocystic breasts; Useful in treating PMS	Cold-pressed vegetable oils, whole grains, dark-green leafy vegetables, nuts, legumes	8-10 IU	200–800 IU

Nutrient	Major Uses	Food Sources	RDA	ODA
Vitamin K	Needed for blood clotting May play a role in bone formation May prevent osteoporosis	Green leafy vegetables		65–80 mcg
B Complex B$_1$ (thiamin); B$_2$ (riboflavin); B$_3$ (niacin, niacin-amide); B$_6$ (pyridoxine)	Maintains healthy nerves, skin, eyes, hair, liver, mouth, muscle tone in gastrointestinal tract B vitamins are coenzymes involved in energy production Emotional or physical stress increases need May be useful for depression or anxiety	Unrefined whole grains, liver, green leafy vegetables, fish, poultry, eggs, meat, nuts, beans	1.2–14 mg	25–300 mg

B$_1$
High-carbohydrate diet increases need
B$_2$
May be useful with B$_6$ for treatment of carpal tunnel syndrome
May prevent cataracts
Increased need with oral contraceptives
Increased need with strenuous exercise
B$_3$
Useful for circulatory problems
Lowers serum cholesterol and triglycerides
B$_6$
May be useful in preventing oxalate stones
May be used as mild diuretic
May be useful for PMS
Increased need with oral contraceptives
May be useful in treating asthma

Nutrient	Major Uses	Food Sources	RDA	ODA
B$_{12}$ (cobalamin)	Needed for fat and carbohydrate metabolism Prevention and treatment of B$_{12}$ anemia Maintains proper nervous system function May be useful for anxiety and depression	Kidney, liver, egg, herring, mackerel, milk, cheese, tofu, seafood	2 mcg	25–300 mcg
Folic acid	Works closely with B$_{12}$ Involved in protein metabolism Needed for healthy cell division and	Beef, lamb, pork, chicken, liver, green leafy vegetables, whole wheat,	180–200 mcg	400–1,200 mcg

Nutrient	Major Uses	Food Sources	RDA	ODA
	replication	bran, yeast		
	Prevention and treatment of folic acid anemia			
	Stress may increase need			
	May be useful for depression and anxiety			
	May be useful in treating cervical dysplasia			
	Oral contraceptives may increase need			
Panto-thenic acid	Needed in fat, protein, and carbohydrate metabolism	Eggs, saltwater fish, pork, beef, milk, whole wheat, beans, fresh vegetables	None	25–300 mg
	Needed for synthesis of hormones and cholesterol			
	Needed for red blood cell production			
	Needed for nerve transmission			
	Vital for healthy function of the adrenal glands			
	May be useful for joint inflammation			
	May be useful for depression and anxiety			
Biotin	Needed for metabolism of protein, fats, and carbohydrates	Meat, cooked egg yolk, poultry, yeast, soybeans, milk, saltwater fish, whole grains	None	25–300 mcg
	Not enough data available, but deficiencies may be implicated in high serum cholesterol, seborrheic dermatitis, and certain nervous system disorders			
Choline and Inositol	Involved in metabolism of fat and cholesterol and absorption and utilization of fat	Egg yolk, whole grains, vegetables, organ meats, fruits, milk	None	25–300 mg
	Choline makes an important brain neurotransmitter			
PABA	Needed for protein metabolism	Liver, kidney, whole grains, molasses	None	25–300 mg
	Needed for folic acid			

Nutrient	Major Uses	Food Sources	RDA	ODA
	metabolism Used topically as a sunscreen			

A combination of all the B vitamins can usually be found in B-complex and multivitamin formulas. If you wish to take any additional B vitamins, please make sure you are taking a complete B-complex first.

Nutrient	Major Uses	Food Sources	RDA	ODA
Vitamin C (ascorbic acid)	Growth and repair of tissues May reduce cholesterol Antioxidant Cancer prevention Enhances immunity Stress increases requirement May reduce high blood pressure May prevent atherosclerosis Protects against pollution	Green vegetables, berries, citrus fruit	60 mg	500–5,000 mg (higher during stress or illness)
Calcium	Needed for healthy bones and teeth Needed for nerve transmission Used for muscle function May lower blood pressure Osteoporosis prevention	Dairy foods, salmon, sardines, green leafy vegetables, seafood	1,200 mg	1,000–1,500 mg
Phosphorus	Necessary for healthy bones Needed for production of energy Used as a buffering agent Needed for utilization of protein, fats, and carbohydrates	Available in most foods; sodas can be very high	800 mg	Generally available through foods: 200–400 mg
Magnesium	Needed for healthy bones Involved in nerve transmission Needed for muscle function Used in energy formation Needed for healthy blood vessels May lower blood pressure	Widely distributed in foods, especially dairy foods, meat, fish, seafood	280–350 mg	500–700 mg

Nutrient	Major Uses	Food Sources	RDA	ODA
Zinc	Needed for wound healing Maintains taste and smell acuity Needed for healthy immune system Protects liver from chemical damage	Oysters, fish, seafood, meats, poultry, whole grains, legumes	12–15 mg	22.5–50 mg
Iron	Vital for blood formation Needed for energy production Required for healthy immune system	Meat, poultry, fish, liver, eggs, green leafy vegetables, whole-grain or enriched breads and cereals	10–15 mg	15–30 mg
Copper	Involved in blood formation Needed for healthy nerves Needed for taste sensitivity Used in energy production Needed for healthy bone development	Widely distributed in foods, copper cookware, and copper plumbing	None	Needs can generally be met through food: 0.5–2 mg
Manganese	Needed for protein and fat metabolism Used in energy formation Required for normal bone growth and reproduction Needed for healthy nerves Needed for healthy blood sugar regulation Needed for healthy immune system	Nuts, seeds, whole grains, avocado, seaweed	None	15–30 mg
Chromium	Required for glucose metabolism May prevent diabetes May reduce cholesterol	Brewer's yeast, beer, meat, cheese, whole grains	None	200–600 mcg
Selenium	Cancer prevention Heart disease prevention	Depends on soil content, may be in grains and meat	55–70 mcg	50–400 mcg (50–100 mcg for those who live in high-selenium areas)
Iodine	Needed for healthy thyroid gland Prevents goiter	Iodized salts, seafood, saltwater fish, kelp	150 mcg	50–300 mcg (50–150 mcg for those who use iodized salt)

Nutrient	Major Uses	Food Sources	RDA	ODA
Potassium	May lower blood pressure Needed for energy storage Needed for nerve transmission, muscle contraction, and hormone secretion	Dairy foods, meat, poultry, fish, fruit, legumes, whole grains, vegetables	None	99–300 mg
Boron	Prevents bone loss May enhance bone density	Fruits, vegetables	None	3–6 mg*
EPA	Prevents heart disease May lower blood pressure May lower triglycerides May lower cholesterol Prevents excess blood clotting May relieve inflammatory and allergic reactions May inhibit cancer May enhance immune system	Coldwater fish	None	250–3,000 mg*
GLA	May prevent heart disease Relieves allergic reactions Relieves eczema Relieves arthritis Relieves PMS symptoms May assist in weight loss	Evening primrose, borage, black currant oils	None	70–240 mg*
Garlic	May lower blood pressure May enhance immune system May prevent heart disease May lower triglycerides May lower cholesterol Antibacterial, antiviral, antifungal Prevents excess blood clotting May prevent cancer	Garlic	None	200–1,200 mg*
Coenzyme Q_{10} (CoQ)	Cell energy and metabolism Prevents cell damage May be useful in heart disease such as angina, congestive	None	None	10–300 mg*

Nutrient	Major Uses	Food Sources	RDA	ODA
	heart failure, arrhythmia, high blood pressure			
	May protect heart muscle and promote faster recovery from heart attack and heart surgery			
Germa- nium	Needed for cell metabolism	A variety of medicinal plants	None	30–150 mg*
	May prevent or slow growth of cancer			
	May enhance immune system			
	May lower blood pressure			
	Relieves pain			

*Figure 19-2 is from *The Real Vitamin & Mineral Book*, by Shari Lieberman (New York: Avery Publishers, 1992). Used by permission.

FIGURE 19-3

24 Good Reasons for Using Vitamin and Mineral Supplements*

1. Poor Digestion

Even when your food intake is good, inefficient digestion can limit your body's uptake of vitamins. Some common causes of inefficient digestion are not chewing well enough and eating too fast. Both of these result in larger than normal food particle size, too large to allow complete action of digestive enzymes. Many people with dentures are unable to chew as efficiently as those with a full set of original teeth.

2. Hot Coffee, Tea, and Spices

Habitual drinking of liquids that are too hot, or consuming an excess of irritants such as coffee, tea, or pickles and spices can cause inflammation of the digestive linings, resulting in a drop in secretion of digestive fluids and poorer extraction of vitamins and minerals from food.

3. Alcohol

Drinking too much alcohol can damage the liver and pancreas, which are vital to digestion and metabolism. It can also damage the lining of the intestinal tract and adversely affect the absorption of nutrients, leading to subclinical malnutrition. Regular use of alcohol increases the body's need for B-group vitamins, particularly thiamine, niacin, pyridoxine, folic acid, and vitamins B_{12}, A, and C as well as the minerals zinc, magnesium, and calcium. Alcohol affects availability, absorption, and metabolism of nutrients.

4. Smoking

Smoking too much tobacco is also an irritant to the digestive tract and increases the metabolic requirements of vitamin C, all else being equal, by at least 30 mg per cigarette over and above the typical requirements of a nonsmoker. Vitamin C, which is normally present in such foods as cabbage, onions, oranges, and grapefruit, oxidizes rapidly once these fruits are cut, juiced, cooked, or stored in direct light or near heat. Vitamin C is important to the immune function.

is normally present in such foods as cabbage, onions, oranges, and grapefruit, oxidizes rapidly once these fruits are cut, juiced, cooked, or stored in direct light or near heat. Vitamin C is important to the immune function.

5. Laxatives

Overuse of laxatives can result in poor absorption of vitamins and minerals from food by hastening the intestinal transit time. Paraffin and other mineral oils increase losses of fat soluble vitamins A, E, and K. Other laxatives used to excess can cause large losses of minerals such as potassium, sodium, and magnesium.

6. Fad Diets

Bizarre diets discard whole groups of foods seriously lacking in vitamins. Popular low-fat diets, if taken to an extreme, can be deficient in vitamins A, D, and E. Vegetarian diets, which exclude meat and other animal sources, must be very skillfully planned to avoid vitamin B_{12} deficiency, which may lead to anemia.

7. Overcooking

Lengthy cooking or reheating meat and vegetables oxidizes and destroys heat susceptible vitamins such as the B-group, C, and E. Boiling vegetables removes water-soluble vitamins B-group and C and many minerals. Light steaming is preferable. Some vitamins, such as vitamin B_6, can be destroyed by microwave irradiation.

8. Food Processing

Freezing food containing vitamin E can significantly reduce its levels once defrosted. Foods containing vitamin E exposed to heat and air can turn rancid. Many common sources of vitamin E, such as bread and oils, are nowadays highly processed, so that the vitamin E content is significantly reduced or missing totally, which increases storage life but can lower nutrient levels. Vitamin E is an antioxidant which defensively inhibits oxidative damage to all tissues. Other vitamin losses from food processing include vitamin B_1 and C.

9. Convenience Foods

A diet dependent on highly refined carbohydrates, such as sugar, white flour, and white rice, place greater demand on additional sources of B-group vitamins to process these carbohydrates. An unbalanced diet contributes to such conditions as irritability, lethargy, and sleep disorders.

10. Antibiotics

Some antibiotics, although valuable in fighting infection, also kill off friendly bacteria in the gut, which normally produces B-group vitamins to be absorbed through the intestinal walls. Such deficiencies can result in a variety of nervous conditions; therefore, it may be advisable to supplement with B-group vitamins when on a lengthy course of broad-spectrum antibiotics.

11. Food Allergies

The omission of whole food groups from the diet, as in the case of individuals allergic to gluten or lactose, can mean the loss of significant dietary sources of nutrients such as thiamine, riboflavin, or calcium.

12. Crop Nutrient Losses

Some agricultural soils are deficient in trace elements. Decades of intensive agriculture can overwork and deplete soils, unless all the soil nutrients, including trace elements, are regularly replaced. Food crops can be depleted of nutrients due to poor soil management. In a U.S. Government survey, levels of essential minerals in crops were found to have declined by up to 68% over a four-year period in the 1970s.

13. Accidents and Illness

Burns lead to a loss of protein and essential trace nutrients such as vitamins and minerals. Surgery increases the need for zinc, vitamin E, and other nutrients involved in the cellular repair mechanism. The repair of broken bones will be retarded by an inadequate supply of calcium and vitamin C and conversely enhanced by a full dietary supply. The challenge of infection places high demand on the nutritional resources of zinc, magnesium and vitamins B_5, B_6, and zinc.

14. Stress

Chemical, physical, and emotional stress can increase the body's requirements for vitamins B_2, B_5, B_6, and C. Air pollution increases the requirements for vitamin E.

15. P.M.S.

Research has demonstrated that up to 60% of women suffering from symptoms of premenstrual tension, such as headaches, irritability, bloatedness, breast tenderness, lethargy, and depression, can benefit from supplementation with vitamin B_6.

16. Teenagers

Rapid growth spurts, such as in the teenage years, particularly in girls, place high demands on nutritional resources to underwrite the accelerated physical, biochemical, and emotional development in this age group. Data from the U.S.A. Ten State Nutrition Survey (in 1968-70 covering a total of 24,000 families and 86,000 individuals) showed that between 30–50% of adolescents aged 12 to 16 had dietary intakes below two-thirds of the recommended daily averages for vitamin A, C, calcium, and iron.

17. Pregnant Women

Pregnancy creates higher than average demands for nutrients to ensure healthy growth of the baby and comfortable confinement for the mother. The nutrients which require increase during pregnancy are the B-group, especially B_1, B_2, B_3, B_6, folic acid and B_{12}, A, D, E, and minerals calcium, iron, magnesium, zinc, and phosphorous. The USA Ten State Nutrition Survey in 1968–70 showed as many as 80% of the pregnant women surveyed had dietary intakes below two-thirds of recommended daily allowances. Professional assessment of nutrient requirements during pregnancy should be sought.

18. Oral Contraceptives

Oral contraceptives can decrease absorption of folic acid and increase the need for vitamin B_6 and possibly vitamin C, zinc, and riboflavin. Almost 22% of Australian women ages 15 to 44 are believed to be on "the pill" at any one time.

19. Light Eaters

Some people eat very sparingly, even without weight reduction goals. U.S. dietary surveys have shown that an average woman maintains her weight on 800 calories per day, at which level her diet is likely to be low in thiamine, calcium, and iron.

20. The Elderly

The aged generally have a low intake of vitamins and minerals, particularly iron, calcium, and zinc. Folic acid deficiency is often found, in conjunction with vitamin C deficiency. Fiber intake is often low. Riboflavin (B_2) and pyridoxine (B_6) deficiencies have also been observed. Possible causes include impaired sense of taste and smell, reduced secretion of digestive enzymes, chronic disease, and maybe, physical impairment.

21. Lack of Sunlight

Invalids, shiftworkers, and people with minimal exposure to sunlight can suffer from insufficient amounts of vitamin D, which is required for calcium metabolism, without which rickets and osteoporosis (bone thinning) has been observed. Ultraviolet light is the stimulus to vitamin D formation in skin. It is blocked by cloud, fog, smog, smoke, ordinary window glass, curtains, and clothing. The maximum recommended daily supplemental intake of vitamin D is 400 i.u.

22. Bio-Individuality

Wide fluctuations in individual nutrient requirements from the official recommended average vitamin and mineral intakes are common, particularly for those in high physical demand vocations, such as athletics and manual labor, taking into account body weight and physical type. Protein intake influences the need for vitamin B_6 and vitamin B_1 is linked to caloric intake.

23. Low Body Reserves

Although the body is able to store reserves of certain vitamins such as A and E, Canadian autopsy data has shown that up to 30% of the population have reserves of vitamin A so low as to be judged "at risk." Vitamin A is important to healthy skin and mucous membranes (including the sinus and lungs) and eyesight.

24. Athletes

Athletes consume much food and experience considerable stress. These factors affect their needs for B-group vitamins, vitamin C, and iron in particular. Australian Olympic athletes and A-grade football players, for example, have shown wide ranging vitamin deficiencies.

---

*Figure 19-3 is from *Fitness: A Complete Guide*, F. C. Hatfield (ed.), ISSA, 1991

Minerals

Until recently, vitamins were thought to be a more important concern in athletic performance than minerals. Through vast research, it is now believed that minerals play a very significant role in various bodily functions essential to physical training. A deficiency in any mineral can be disastrous to peak performance. Iron and calcium, for example, are minerals commonly lacking in most diets. Failure to consume adequate levels of these two minerals can result in fatigue, weakness, and injury. Women tend to be more likely to experience such deficiencies than men.

Minerals are found in plants and animal foods along with your drinking water. Most often, though, the quantities of minerals found in these sources are too little. Since the stresses associated with intense training promote the loss of various minerals, it becomes more important to increase your mineral intake.

Some of the minerals important to intense physical training are
Calcium: The most abundant mineral in your body. It helps to
make up your teeth and bones and is needed for
muscle contractions. According to reliable sources,

only about 10 percent of the calcium in dairy
products is absorbed in your body—no wonder many
people are deficient in this mineral. This is part of the
basis for athletes often experiencing stress fractures.
Good sources of calcium are dairy products and
calcium carbonate supplements.

Magnesium: Another mineral essential to muscle contraction,
notably in the relaxation phase. Lack of magnesium
will result in fatigue, spasms, muscle twitching, and
muscle weakness. Foods that provide you with quality
magnesium are soybeans, leafy vegetables, brown rice,
whole wheat, apples, seeds, and nuts.

Phosphorus: The second most abundant mineral in your body.
It's involved in muscle contractions and helps in the
utilization of foodstuffs. By consuming large
quantities of phosphorus you might experience a
depletion of calcium and magnesium in your bones,
muscles, and organs, resulting in weakness. Fish and
poultry contain quality phosphorus.

Iron: Essential in making hemoglobin or oxygen in your blood
and crucial in the transportation of oxygen during
endurance activities. An intake of more than 50
milligrams a day for prolonged periods can be toxic.
Interestingly, coffee and tea consumption can limit the
absorption of iron. The best source of iron is red meat.
Even cooking in an iron skillet can increase the iron
content in your food.

Copper: Helps convert iron to hemoglobin and promotes the
use of vitamin C. Many foods have copper in them,
but often in small quantities.

Zinc: Responsible for cell growth by acting as an agent in
protein synthesis, therefore vital for tissue repair, and
aids in the use of vitamin A and B-complex. It
prolongs muscle contractions and therefore increases
your endurance. Sources include eggs, whole grains,
and oysters.

Manganese: A mineral essential in numerous functions,
including glandular secretions, the metabolism of
protein, and brain function. Too much manganese can
inhibit the absorption of iron. Food sources are tea,
leafy green vegetables, and whole grains.

Sodium and Potassium: Minerals that need to have a balance
in order to be capable of maximal muscular power.

These minerals are needed in the transmission of nerve impulses. Deficiencies will produce cramping and weakness. Good sources are green leafy vegetables, bananas, citrus, and dried fruits. Incidentally, salt tablets for sodium intake are a no-no!

Bodybuilders vary in the amounts of extra minerals needed. Much depends on your age, sex, genetics, medical history, and level of training. In practical terms, estimates of daily requirements provide guidelines only, not concrete recommendations.

SELECTING YOUR FOOD SOURCES

As a serious bodybuilder, you need to make careful decisions about the various sources of nutrients in your diet and the calories they supply in carbohydrates, protein, fiber, and fat. Figures 19-4 and 19-5 list the best grains and legumes for high complex carbohydrate, high protein, low fat, and sufficient fiber content.

Remember that you're trying to get about 50–60 percent of the calories in your diet from complex carbohydrates. The actual level of energy-supplying carbs may be closer to about 40–50 percent because undigestible fiber comprises part of the carbohydrate source. Undigestible fiber will not supply your body with calories.

NUTRIENT SYNERGY

As a bodybuilder, you have a basic need to increase energy in all areas of physical endeavor. Your most important outlet is anaerobic strength endurance, as this is essentially what you need to get you through your weight training sessions.

There is no one food or food group that is going to supply you with the exact kind of energy you need. Rather, a balanced combination of food and nutrients—along with certain vitamin and mineral supplements—will interact with one another in a process known as synergy. From this synergy of various nutrient sources, you'll derive the kinds of energy that you need for strength endurance.

Synergy refers to the fact that every known nutrient may affect the action of any other. In nutrition, substances interact in multiples to produce biological functions. In other areas of science, one single substance may create one single condition, but not in nutrition. Nutrients team up, combining in different ways to cause different effects.

FIGURE 19-4

Top 20 Grains and Legumes for Bodybuilders

TOP PROTEIN SOURCES	TOP CARBOHYDRATE SOURCES
Over 20% protein	**Under 5% fat**
Under 20% fat	**Over 70% carbohydrate**
Soybeans	Brown rice
Split peas	Whole barley
Kidney beans	Whole buckwheat
Dried whole peas	Whole rye
Wheat germ	Foxtail mullet
Lima beans	Wild rice
Black-eyed peas	Whole corn
Lentils	Pearl millet
Black beans	Whole wheat
Navy beans	Rolled oats

FIGURE 19-5

The Fiber "10" Chart for Bodybuilders

EACH CONTAINS 10 GRAMS OF DIETARY FIBER

Grains	Vegetables	Fruits
½ cup All Bran	½ cup mixed beans	3 pears
1 cup rolled oats	½ cup peas, lentils	3 bananas
1 cup whole-grain cereal	1 cup peanuts	4 peaches
2 cobs sweet corn	2 cups soybeans	4 oz. blackberries
3 slices whole rye	3 cups steamed veg.	5 apples
3 cups puffed wheat	4 servings mixed salad	6 oranges
4 slices whole-wheat bread	4 large carrots	6 dried pear halves
4 Shredded Wheat	4 cups sunflower seeds	10 dried figs
4 oz. bag of popcorn	5 cups raw cauliflower	20 prunes

20

FAD DIETS AND BODYBUILDING

Many people are very conservative in their beliefs and prejudices regarding nutritional practices. More than any other group of athletes, bodybuilders are continually looking for special foods and diets that will help increase their muscle mass or shed fat. Unfortunately, most are not knowledgeable about nutrition and therefore fall victim to those who market so-called anabolic supplements under false pretenses.

Even the most well-balanced diet cannot account for full replenishment of vitamins, minerals, and foodstuffs used up by bodybuilders. Proper supplementation is most often necessary. But supplementation with *what*?

The old shotgun approach has been disclaimed as a bad practice for full effects of nutritional supplementation. Because your body goes through various phases of breakdown and rebuilding, supplements used for rebuilding are best taken when your body is capable of using them, and some supplements do not react well with others. This is when we look for information from an experienced and educated sports nutritionist.

When you pick out what is fact from what isn't, you must know the purpose of proper nutrition and supplementing. Your nutrition and nutritional supplements should be taken for enhanced metabolic processes (including both anabolism and catabolism), adaptation, improved work capacity, and a speedier recovery, not solely to compensate for used energy.

When you plan to follow sound nutritional practices or to supplement smartly, you need to take a programmed, integrated approach. Remember, the shotgun approach is not a sound means to maximizing your full potential. A proper combination of food types can be crucial to supplying ample energy for your particular physical demands. Not all athletes require the same nutrition, and bodybuilders are no exception. Without good nutrition and proper supplementation, you will find it quite difficult to improve on your physique.

THERE'S NO SUCH THING AS A FREE LUNCH

Many people want something for nothing. This attitude also applies to those wishing to lose fat weight, gain muscle mass, or improve their physical fitness or sports performance. Unfortunately, for those who fall victim to fad diets, there is no miracle means to good nutritional practices. For bodybuilders attempting to cut fat just before a contest or put on more muscle in the shortest possible time, fad diets and misleading claims made by advertisers often look great.

Carbohydrate-Restricted Diets

Fad diets almost always severely cut carbohydrate foods from their lists of recommended consumption. Not only does this leave you with severely diminished energy, but it can produce a frequently fatigued body not capable of performing anywhere near maximal potentials. The fact is you need carbohydrates for your brain, heart, and muscles, among other vital organs. By limiting your carbohydrate consumption too much, you are defeating your purpose of attaining physical greatness.

Protein-Restricted Diets

Diets that drastically cut protein are another culprit. By having an intake low in protein when you are an active bodybuilder, you are simply asking for trouble. Muscle soreness, general fatigue, and overall weakness accompany too-low protein consumption.

Fat-Restricted Diets

Although diets that notably cut fat intake are usually healthy diets, those who reduce their levels of unsaturated fat to nearly nothing are also asking for trouble. Not only does fat act as a carrier for the four fat-soluble vitamins (A, D, E, and K), but it helps cushion your kidneys, liver, and nerves. For women, fat is essential to insulate and pad female reproductive organs and mammary glands. Research has shown that an extremely limited intake of unsaturated fat can result in elevated cholesterol—a condition that can lead to a heart attack or stroke.

Calorie-Restricted Diets

Since most diets limit your number of calories per day, it is highly unlikely that full vitamin and mineral replenishment will take place. Even the ballyhooed balanced diet is a myth, as it's impossible to achieve, particularly by bodybuilders in heavy training and contest preparation. Certain supplements must be taken at specific times in order to maximize their effects on your body. Usually, this is done during the restorative processes following exercise.

21

YOUR METABOLIC RATE

Your BMR is your basal metabolic rate. This is the measure of total energy expended for normal maintenance, repair, and function of your body if you were lying down and resting (not sleeping) during a 24-hour period. The higher your basal metabolic rate, the faster and more continuously you'll burn calories, even while in a rested or relaxed state.

New knowledge confirms that people who exercise aerobically for 30–45 minutes at 75 percent of their capacity will continue to burn calories at an increased rate for several hours after exercising. If you're a bit overweight from carrying too much fat on your body, consider getting in about three aerobic workouts a week until your fat level comes down to an acceptable point. Elite bodybuilders should eschew long, tedious aerobic training. It's muscle-wasting. Instead, practice discipline in the off-season so you don't get fat in the first place.

After beginning or resuming a rigorous training program, your BMR will actually increase after a few weeks. Bodybuilders generally have a higher resting metabolism than the average sedentary person.

You can estimate your metabolic rate for various activities by comparing it to that of a 154-pound man (the so-called average American man). A 154-pound man burns about 70 calories per hour sleeping, or 560 calories in an eight-hour cycle. Add light activity, and it goes up to 100 calories per hour and 800 calories over an eight-hour cycle.

Consider what you do all day. You can adjust for differences in body weight (compared to the 154-pound man) by adding or subtracting 10 calories per hour per activity for each five pounds' difference (from the 154-pound man). Other factors must also be considered, as everyone has individual metabolism and metabolic functions. Age, sex, body size, and body weight, as well as your endocrine system (hormones) function, are some of the variables influencing your BMR.

FIGURE 21-1

Formulas for Estimating Your Basal Metabolic Rate (BMR)

Men's BMR = $1 \times$ body weight (kg) $\times 24$
Women's BMR = $.09 \times$ body weight (kg) $\times 24$

Remember, your body is never totally at rest. Your body is constantly busy building, maintaining, or repairing cells, maintaining body and muscle tissue, and carrying on an assortment of vital organ functions, breathing, and digestion. You're constantly burning calories. The more efficiently your body does its work—its basic survival work—the higher your BMR will become. The higher your BMR, the quicker you shed unnecessary fat, and the sooner your muscles will become stronger, bigger, and more visible.

FIGURE 21-2

Energy Costs of Various Activities

PHYSICAL ACTIVITY	ESTIMATED CALORIES PER HOUR	PHYSICAL ACTIVITY	ESTIMATED CALORIES PER HOUR
Archery	270	Running (7-min. mile)	950
Badminton	400	Singing	120
Basketball	560	Sitting in class	90
Billiards	235	Skating	470
Bowling	215	Skiing (Nordic)	1,080
Bull Session	90	Skipping rope	800
Calisthenics	200	Sleeping	70
Cleaning	185	Soccer	540
Cooking	240	Softball	280
Cycling (5 mph)	300	Squash	650
Disco	450	Studying/Reading	105
Dressing	200	Swimming	500
Driving to class	180	Table tennis	280
Field Hockey	560	Tennis	450
Gardening	295	Volleyball	255
Golf	340	Walking to class	300
Gymnastic	257	Walking up stairs	180
Jogging	750	Washing and shaving	150
Lying quietly	80	Watching TV	90
Marathon running	990	Weight training	550
Playing cards	140	Wood chopping	560
Racquet sports	870	Wrestling	790
Rowing (6 mph)	900		

22

THE GLYCEMIC INDEX

The glycemic index is an important scientific development for body-builders. Through the use of this index, you can determine what kind of fuel you get from what kinds of foods.

Remember, not all carbohydrates have the same effect on your blood sugar. Some take longer to break down than others. For example, apples and oranges are converted to blood sugar at relatively slow rates. Most fruits and beans are extremely slow to convert, that makes these foods desirable fuel sources before games or workouts. Whole wheat, oats, and brown rice are also good athletic choices for energy from the carbohydrate category.

You may notice some surprising statistics as you check over the glycemic index. Carrots, white potatoes, bananas, and white rice have high glycemic values and cause a rapid rise and fall in your blood-sugar levels. You may have previously thought of some of these as healthy foods—the truth is, you should actually avoid these items before training. Eat them on off-days or after workouts. Your pre-workout meal should be comprised of foods that have a glycemic index under 50 or so. This will ensure long-lasting energy for the tough workout ahead.

Study Figure 22-1 to learn the glycemic indexes of various foods. Remember, the higher the count, the less desirable that food is as a source of energy for training. Don't consume it during your preworkout meal. You should include wholesome (nutrient-dense) high-glycemic index foods in other meals, though.

Figure 22-2 is a graphic representation of how blood sugar reacts to foods of differing glycemic indexes.

FIGURE 22-1

The Glycemic Index of Various Foods
Recommended for Fat Loss and Preworkout Diets

EAT LESS OF THESE		EAT MORE OF THESE	
Food	**Glycemic Index**	**Food**	**Glycemic Index**

Sugars

Glucose	100	Fructose	20
Honey	87		

Vegetables

Parsnips	98	Soybeans	15
Carrots	90	Kidney beans	30
White potatoes	70	Lentils	25
Mashed potatoes	80	Sweet potatoes	48
Broad beans	75	Yams	45

Fruits

Bananas	65	Apples	36
Raisins	68	Oranges	40
Equatorial fruits	60–70	Northern fruits	30–40
Dried fruits	65–70		

Grains and Pasta

White flour spaghetti	56	Whole-wheat spaghetti	40
Cornflakes	85	Oats	48
White rice	70	Brown rice	60
White flour pancakes	66	Buckwheat pancakes	45
White bread	76	Whole-wheat bread	64

Lean Meats, Fish, Fowl, Milk, Eggs, Dairy

Milk, cheese, yogurt, and meats all have glycemic indexes in the 30–40 range. Ensure that these high protein foods are carefully chosen for their low fat content.

These are your primary protein sources. As such, they are not eaten so much for energy as they are for growth and tissue repair. Eat as normally indicated, reducing your intake a bit before intense training sessions.

FIGURE 22-2
Blood-Sugar Reactions at
Different Glycemic Indexes

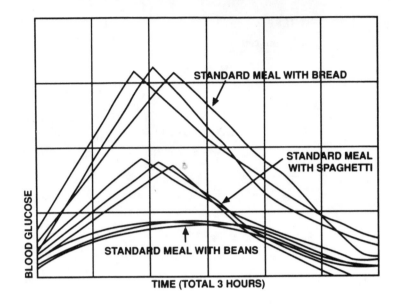

23

SUPPLEMENTS

Vitamins and minerals aren't the only supplements with the ability to assist you in maximizing your training efforts. Many supplements both improve the nutritional quality (biological activity or assimilability) of your food and are capable of amplifying many of your own body's important functions.

Many esoteric substances on the market promise miracles in your performance capabilities. Most do not provide any such thing. On the other hand, some are effective in some regards, and you may find them quite beneficial in promoting improvements in your training and sports performance over the long run.

The supplements listed below are among the best of the hundreds you will see on the health-food-store shelves. Don't be misled by the outrageous claims appearing in many muscle magazines. Most of those claims are either false or grossly exaggerated, designed to seduce you into spending your hard-earned money. Each of the training programs outlined in Part Two includes several of these important substances in the "daily clocks."

ESSENTIAL AMINO ACIDS

The essential amino acids are those which must be derived from food because your body cannot manufacture them for you. Taking a supplement of essential aminos before each meal can improve the quality of the protein in your meal, thereby allowing you to get more out of each meal.

Meat and milk, for example, are only about 60–70 percent assimilable because certain essential aminos are in short supply. None of the remaining aminos can be used if even one of the essential ones runs out. The leftover aminos are relegated to use as simple energy—a poor substitute for carbohydrates.

In order to get ample protein for growth and repair, you'll have to ingest about 30 percent more calories in the form of protein. If you're on a calorie-restricted diet, as most bodybuilders are during the precontest phase of their training mesocycle, those added calories can spell defeat.

THE BRANCHED-CHAIN AMINOS

Leucine, isoleucine, and valine (the "branched chain" aminos) are three of the essential amino acids. They're critically important for muscle repair and muscle growth following heavy training. Branched-chain aminos (BCAAs) comprise fully 70 percent of your body's protein. Fifty percent of all posttraining amino acid needs must be filled by these workhorses. They also supply 10–20 percent of your high-intensity–workout energy. Even during the day, they supply one third of your amino needs.

During times of stress, injury, or extreme exertion, your body mobilizes the BCAAs to synthesize glucose (blood sugar) in the liver, a process called gluconeogenesis. This function has the express purpose of sparing muscle protein from being cannibalized for energy. Thus, the BCAAs are said to be anabolic agents.

GLUTAMINE

L-glutamine, one of the nonessential amino acids, is important both during and following training because it tends to neutralize the catabolic effects of cortisol, a corticosteroid formed during and after intense training. Cortisol causes a breakdown of protein in your muscles. Increased cortisol secretion acts as an insulin antagonist by inhibiting glucose uptake and utilization. This fact is significant to bodybuilders because glucose is protein-sparing. If your muscles can't use blood sugar (glucose) to replace muscle glycogen, they have to get their energy from "stored" protein (your muscles!).

L-glutamine is found more abundantly in your blood than any other amino acid. Its presence there is critical for regulation of your body's acid-base balance, regulation of your body's electrolyte levels, removal of ammonia (a caustic byproduct of protein metabolism), and important neurotransmitter functions.

L-glutamine is interconvertable with glutamic acid (another nonessential amino acid). Vitamin B_6 is needed in abundance in order for L-glutamine to work properly in the body.

PROTEIN POWDER

Sometimes, your meal may be too low in protein. In such cases, a protein shake can supplement your meal very well without the nuisance of having to ingest too much fat. Recall that protein is essential for tissue repair, tissue growth, and improved metabolism.

INOSINE

Inosine has been found to be effective in promoting rapid anaerobic energy. That means that energy for explosive and middistance type athletes can be slightly augmented both in workouts and during competition.

MEAL-REPLACEMENT DRINKS

If you need an aggressive fat-loss program, meal-replacement drinks may help control your caloric intake while at the same time provide a very good balance of essential fats, protein, carbohydrates, vitamins, and minerals.

Such a drink should never completely take the place of real food, however. Of your five daily meals, one or two may, for a short time, be replaced with a liquid meal, but stop using the drink when your target weight is attained.

ANTIOXIDANTS

According to emerging research into their miraculous benefits antioxidants are vital for improving your general health over a lifetime—not just for sports training. In fact, vitamins A, E, and C are among the important antioxidants. Glutathione, selenium, superoxide dimutase (SOD), and certain herbs are also included amongst the antioxidants. All combat the long-term damage taking place inside your body from free radicals which are formed by air pollution, processed foods, many environmental toxins, and even strenuous exercise itself.

In Part Seven, there's an extended discussion of antioxidants and their importance to bodybuilders.

ENDURANCE SUPPLEMENTS

DMG (dimethylglycine), Octacosanol, and Coenzyme Q_{10} (CoQ_{10}) are three substances that have been shown to improve both anaerobic and aerobic strength endurance. However, none appears to be effective after you're in great shape; they only appear to be assistive during the early stages of your training. None is a miracleworker.

You won't bring your mile time down from 8 minutes to 4 minutes, or your marathon time down from 4 hours to 2½ hours by taking these endurance supplements, but you may be able to improve your energy output for extended workouts. If for scheduling reasons you can't engage in double or triple variable split training, each of your daily workouts will be longer than optimal, and such supplements may be assistive.

GLUCOSE TOLERANCE FACTORS

Chromium polynicotinate (ChromeMate: chromium bound to niacin) and chromium picolinate (chromium bound to zinc) have made big news in the world of sports nutrition. They've been widely touted as viable steroid replacements because of their reported anabolic effects.

Their major value, however, is in providing a stabilizing influence on your insulin levels. That makes them excellent supplements for appetite control (i.e., fat-loss programs). It also makes them excellent for prolonged workout energy.

VARIOUS HERBAL PREPARATIONS

Herbs have been used for their curative powers for thousands of years. They're so important, in fact, that they deserve a special section in this book. Refer to Chapter Thirty for a detailed discussion on this intriguing, often overlooked aspect of bodybuilding science.

REHYDRATION DRINKS

Water is the most abundant and most important nutrient in your body. You cannot live without it. For any athlete who trains regularly, water is even more important.

Some time ago, scientists discovered that not only water was lost through sweating, but valuable minerals, too. This was the basis for various types of rehydration drinks. The solutions that make up these drinks not only provide fluid replacement, but include electrolytes and some sugar for energy.

FIGURE 23-1

Supplements and the Uses to Which They Are Often Put

Key
★—Highly effective
1—Effective
2—Possibly effective
3—Probably not effective
4—Not effective

Supplement	Strength	Fat loss	Size	Pain	Mental concentration	Anaerobic energy	Aerobic energy	Workout recovery	Tissue repair	General health
PROTEIN/AMINOS	1	3	1	4	4	3	3	2	2	1
VITAMINS/MINERALS	1	3	1	4	4	3	3	1	1	1
BCAAs	2	3	2	4	3	1	1	★	1	3
INOSINE	2	2	2	4	4	1	2	2	2	2
L-CARNITINE	3	1	3	4	4	2	2	2	2	2
GAMMA ORYZANOL (FERULIC ACID)	2/1*	2	2/1*	4	4	4	3	3	2	2
DMG (BETAINE)	3	3	3	4	1	1	2	2	2	1
CAFFEINE/MATE	2	2	4	3	1	2	2	3	3	4
MAHUANG	2	4	4	4	1	4	4	4	4	4
MUMIE	4	4	4	1	4	4	4	★	★	1
ASPIRIN (AND SALICILATES)	4	4	4	★	4	4	4	★	★	★
BORON	2	4	2	4	4	4	4	2	2	2/1*
GROWTH HORMONE RELEASERS	1	1	1	4	4	4	4	1	1	2
GLUCOSE POLYMER DRINKS	4	2	3	4	3	1	★	1	3	2
MUSCO MXT	4	4	4	4	4	4	4	4	4	4
ELEUTHEROCOCCUS	2	3	3	4	2	3	3	1	1	1
DLPA	4	4	4	1	4	4	4	3	3	3
GLANDULARS	2	4	2	4	3	2	2	2	2	3
BETA SITOSTEROL	3	4	3	4	4	3	3	2	3	2
SMILAX OFFICIANALIS	3	4	3	4	4	4	3	3	3	4
BREWER'S YEAST	3	4	3	4	4	3	3	3	2	2
ROYAL JELLY	3	4	3	4	2	3	2	4	2	3
WHEAT GERM	3	4	3	4	4	3	3	3	3	2
OXYGEN (INGESTED)	2	4	3	4	2	1	1	3	3	4
OXYGEN (BREATHED)	3	4	4	3	2	2	2	4	4	4
OCTACOSANOL	3	2	3	4	2	1	★	1	3	2
CHROMIUM POLYNICOTINATE	1	★	★	4	4	2	1	1	★	★
CHROMIUM PICOLINATE	2	1	1	4	4	2	2	2	2	4
AMMONIA SCAVENGERS	2	3	2	4	2	3	★	1	1	1
COENZYME B12 (DIBENCOZIDE)	1	4	1	4	4	3	3	2	2	3
COENZYME Q10 (UBIQUINONE)	2	4	4	4	4	4	1	1	1	1
LACTATE	4	4	3	4	3	★	1	1	4	3

*2 = males, 1 = females
Ratings based both on research and logical inference from theory and practice.

Endurance athletes have a special problem because of the long training sessions they undergo. Using only water for fluid replacement can result in low blood-sugar levels. This produces early fatigue and low endurance.

Because your small intestine absorbs fluids from a glucose/sodium solution quite rapidly, solutions containing these two minerals are best. The glucose stimulates sodium uptake in your small intestine, which markedly increases fluid absorption. For this reason alone, rehydration drinks containing carbohydrates and sodium are effective fluid replacement drinks.

The effectiveness of sports drinks for fluid replacement depends on their ability to reduce feelings of fatigue, soreness, and possible stiffness following prolonged training sessions. To be efficient, the drinks must be capable of getting into your blood at a quick rate. A new method permitting quick absorption in your stomach is the bonding together of several glucose molecules.

Fluid replacement drinks that contain a low glycemic index provide you with stable levels of blood sugar along with fluids and minerals.

Drinks like Gatorade (to name one of dozens on the market) are actually quite good at replacing fluids lost in sweat; replacing sodium, potassium, calcium, and magnesium lost in sweat; and providing a very excellent source of both short-term and long-term energy for grueling sports competition and training sessions—but then, so are most of the foods you'll be eating as a serious bodybuilder. Besides, drinking sugar water during and following training has its disadvantages.

Your preworkout meal, being comprised of low glycemic index foods, should be more than adequate to carry you through even the most grueling workout. If you haven't eaten correctly prior to training, a sports drink may be the best thing for you. Also, remember that taking in sugar will cause your blood sugar (and, therefore, your insulin level) to skyrocket. If this happens after a workout, you may be able to replenish spent energy stores, but you're certainly not going to get a significant growth hormone (GH) response from your training. The high level of insulin that invariably accompanies increased blood sugar will suppress GH secretion. No GH, no growth and repair! Remember, GH is the anabolic substance your body needs following intense training in order to force an adaptive (anabolic) response.

Be aware that some sports drinks are better than others. Be discerning, and figure out which ones are best for you and when it is best to take them.

OTHER BODYBUILDING SUPPLEMENTS

There are many more excellent supplements—indeed, far more than the scope of this book warrants for detailed discussion. Figure 23-1 and Chapter Thirty's discussion on nature's medicine chest (herbs) provide guidelines for choosing which ones are suitable for you right now, during this mesocycle of your training. Educate yourself on those which seem to fit.

Remember, use only those supplements that are supportive of your short-term goals.

- You don't need all of them all the time
- You don't have enough room in your belly for all of them all the time
- You can't afford to buy all of them all the time
- Most aren't capable of delivering the benefits they claim to be able to anyway

An integrated, scientific approach is the only way to ensure optimal use of nutritional supplements.

Do not take the advertising hype you'll see in bodybuilding magazines as gospel. There are a few excellent books on the subject of sports nutrition; just be sure that the book you choose isn't one of the many books written by an author hired by a sports-nutrition company to make illegal claims seem respectable. Remember, making medical claims for food supplements is against the law— it's called advertising extension. Writing a book is a "safe" way of circumventing this law.

PART SIX

BODYBUILDING AND THE ENDOCRINE SYSTEM

DEDICATED TO JIM QUINN

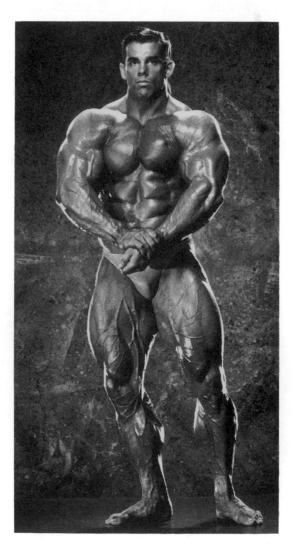

Jim Quinn

24

YOUR HORMONES

Let's set the record straight right now on the importance of your hormones. Every morsel of food you eat, every supplement you ingest, every training act you perform in the gym—practically everything you do—is modified in some way by the hormonal interactions each act instigates. You are virtually captive to your hormones.

Indeed, fellow iron freaks, your very existence and your future training progress are so totally controlled by your hormones that you had better start learning more about your endocrine system now. This is a new age of bodybuilding. It must, by law, by popular demand, and by every moral standard of society ever written, be drug-free.

A PRIMER ON HORMONES

Everybody talks about hormones, but few people really know what they are or where they come from. Fewer still have any clue on what they do.

Hormones are secreted by various glands comprising the endocrine system. The two types of hormones, steroids and polypeptides, diffuse into the blood, course through your body, and eventually act upon a target organ. The problem is, according to scientists, that we have only a minute clue as to what actions each have individually, and practically no clue as to how they interact.

Steroidal hormones are produced from cholesterol in the gonads and the cerebral cortex, while polypeptide hormones are manufactured in the many other glands (see Figure 24-2) from various amino acid combinations.

Hormones regulate almost all your bodily functions. They regulate growth and development, help you cope with both physical and mental stress, and regulate all forms of training responses, including protein metabolism, fat mobilization, and energy production. In a nutshell, they do it all.

It is most important to remember that endocrine function cannot be discussed apart from nervous system function. These two systems act together as synergists in hormonal regulatory functions. Thus, fright, pain, cold, and all of your other senses of both environmental and bodily happenings will activate hormonal responses in an intimidatingly complex array.

The hormones will act in three different ways, basically. They can alter the rate of synthesis of your cellular protein, change the rate of enzyme activity, or change the rate of transport of nutrients through the cell wall.

Although the effects that hormones exert directly upon your various bodily functions are complicated to understand, the resultant effects—the indirect effects—are often of greatest concern to you as a bodybuilder. It's like a cue ball hitting another ball which, in turn, causes yet a third ball to go into the pocket. The cue ball had a direct effect upon ball number two but an indirect effect upon ball number three.

For example, insulin, a hormone released from the beta cells in the islets of Langerhans in your pancreas, increases cellular uptake of glucose, which in turn causes increased synthesis of muscle glycogen. This leads to a decrease in blood-borne glucose, which in turn causes a decrease in insulin production. During prolonged workouts, this reduction in blood glucose and the attendant decrease in insulin production causes an increase in the mobilization of stored fat.

The lowered blood glucose also stimulates another hormone to be released—glucagon, also manufactured in the islets of Langerhans (the alpha cells) in the pancreas—which performs the opposite function of insulin. Glucagon stimulates both glycogenolysis and gluconeogenesis in the liver. The glucose generated in this fashion is released into the bloodstream, thereby once again raising the insulin levels.

The process of gluconeogenesis—the conversion of liver glycogen into glucose—activates yet another process. Blood-borne amino acids taken up by the liver can adversely affect your ability to grow because of the reduced availability of the amino acids during protein turnover promoted by exercise.

The cycle of activity is never-ending. It makes you wonder

whether it can be controlled or whether you'd even care to try.

The chain of events shown in Figure 24-1 is quite controllable, as it happens, by merely keeping your workouts short, intense, and more frequent—a good reason to engage in the double variable split training discussed in Part Two.

FIGURE 24-1

Just One of Thousands of Hormonally Controlled Reactions

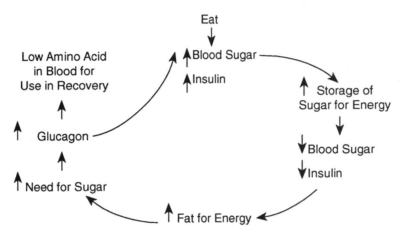

MUSCLE GROWTH AND HORMONAL REGULATION

The point of bodybuilding is to get bigger muscles—period. That singular objective should be accomplished while maintaining good health. I fear that this is not often the case, due in part to the unwise (and certainly naive) use of multiple drugs which induce hormonal activity beyond reasonable bounds.

More than one bodybuilder has died from trying to fool Mother Nature. Indeed, one champion bodybuilder recently died from what was reported to be insulin shock—he had apparently injected insulin into his body under the foolish notion that he would get more muscle and less fat by doing so. Bodybuilding officials initially insisted that his death was the result of his abuse of diuretics (drugs that cause your body to excrete water) to get rid of cuts-masking extracellular fluid. Either way, he was a fool. There is no such thing as a free lunch when it comes to these kinds of dangerous drugs, folks! One way or the other, you'll pay a price. The price of death is too dear.

The fact that several hormones can be safely and healthfully regulated in large measure through carefully constructed training and a smart regimen of supplementation is reason enough to avoid the use of drugs. Let's explore a few alternatives.

Growth Hormone

By stimulating growth hormone release from your anterior pituitary gland, you will

- Increase protein synthesis
- Decrease carbohydrate utilization for energy
- Increase the mobilization of stored fat
- Promote cell division and cell proliferation

Scientists believe that growth hormone (GH) is released as a result of neuronal signals—your nervous system—such as anxiety and stress of the type caused by exercise. Neural input to the hypothalamus causes a hormone-releasing factor to be secreted, which in turn causes GH to be released. Of course, amino acids such as arginine, ornithine, glycine, and others are known to have GH-releasing properties as well, but only after they're converted biochemically.

It's well known that your GH response will be improved with intense exercise as opposed to low-intensity training. You should avoid prolonged training because of the problem noted earlier of promoting an insulin response. Prolonged training is sometimes OK for aerobic athletes but rarely for bodybuilders or other anaerobic athletes.

The Thyroid Hormones

Your anterior pituitary—sometimes referred to as the "master gland" because of all the important hormones it produces—releases a substance called thyroid stimulating hormone (TSH). The thyroid gland, located in your neck, releases two hormones, thyroxine (T_4) and triiodothyronine (T_3). Your T_4 raises the metabolic rate of all cells by as much as four times; thus, carbohydrate and fat metabolism is greatly facilitated by thyroxine. Conversely, obesity can result from abnormally low thyroid activity. This is only responsible for under 3 percent of all cases of obesity, however, so it's not to be taken as an excuse for one's gustatory slovenliness, generally speaking.

It's believed that over the course of time, careful eating and exercise patterns will increase your metabolic rate by some sort of set-point calibration mechanism.

The Adrenal Hormones

Your adrenal glands are comprised of two parts, the cortex (outer layer) and the medulla (inner). Both are important to you. Exercise dramatically increases output of epinephrine, which in turn causes increased blood flow to working muscles, enhanced cardiac output, the mobilization of energy substrate, glycogenolysis, fat mobilization, and other "gearing up for stress" functions.

Your cortex releases a group of hormones called the adrenocortical hormones (mineralocorticoids, glucocorticoids, and androgens). Your mineralocorticoids—there are three—are comprised chiefly of aldosterone.

Aldosterone regulates the reabsorption of sodium in the distal tubules of the kidney. High levels of aldosterone cause sodium in the kidneys to be reabsorbed into the blood instead of being excreted with the urine. Low aldosterone, on the other hand, causes sodium to be excreted in large amounts through the urine. Thus, aldosterone is responsible for controlling sodium balance in your body and directly impacts upon whether you're holding water.

But watch out! A disrupted sodium balance can cause an increase in blood volume, which in turn causes increased cardiac output and blood pressure. During exercise, there's a constriction of blood vessels to the kidneys, so the kidneys are forced to release an enzyme called renin into the bloodstream.

Renin then stimulates the release of yet another kidney enzyme called angiotensin, which stimulates the adrenal cortex to release aldosterone.

Another corticosteroid, cortisol, is of interest to you and your training efforts. Cortisol is pretty nasty stuff. It's catabolic, meaning it causes a breakdown of protein in your muscles. Increased cortisol secretion also acts as an insulin antagonist by inhibiting glucose uptake and utilization.

High cortisol levels cause your liver to split the fat molecules that are mobilized via cortisol activity into ketoacids. High levels of these ketoacids in the extracellular fluid can cause a dangerous situation called ketosis. This is common among those of you who have been on a carbohydrate-restricted diet (such as before a bodybuilding contest or to make weight) and is a good reason to do your dieting well in advance of your competition.

FIGURE 24-2

Your Hormones and Their Functions

HOST GLAND	HORMONE	HORMONE FUNCTIONS	CONTROL OF HORMONE SECRETION	↑ EXERCISE EFFECTS ON HORMONE SECRETION
Anterior pituitary	Growth hormone (GH)	Stimulates tissue growth; mobilizes fatty acids for energy; inhibits CHO metabolism	Hypothalamic releasing factor (GHRF)	↑ with increasing exercise
	Thyrotropin (TSH)	Stimulates production and release of thyroxine from thyroid gland	Hypothalamic TSH-releasing factor; thyroxine	↑ with increasing exercise
	Corticotropin (ACTH)	Stimulates production and release of cortisol, aldosterone, and other adrenal hormones	Hypothalamic ACTH-releasing factor; cortisol	?
	Gonadotropin (FSH and LH)	FSH works with LH to stimulate production of estrogen by ovaries; LH works with FSH to stimulate production of estrogen and progesterone by ovaries and testosterone by male testes	Hypothalamic FSH and LH releasing factor; female—estrogen and progesterone; male—testosterone	No change
	Prolactin (PRL)	Inhibits testosterone; mobilizes fatty acids	Hypothalamic PRL-inhibiting factor	↑ with increasing exercise

HOST GLAND	HORMONE	HORMONE FUNCTIONS	CONTROL OF HORMONE SECRETION	↑ EXERCISE EFFECTS ON HORMONE SECRETION
	Endorphins	Blocks pain; promotes euphoria; affects feeding and female menstrual cycle	Stress— physical/ emotional	↑ with long-duration exercise
Posterior pituitary	Vasopressin (ADH)	Controls water excretion by kidneys	Hypothalamic secretory neurons	↑ with increasing exercise
	Oxytocin	Stimulates muscles in uterus and breasts; important in birthing and lactation	Hypothalamic secretory neurons	?
Adrenal cortex	Cortisol Corticosterone	Promotes use of fatty acids and protein catabolism; conserves blood sugar–insulin antagonist; has anti-inflammatory effects with epinephrine	ACTH; stress	↑ in heavy exercise only
	Aldosterone	Promotes retention of sodium, potassium, and water by the kidneys	Angiotensin and plasma potassium concentration; renin	↑ with increasing exercise
Adrenal medulla	Epinephrine Norepinephrine	Facilitates sympathetic activity, increases cardiac output, regulates blood vessels, increases glycogen catabolism and fatty acid release	Stress stimulated hypothalamic sympathetic nerves	Epinephrine, ↑ in heavy exercise Norepinephrine, ↑ with increasing exercise

HOST GLAND	HORMONE	HORMONE FUNCTIONS	CONTROL OF HORMONE SECRETION	↑ EXERCISE EFFECTS ON HORMONE SECRETION
Thyroid	Thyroxine T_4 Triiodothyronine T_3	Stimulate metabolic rate; regulate cell growth and activity	TSH; whole body metabolism	↑ with increasing exercise
Pancreas	Insulin	Promotes CHO transport into cells; increases CHO catabolism and decreases blood glucose; promotes fatty acid and amino acid transport into cells	Plasma glucose levels	↑ with increasing exercise
	Glucagon	Promotes release of glucose from liver to blood; increases fat metabolism	Plasma glucose levels	↑ with increasing exercise
Para-thyroid	Parathormone	Raises blood calcium; lowers blood phosphate	Plasma calcium concentration	?
Ovaries	Estrogen Progesterone	Controls menstrual cycle; increases fat deposition; promotes female sex characteristics	FSH, LH	↑ with exercise; depends on menstrual phase
Testes	Testosterone	Controls muscle size; increases RBC; decreases body fat; promotes male sex characteristics	LH	↑ with exercise
Kidney	Renin	Stimulates aldosterone secretion	Plasma sodium concentration	↑ with increasing exercise

FIGURE 24-3

Hormones and Their Response to Exercise Training

HORMONE   **TRAINING RESPONSE**

Hypothalamus-Pituitary Hormones

Growth hormone   No effect on resting values; trained tend to have less dramatic rise during exercise
Thyrotropin   No known training effect
ACTH   Trained have increased exercise values
Prolactin   Some evidence that training lowers resting values
FSH, LH, and   Trained females have depressed values
Testosterone   Trained males have depressed testosterone, with probably no change in LH and FSH

Posterior Pituitary Hormones

Vasopressin (ADH)   Some evidence that training results in slight reductions in ADH at a given workload
Oxytocin   No research information available

Thyroid Hormones

Thyroxine   Reduced concentration of total T_3 and an increased free
Triiodothyronine   thyroxine at rest. Increased turnover of T_3 and T_4 during exercise

Adrenal Hormones

Aldosterone   No significant training adaptation
Cortisol   Trained exhibit slight elevations during exercise
Epinephrine   Decrease in secretion at rest and same exercise intensity
Norepinephrine   after training

Pancreatic Hormones

Insulin   Training increases sensitivity to insulin; normal decrease in insulin during exercise is greatly reduced in response to training
Glucagon   Smaller increase in glucose levels during exercise at both absolute and relative workloads

Kidney Hormones

Renin   No apparent training effect
Angiotensin

Figures 24-2 and 24-3 are from *Exercise Physiology: Energy, Nutrition, and Human Performance*, 2nd ed., by W. D. McArdle, F. I. Katch, and V. L. Katch (Philadelphia: Lea and Febiger, 1986). Used with permission.

25

THE GROWTH
HORMONE RESPONSE

In bodybuilding today, *drugs* is a dirty word. Massive media coverage has made performance-enhancing drugs like steroids and growth hormone infamous. In fact, the media's widespread coverage, not to mention their zeal for sensationalism, of these substances was largely responsible for making the use of these drugs against the law.

Nowadays, elite athletes in every sport are pushing the frontiers of science in their bid to find safe and effective ways of getting bigger, faster, and stronger—without having to resort to the use of drugs. That's perhaps more true in bodybuilding than in any other sport. Bodybuilders have always been at the fore when it comes to the application of cutting-edge science to training practices.

One way of improving performance that's showing promise is in stimulating a natural growth hormone response. Growth hormone is one of the most important factors in getting big and getting strong. Growth hormone is manufactured in your anterior pituitary gland, at the base of your brain. This amazing morsel of your anatomy is less than one centimeter in diameter and weighs less than one-half gram. It takes its orders from hormones produced in your hypothalamus, also at the base of your brain. Much of what a bodybuilder does in order to achieve that characteristic look of being massive and cut to ribbons is controlled by hormones.

Your hypothalamus receives signals from almost all possible sources in your nervous system. Pain, excitement, depression, smells, even the concentration of nutrients, electrolytes, water, and blood-borne hormones are sensed by the hypothalamus. A lot of heavy weight-training stress? The hypothalamus tells the anterior pituitary to secrete some growth hormone.

Haven't eaten in awhile? The hypothalamus tells the pituitary to secrete hormones that will either cannibalize a bit of your muscle tissue for life-sustaining energy or to save that tissue and instead mobilize some fat for energy.

Tissue bloat? Leave it to the good ol' hypothalamus to tell the posterior pituitary to get rid of some of the excess fluid.

All of these activities are interrelated, and all are to some degree controllable by your actions. Since we're focusing on growth hormone and its ability to affect metabolic functions important to bodybuilders (especially protein synthesis), let's look at some of the benefits of stimulating a growth hormone response and some of the ways you may be able to stimulate it. Growth hormone increases protein production, decreases your use of carbohydrates for energy, increases your use of stored fat for energy, and promotes muscle growth.

You may be able to more effectively stimulate growth hormone production.

1. Training two or three times daily in shorter, more intense bursts will provide several growth hormone responses.

2. Avoiding food for about 45–60 minutes following intense training (until your blood sugar is low from replenishing spent muscle glycogen stores) will ensure a more prominent growth hormone response.

3. Make sure the temperature in your gym is very warm. If it isn't, wear warm clothing. And, unless your training session lasts over 90 minutes, which it shouldn't, don't rehydrate until after training. You'll get a better growth hormone response that way.

4. Taking a sauna each day can provide a growth hormone response. Again, be sure to replace the water and electrolytes you've lost from sweating well after showering.

5. Sleep at night (during the first hour or so) is accompanied by a growth hormone response. So are naps during the day, provided they're good quality naps. They needn't be greater than 30 minutes in duration.

6. Certain amino acids (typically, ornithine and arginine) are often used by athletes in the hopes of getting a growth hormone response. It's only speculative whether the growth hormone response is significant enough to promote added muscle growth (reports are largely anecdotal).

7. There is some striking evidence that the balance of fats, proteins, and carbohydrates in your diet can be fine-tuned to ensure greater growth hormone output. It appears that your body finds ways of adjusting its hormone output based on nutrient intake to maximize the training effect.

8. One of the reasons that bodybuilders eat 5–7 times daily is they can get bigger and more cut that way. Some scientists concur that eating more frequent meals is a great way to stimulate growth hormone responses.

Scientists aren't in total agreement as to how many growth hormone peaks per day is most effective. Swedish scientists working with rats have shown that four to six peaks are optimal and that less growth occurred with ten peaks per day. In contrast, a U.S. research study, which also used rats, showed that nine peaks produced the greatest growth.

When scientists have looked at growth hormone output every 10–15 minutes (instead of their normal practice of only once per hour), they've noticed peaks superimposed upon peaks. They aren't sure what this means or whether stimulating greater secretion now will result in less later (in a balancing effect). Research is clearly needed.

In the meantime, we can safely speculate that promoting growth hormone release naturally may indeed be of significant benefit to you in your bodybuilding efforts. I hasten to add that, considering the interaction of your body's functions—especially the multiple functions of the pituitary gland and the hypothalamus to which it is subordinate—shotgunning your training methods or nutrient intake is *not* the way to go.

It is very clear to me from all this that timing appears to be very important and that multiple training, eating, and sleeping bouts daily is probably better than the old way.

Refer again to the daily clocks presented in Part Two. Every minute of the day should be carefully scheduled in order to maximize the effects of your activities on growth hormone secretion. Everything you do in the way of training, therapy, sleeping, and eating is done so that you can take advantage of your own body's biochemistry.

Of course, the point of bodybuilding is to get bigger muscles and less fat. Through carefully constructing your training, diet, and supplementation regimen, you can effectively regulate the entire hormonal process that'll make this happen.

FIGURE 25-1

Nondrug Stimuli Affecting hGH Release

STIMULUS	RELEASER	INHIBITOR
Training	Intensity	Overtraining
	Frequency	Overstrain
	Duration	Training sessions longer than an hour
Stress	Pain	Comfort
	Anxiety	Calm
	Heat	Cold
Diet*	Balanced	Unbalanced
Sleeping	Deep sleep	Disturbed sleep

---

*Your muscles' insulin sensitivity appears to be affected.

26

YOUR MUSCLES' HYPERTROPHY PROCESS

Why is weight training the best way to make your muscles grow bigger? How does it happen? More important, if you knew the answers to these two questions, would your knowledge aid you in improving the efficiency of the hypertrophy process?

"Who cares, Dr. Squat! Just gimme a barbell, let me lift it, and to hell with all this science!" is the pragmatic response I get from bodybuilders who are into lifting for lifting's sake. That's OK. But, since you've gotten this far along in reading this book, I'm certain that you've already learned the answer to the third question posed in paragraph one.

In a word, yes.

Let's have a look at the structural elements comprising a muscle cell. Then you'll be able to more clearly visualize how you, the architect, can build more muscle by manipulating the stresses you apply to them during intense training.

YOUR MUSCLES' STRUCTURE AND FUNCTION

Inside every muscle cell there are thick filaments (myosin) and thin filaments (actin). They are the contractile elements in your cells. These are the proteins which, when they are forced to contract, cause the growth process to occur. The breakdown of ATP (adenosine triphosphate) molecules causes the thick filaments to slide across the thin filaments.

How do we get the ATP to break down? An enzyme called

myosin ATPase is secreted from the tiny hairlike structures (called *cross bridges*) of the thick filaments and interacts with the ATP, causing it to break down. This interaction liberates energy for contraction.

Now, let's back up for a moment. Remember that you have red (slow-twitch) and white (fast-twitch) muscle fibers. They're so named because of their inherent contraction speed and resistance to fatigue. Scientists called the slow-twitch (fatigue-resistant) fibers *Type I fibers* and the fast-twitch fibers *Type II fibers*. The fast-twitch fibers are the ones that have the greatest capacity for hypertrophy and are divided into two specific groups: Type IIa fibers (which are both fast-twitch and highly fatigue–resistant) and Type IIb fibers (very low resistance to fatigue).

Each one of these fiber types has its own unique form of ATPase. Whether a muscle cell becomes a Type I, Type IIa, or Type IIb fiber is largely a result of the specific form of ATPase the myosin filaments' cross bridges secrete.

FIGURE 26-1

An Electron Micrograph of a Muscle's Cross-Section

F = Type IIb Fibers (fast-twitch, low oxidative capacity)
S = Type I Fibers (slow-twitch, high oxidative capacity)
I = Type IIa Fibers (fast-twitch, high oxidative capacity)

Remember that bodybuilders and explosive athletes want to preserve their Type IIb fibers, glycolytic athletes opt for Type IIa fibers, and endurance athletes require Type I fibers.

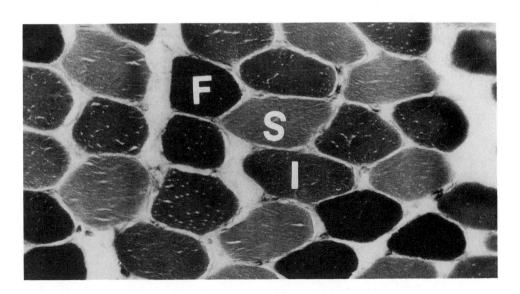

FIGURE 26-2

Muscle-Fiber Types and Their Functions

FIBER TYPE	FUNCTION AND TRAINING ADVICE
Type I	Slow-twitch, oxidative (highly fatigue-resistant), little capacity for exercise-induced hypertrophy (however, hypertrophy pronounced with anabolic steroid use), high resistance to exercise-induced structural damage

All Training Periods

Responds best to high-repetition training with lighter weights and slow, continuous tension movements

Type IIa	Fast-twitch, oxidative (highly fatigue-resistant), high capacity for exercise-induced hypertrophy, moderate resistance to exercise-induced structural damage

During High-Intensity Period

Responds best to medium-rep training with moderate weight and fast concentric movements but slow, deliberate eccentric movements

During Low-Intensity Period

Delete eccentric phase

Type IIb	Fast-twitch, glycolytic (low oxidative capacity, highly susceptible to fatigue), great capacity for exercise-induced hypertrophy, great susceptibility to exercise-induced damage

During High-Intensity Period

Responds best to explosive training with heavier weights, deliberate eccentric

During Low-Intensity Period

Delete eccentric phase

THE IMPORTANCE OF THE ECCENTRIC PHASE OF CONTRACTION

For explosive athletes whose sport-related skills are predominantly restricted to the ATP/CP pathways of muscle energetics (see Part Four for a discussion of the pathways of muscular energetics), avoidance of eccentric training is usually advised. This is because microtrauma to the thick and thin myofibers invariably accompanies such forced elongation of the myofilaments. However, for the purpose of inducing hypertrophy—a unique requirement of bodybuilding—the eccentric phase is critical.

"Whoa! Do you mean that I have to *purposely* inflict damage to my muscle cells?"

Yep.

"Why?"

Dr. Scott Connelly, in an erudite explanation of the hypertrophy process which appeared in *Muscle Media 2000* magazine, explained why. He elaborated on the process of doing several reps in order to exhaust the ATP regeneration process so that the muscle would cease to contract. At that point, said he, "stretching a myofiber in this [fatigued] condition as would occur on the subsequent eccentric phase of the next rep would be predicted to 'tear' the sarcomere [the actin/myosin filaments] at its weakest link. . . . This would be expected in Type IIb fibers with the least total oxidative capacity."

Dr. Connelly went on to explain a relatively new concept in bodybuilding, which involves a muscle cell's switching to a different form of ATPase (the enzyme that breaks ATP down in order to liberate energy for muscle contraction). According to his theory, the replacement of Type IIb ATPase with the Type IIa variety is caused by heavy use of exhausting eccentric training.

This, in turn, increases your muscles' population of Type IIa fibers at the expense of Type IIb fibers. The theory, of course, is that by inflicting such exhausting stress on your muscles, they adapt to the increased energy and repair needs by switching to the ATPase isomer form that Type IIa fibers possess (remember, they're more fatigue- and injury-resistant) or reducing the population of the more injury-prone Type IIb fibers.

The steps through which this entire process progresses are damage (microtrauma stemming from eccentric contraction), inflammation, repair (protein turnover and elimination of destroyed tissue), and tissue remodelling (adaptive growth).

The most interesting element of Dr. Connelly's theory is that, upon damaging the cells' membranes through eccentric contraction while the cell is in a fatigued state, certain protein growth factors are liberated in the interstitial spaces surrounding the injured cell. Called FGF (fibroblast growth factor—fibroblasts are newly forming cells), IGF-I (insulinlike growth factor, type one) and IGF-II (insulin-like growth factor, type two), these growth factors are known to stimulate the development of noncontractile satellite cells and cause the conversion of satellite cells to become part of the neighboring contractile cell in order to give it greater protection from stress. This, Dr. Connelly reasons, is what causes hypertrophy of the contractile cell.

FIGURE 26-3

Schematic Representation of a Muscle's Organization

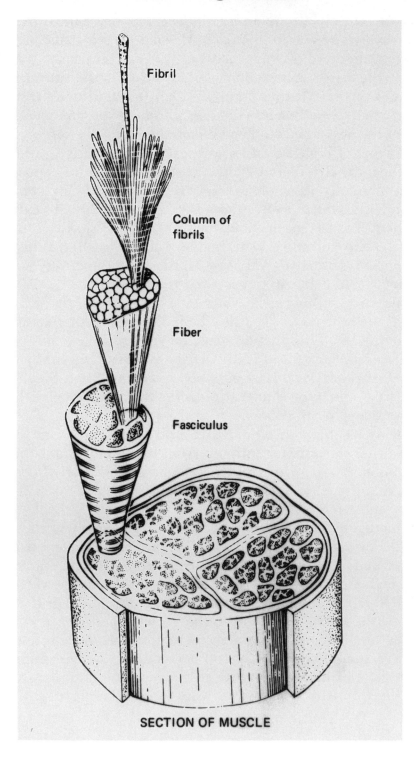

Fibril

Column of fibrils

Fiber

Fasciculus

SECTION OF MUSCLE

This is a revolutionary concept, folks!

Trouble is, if this process were to continue for any length of time, pretty soon all of your Type IIb fibers would be gone—converted to Type IIa fibers. This is not good news. Theoretically, when that happens, further hypertrophy would be impossible. This situation may well be what all of us have, for many years, called plateauing.

This is the most compelling rationale for applying periodization to your bodybuilding program. Refer back to Part Two and read the rationale for applying an "ABC" system to your training intensity. It will now make far more sense to you.

By varying the intensity—balancing high-intensity periods with low-intensity periods—it's reasonable to speculate that carefully alternating both your training intensity and the application of eccentric movements, two very important things will happen: you can limit the amount of (unwanted) conversion of Type IIb to Type IIa fibers that takes place as an adaptive response to training, and you'll continue to develop more satellite cells (whose ultimate destiny is to become part of the contractile cell), thereby forcing hypertrophy to continue.

PART SEVEN

DRUGS AND OTHER SUBSTANCES

DEDICATED TO MIKE CHRISTIAN

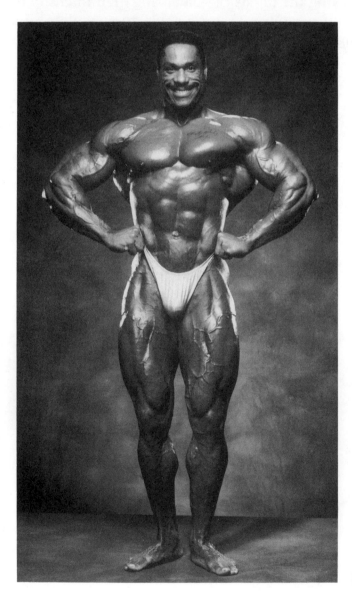

Mike Christian

27

SUBSTANCES TO LOOK OUT FOR

As a bodybuilder, you must know the substances to stay away from as well as those to take. Many of these substances are drugs; some are simply thought of as drugs. What you must realize is that many of these substances are commonly used among athletic competitors who don't know the serious side effects or, more commonly, don't know that their net effects are hampering their bodybuilding efforts.

I hasten to add that I do not want to be guilty of preaching about the obvious dangers of drug misuse and abuse. My principal intent is to aid you in becoming a better bodybuilder.

THE EFFECTS OF ALCOHOL

Many athletes think it is macho to drink a mug of beer before competitions like arm-wrestling or other similar strength events. Truth be known, it's not.

Consuming alcohol before your training or prior to a competition is both unproductive and potentially dangerous. Although small amounts of alcohol consumption have been shown to increase muscular endurance and strength output, these benefits are very short-lived—for, say, twenty minutes—then problems occur.

The numerous negative side effects of alcohol undoubtedly outweigh its possible benefits to any athlete. Since alcohol is a toxin (poison), a host of physical abnormalities can persist. These abnormalities can reduce your strength, endurance, recovery capabilities, aerobic capacity, and ability to metabolize fat and can interfere with muscle growth.

Alcohol can also affect your nervous system and brain. With long-term alcohol use, a severe deterioration of your central nervous system is possible. With short-term use, nerve-muscle interaction can be reduced. This will result in a loss of strength.

Other dangerous effects include reduced hand-eye coordination and balance and longer periods required for healing of injuries. Alcohol has been responsible for a number of sexual dysfunctions including loss of libido, reduced sperm formation, menstrual irregularities, and shrinkage of sexual organs.

When alcohol reaches your muscle cells, it can damage them. Inflammation of the muscle cells is common among alcohol users. When alcohol consumption is practiced for a long time, some of these damaged cells can die, resulting in less functional muscle contractions. In any event, the alcohol will leave you with more muscle soreness following training, requiring additional time for recuperation.

Alcohol's negative effects on your heart and circulatory system are numerous. You can experience a reduction in your endurance capacities when you drink alcohol, especially in large quantities. When consuming alcoholic beverages, your heat loss increases because alcohol stimulates your blood vessels to dilate. When the vessels under your skin dilate, heat loss increases. This can cause your muscles to get cold and, as a result, be slower and weaker during contractions.

In addition, alcohol can cause several gastric, digestive, and nutritional irregularities. This drug causes a release of insulin that will in turn increase the metabolism of glycogen, thereby sparing fat, making it more difficult to lose fat. Since alcohol consumption can interfere with the absorption of many nutrients, it is possible to become somewhat anemic and deficient in the B vitamins.

Because your liver is the organ that detoxifies alcohol, the more alcohol you consume, the harder your liver has to work. This additional stress on your liver can damage and even destroy some liver cells.

Since alcohol acts as a diuretic, large amounts of alcohol can place undue stress on your kidneys. With a diuretic action, large amounts of antidiuretic hormone (ADH) are excreted. This can result in elevated water retention, something no athlete can afford to have happen.

Alcohol is not a drink for athletes. Its effects on strength, reaction time, skill, and heart function are less than desirable. In fact, alcohol is not a nutritional source of energy even though it contains seven calories per gram.

THE EFFECTS OF NICOTINE

The active ingredient in tobacco is nicotine. Although this substance stimulates your adrenal glands for increased energy, the long-term negative side effects by far outweigh any possible benefits.

When you inhale smoke, your heart has to work harder. You can see this by monitoring the pulse of smokers after they puff on a cigarette. Your heart actually beats faster and harder. In many who smoke, this effect causes irregular heart contractions that can persist for thirty to forty-five minutes. Together with increased heart rate comes an elevation in blood pressure and more resistance in your airway. It then becomes more difficult to breathe. Your arteries constrict and cause pressure to build up in them. This, of course, causes higher blood pressure. These effects also occur in the arteries of your heart, causing less blood flow to the heart muscles.

One by-product of smoking is carbon monoxide. This substance easily attaches to oxygen and leaves less oxygen available for the working muscles. This reduces your endurance tremendously.

The oxygen in your lungs also decreases with smoking by nearly half. The numerous toxic by-products of smoking have been associated with cancer, heart disease, and other degenerative illnesses.

Skin temperature can drop due to smoking. This can cause an athlete to feel cold and be less functional during training and competition.

Other forms of tobacco use include snuff and chewing tobacco. Both forms are not without bad side effects. In addition to the nicotine that ends up in your saliva and down your throat, many forms of mouth cancer are caused from these practices.

THE EFFECTS OF CAFFEINE

Make no mistake about it, caffeine is a powerful drug. It is easily obtained in many food products including coffee, tea, chocolate, many soft drinks, analgesics, and diet aids.

This drug has been proven to stimulate your central nervous system, mobilize free fatty acids, improve muscle contractions, mobilize various hormones and substrates essential to metabolism, and mobilize carbohydrates for energy. But how you use it is crucial to the possible benefits it might permit.

If you have a high tolerance to caffeine, its use in sports can be beneficial. But if you have a low tolerance to caffeine, its consumption can leave you less than ready for competition.

Reaction time can be improved with caffeine providing the

caffeine is in moderate dosages, say two cups of black coffee one hour before the event. The effect can last for roughly two to two-and-a-half hours. Heavy coffee drinkers who consume two to six cups a day might be forced to stop drinking coffee a few days prior to competition, only so they can get an effect from it when they consume it just prior to the competition. If abstinence is not practiced in these cases, reaction time can be unchanged.

As most of us already know, caffeine has the power to reduce drowsiness, increase alertness, and reduce our perception of fatigue. Dosages of approximately 3.0 milligrams of caffeine per kilogram of body weight are shown to be beneficial. Anything less might be unproductive, while more can decrease performance. The loss of fat is also increased with the use of caffeine before training.

In athletes who participate in activities that require explosive and powerful movement, like sprinting, weightlifting (including bodybuilding), and football, caffeine appears to be of no advantage. The only possible benefit is that caffeine consumption might get you up, with an elevated heart rate, and perhaps prepare you for the event.

In endurance sports like long distance running, cycling, and cross-country skiing, caffeine can help. It will aid in mobilizing energy stores responsible for enduring muscle work (fat deposits). This can promote the uptake of free fatty acids by your muscle cells along with the increased use of muscle triglycerides during endurance events. This will spare glycogen use for more intense activity at a later time.

It is important to remember, however, that if you are not accustomed to consuming food products containing caffeine, attempting to benefit from their use prior to a competition can be either good or bad. You need to know your tolerances before you reach the point of competition.

28

ASPIRIN: THE BEST SUPPLEMENT OF ALL?

Let me start by giving you the bottom line. Aspirin can be the single most important supplement you can use as an athlete or body-builder. There are many reasons why this may be true. If you haven't been using aspirin regularly, that bit of Dr. Squat wisdom may be good news.

However, let me give you the bad news about aspirin. Taking too many at one time—three or more—can be dangerous for some individuals. The first signs of overdose are ringing in the ears, nausea, constipation, heartburn, and indigestion. Overuse of aspirin is linked to Reye's syndrome in children and teenagers. The first two trimesters of a pregnancy are definitely not the best times to use the stuff, and it can cause bleeding in the third. Those suffering from digestive tract ailments such as bleeding ulcers are usually advised by their family doctor to avoid aspirin altogether. Others with stomach problems may be advised by their physician to use only coated aspirin when needed.

Now for the good news. Most, if not all, of these potentially serious side effects can be avoided by going back to nature. The original source of aspirin's active ingredient, salicin, is white willow bark. It's still widely available as an herbal preparation.

If you opt for commercially available aspirin, then have a gander at what scientists claim as its benefits:

- It can dramatically reduce the risk of heart attacks and certain types of stroke

- It can prevent cataracts
- It can decrease frequency and intensity of migraines
- It can augment certain types of cancer treatments
- It can prevent eclampsia during late pregnancy
- It is believed to be effective in combating colds
- It allows most vaccines to work better
- It reduces the production of prostaglandins, released when cells are damaged, causing inflammation, fever, and blood clotting by destroying the enzyme cyclo-oxygenase. (Note: This activity is responsible for its anti-inflammatory, anti–blood clotting, and (indirectly) anti–heart attack benefits.)
- It is believed to prevent colon cancer
- Because it stimulates production of interleukin-2 and gamma interferon, aspirin is an immune system booster. This action opens the door for a host of synergistic applications involving all forms of diseases affecting the immune system, such as colds, AIDS, and diabetes (Note: This immune-system booster activity appears to lessen with continued use of aspirin, meaning that you develop a tolerance to it. You have to take it only when you know you need the boost.)

All of these possibilities are interesting, healthful, positive, and downright amazing. But, other than the obvious health benefits, what does it have to do with bodybuilders in heavy training?

1. Heavy training causes your blood to thicken (when sweating, fluids are taken from the blood)
2. Heavy training damages cells, causing inflammation
3. Inflammation, coupled with less viscous blood, means that the recovery process will be impeded by a substantial margin because it's more difficult to get nutrients in and wastes out
4. Aspirin quells nagging pains associated with the trauma of heavy training; assists in reducing inflammation; assists in thinning the blood, making it easier for nutrient-rich blood to flow to the muscles you've just stressed; and improves your general recuperative/anabolic responses to heavy training

These potential sports-related uses of aspirin are, in my opinion, ample justification for you to seriously consider aspirin as one of your most important OTC (over-the-counter) sports supplements. A few very important cautions, however, are in order.

- Do so only upon clearance from a competent sports physician. *Never* self-administer *any* drug
- Consider using white willow bark instead of the more potent commercial form
- Cycle your use of aspirin, ensuring that a tolerance to the substance does not occur. You may want to use it only for extremely intense workouts, for example
- Dosages of aspirin will vary according to your lean body-weight (250–500 mg per 50 kg of lean body weight is considered a safe dosage, assuming you're past your teen years)
- Never use aspirin if you are pregnant or under the age of 21 unless your physician says it's OK
- It's advisable to use a buffered form of aspirin or, alternatively, a stomach-coating substance such as Maalox prior to use. Another good idea is to pulverize the tablets (crush them between two spoons) and mix them with about 2–4 ounces of milk prior to taking them

29

OTHER DRUGS

Bodybuilders and other athletes have used many, many drugs over the past few years. It is not within the scope of this book to discuss them all. Many excellent books on the market discuss drug abuse in sports. By far the most definitive work ever written is the series by Dr. Mauro DiPasquale. (His works are listed in the Bibliography.)

As a cursory overview of the many pitfalls awaiting drug abusers, carefully examine Figure 29-1. It lists the myriad interactions you can expect—or not expect, as the case may be. The point is that drugs often interact in dangerous and unpredictable ways.

I happen to believe strongly that you can achieve bodybuilding greatness without drugs.

"I know, I know, Dr. Squat!" you may lament. "How can you claim that a bodybuilder can get as big and cut off steroids as he can on?"

Do me a favor. Do yourself a favor. Go back to Part Two and have another look at the gains you can expect through drug-free integrated training. Reread the chapter on ICOPRO's ABC experiment. I tell you, it can be done. It's tough, it takes discipline and fastidiousness, and it takes passion.

FIGURE 29-1
Drugs and Their Interactions

STEROIDS

NAME	CLINICAL USE	BODYBUILDERS USE	CONTRAINDICATIONS	SIDE EFFECTS
1. Testosterone (propionate, enanthate, cypionate, methyltestosterone)	Male hypogonadal states	"Strength/size" drug "androgenic phase" of steroid program	Male breast cancer, prostate cancer, liver disease, kidney disease, pregnancy	Acne, hirsutism in females, water/sodium retention, decreased sperm formation, increased arteriosclerosis, liver disease, neoplasm promotion, gynecomastia
2. Nandrolone decanoate (Deca-Durabolin)	Weight gain promotion after surgery, severe trauma, offset protein catabolism associated with corticosteroids	Injection anabolic, used primarily before contests to promote size/ muscularity	As in 1.	As in 1.
3. Nadroline Phenylpropionate (Durabolin)	Shorter acting version of Deca-Durabolin	As for Deca-Durabolin	As in 1.	As in 1.
4. Oxandrolone (Anavar)	As in 2., plus relief of bone pain in osteoporosis	Anabolic "cutting" drug, power drug supposedly increases strength	As in 1.	As in 1.
5. Oxymetholone (Anadrol 50)	Treatment of anemias due to deficient RBC production, bone marrow failure	Androgenic strength/ bulking drug, adds size and strength	As in 1.	As in 1.

STEROIDS

NAME	CLINICAL USE	BODYBUILDERS USE	CONTRAINDICATIONS	SIDE EFFECTS
6. Stanzolol (Winstrol, Stromba, Stromba Set, Winstrol V)	Hereditary angloedema (hereditary immune system malfunction)	Anabolic cutting-up drug	As in 1.	As in 1.
7. Methandrostenolone (Dianabol)	As for Durabolin	Anabolic to promote weight gain, size increases	As in 1.	As in 1.
8. Methenolone (Primobolin)	As for Durabolin—not available in USA	Anabolic to promote weight gain, size increases	As in 1.	As in 1.
9. Boldenone Undecylenate (Equipoise)	Post-op convalescence of older HORSES (veterinary drug)	Size, strength increase	As in 1.	As in 1.
10. Sustanon 250 (testosterone injection)	Four testosterones in one injection; promotes even blood androgen level	Size/strength bulking drug	As in 1.	As in 1.

GROWTH HORMONE STIMULATORS

NAME	CLINICAL USE	BODYBUILDERS USE	CONTRAINDICATIONS	SIDE EFFECTS
1. Human growth hormone (protropin, asellincrin, cresorman)	Treatment of growth disorders in children due to genetic lack of hGH	Anabolic agent to promote size/strength increase, lipolytic (fat burning) agent	Prepubertal use may produce "giantism," known neoplasms, pituitary tumors	Acromegaly (excessive growth of jaw, hands, feet, tongue, forehead, etc.) diabetes, promotes neoplasm
2. L-dopa	Parkinson's disease	To promote release of growth hormone	Skin cancer (melanoma)	Cardiac effects, gastrointestinal discomfort, psychosis

NAME	CLINICAL USE	BODYBUILDERS USE	CONTRAINDICATIONS	SIDE EFFECTS
THYROID				
1. Triacana (thyroid)	Hypothyroid states (low thyroid)	Cutting-up agent used to hype "metabolism"	Hyperthyroidism, heart disease	Excessive cardiac stimulation, nervousness, tremors, excessive sweating, muscle loss
2. Cytomel (T3 Thyroid)	As for Triacana	Cutting-up agent used to hype "metabolism"	Hyperthyroidism, heart disease	Excessive cardiac stimulation, nervousness, tremors, excessive sweating, muscle loss
3. Synthroid (TY Thyroid)	Longer acting version of thyroid	Cutting-up agent used to hype "metabolism"	Hyperthyroidism, heart disease	Excessive cardiac stimulation, nervousness, tremors, excessive sweating, muscle loss
ESTROGEN BLOCKERS				
1. Nolvadex (Tomoxifen Citrate)	Anti-estrogen agent for breast cancer, male infertility	Prevention and ameloriation of gynecomastic "bitch tits"; cutting agent for females	None known	Promotion of eye diseases; in women, "chemical menopause" hot flashes, nausea, vomiting
2. Testlax (Testolactone)	Anti-tumor agent for breast cancer	Estrogen blocker prevents "bitch tits"	Breast cancer in males	High blood pressure, edema, nausea

AMPHETAMINES

NAME	CLINICAL USE	BODYBUILDERS USE	CONTRAINDICATIONS	SIDE EFFECTS
1. Dexedrine (Dextroamphetamine)	Narcolepsy, attention deficit disorder, antiobesity	"Speed" energy enhancement, anorexic to reduce appetite	Arteriosclerosis, cardiovascular disease, hypertension, hyperthyroidism, glaucoma	Increased body heat, high blood pressure, amphetamine "psychosis," cardiovascular effects, acute mental confusion
2. Methamphetamine	Narcolepsy, attention deficit disorder, antiobesity	"Speed" energy enhancement, anorexic to reduce appetite	Arteriosclerosis, cardiovascular disease, hypertension, hyperthyroidism, glaucoma	Increased body heat, high blood pressure, amphetamine "psychosis," cardiovascular effects, acute mental confusion
3. Ritalin (Methylphenidate)	Narcolepsy, attention deficit disorder, antiobesity	"Speed" energy enhancement, anorexic to reduce appetite	Arteriosclerosis, cardiovascular disease, hypertension, hyperthyroidism, glaucoma	Increased body heat, high blood pressure, amphetamine "psychosis," cardiovascular effects, acute mental confusion

ANTI-INFLAMMATORY

NAME	CLINICAL USE	BODYBUILDERS USE	CONTRAINDICATIONS	SIDE EFFECTS
1. Lasix (Furosemide)	Diuretic-edema, hypertension, pulmonary edema	Diuretic to eliminate sodium and water retention especially before a contest	Kidney failure	Hypokalemia (low blood potassium), nausea, vomiting, dizziness, vertigo, cardiovascular complications
2. Spironolactone (Aldactone)	Diuretic-hypertension hyperaldosteronism	Diuretic blocks sodium retention	Kidney failure, high blood potassium levels	Gynecomastia, cramps, diarrhea, high potassium levels

FIGURE 29-1

Drugs and Their Interactions

	NAME	CLINICAL USE	BODYBUILDERS USE	CONTRAINDICATIONS	SIDE EFFECTS
ANTI-INFLAMMATORY	Non-Steroidal Anti-inflammatory (aspirin)	Reduce inflammation, pain, arthritic states	Same as clinical use	Allergic reactions to these drugs	Gastrointestinal pain, edema, tinnitus, nervousness
	Cortisone (Decadron, Aristocort, Depo-Medrol, etc.)	Adrenal insufficiency, rheumatic disorders, collagen diseases, skin diseases, allergic states	Pain/inflammation, use to treat joint/tendon injuries	Systemic fungal infections, drug hypersensitivity	Sodium/water retention, potassium/calcium loss, muscle catabolism, peptic ulcers, pituitary suppressant
HCG	Human chorionic gonadotropin (Pregnyl)	Cryptochidism, hypogonadal states, female infertility	Promotes fat loss (unproven); stimulates endrogenous testosterone production	Precocious puberty, prostate cancer, other androgen-dependent tumors	Headache, irritability, fatigue, restlessness, depression, edema, gynecomastia

WHAT ALTERNATIVES DO ATHLETES HAVE?

I still believe that natural means of stimulating hGH release is the most beneficial alternative to shooting up.

1. Exercise stimulates hGH release. So do high temperatures. I recommend training in a warm gym—above 74°–76°.

2. Pain and extreme stress both release beta-endorphins into the bloodstream. Thus, make your training more productive in its hGH-releasing capacity by avoiding pain and unnecessarily high-stress exercises. Extreme effort and extreme stress are not the same. Effort, yes. Pain or unnecessary stress, no.

3. Avoid training or going to bed with a bellyful of carbohydrates. High blood glucose will inhibit hGH release exactly when you need it most.

4. Avoid doing the same old exercises or training protocol all the time. Changing routines will inject new adaptive stress, of the positive kind, into your training and in so doing will promote hGH release. If your body has already "adapted" to the stress provided by your old system of training, there will be no further adaptation. This is sometimes referred to as *habituation*.

5. Use arginine/ornithine supplements before training and before going to bed (about one hour before training and immediately before going to bed).

6. Go to bed with little to eat, especially carbs, in order to keep blood sugar in the normal-to-low range.

7. Train with just enough blood glucose to get you through your training and to replace spent stores immediately after training. Training with high blood sugar, remember, inhibits hGH release.

8. The fatter you are, the lower your hGH response to exercise will be (Daugheday, 1985; Galbo, 1983; Marimee, 1979). If you're fat—with a percent of body fat above 15% (men) or 20% (women)—get rid of the baggage, and you'll begin making better muscular gains.

9. Women tend to have higher hGH responses to exercise than men, presumably because of their higher estrogen levels, because they're generally less fit than their male counterparts, or because they respond psychologically to exercise with more stress than men (Shepherd & Sydney, 1975; Galbo, 1983).

30

HERBS: NATURE'S SPORTS PHARMACY

One very important caution has to be mentioned up front. When taken in excess or when combined with other substances or herbs, some herbs can be dangerous, so never assume that "more is better." Seek the advice and guidance of your coach before using herbs. In fact, talking to your family doctor first is a good idea.

Not too long ago, there was no such thing as drugs. Throughout the history of mankind on planet Earth, on into the twentieth century, medical practitioners relied on the bounties provided by Mother Nature for their curative potions. Every species of flower, root, fruit, leaf, bark—even microscopic algae—had long since been exploited by ancient man for its medicinal properties. But the exploitation of Earth's botanical bounty was not limited to medicinal purposes.

No, indeed! Man, you see, has always been ascendant in his thinking. Good health and freedom from disease were not enough— he wanted more than he was born with. He wanted greater powers of concentration, stronger muscles, heightened awareness, and keener survival skills of various sorts. And he wanted to have fun— to play and to make sport.

The wherewithal to improve his physical and mental powers and to engage in sporting endeavors, and thus improve his lot in life, has, since time immemorial, been amplified and supported by powerful substances contained in the plant life of this world. Botanicals— herbal medicines—are man's gift from the Creator. That they are effective is self-evident. Millennia of use by man and thousands upon thousands of research projects give testament to this fact. A vast majority of today's powerful drugs are directly botanical in origin.

It is curious that no one in the history of elite sports has ever combined the power of age-old herbal substances with the technologically advanced nutritional wizardry of our modern age. No one, that is, until now.

Surely, the future of maximum sports performance and bodybuilding excellence is grounded in both the wisdom of the past and the magnificent technological achievements of our scientific age. Powerful and effective herbs have always been here and are here to stay. When they've been programmatically incorporated into scientifically devised training and nutritional regimens, the results have proved astounding indeed.

Over the centuries, man has devised countless botanical preparations. Recent studies have provided us with the knowledge of how many of these substances affect our bodies' functions. Athletes from all sports, including bodybuilders, have found certain herbs and mixtures of herbs to be assistive in their training programs. Here's what they can do for you:

1. Assist in establishing a more conducive systemic and biochemically receptive bodily foundation upon which you can build
2. Help develop the ability to both restore from and adapt to the stresses of intense training, which in turn allows you to then amplify the training for speedier and continued adaptation
3. Effectively assist in building muscle mass
4. Effectively assist in improving your strength levels
5. Assist in improving upon both your oxygen delivery and utilization systems for greater levels of endurance

Few herbs have the power to accomplish these goals by themselves. Most herbs work best when they're combined with others that act as their support systems. The science and art of blending herbs has been with us as long as recorded history. Here is a brief description of what scientifically blended herbal preparations can do for you.

DEVELOPING A FOUNDATION

The word *foundation* says it all. The first step in establishing a firm foundation upon which you build your sports or bodybuilding career is to prepare your body for better use of supplements and dietary intake. In this way, you will find it easier to recover and grow in response to your heavy training loads. This is done through a cleansing formula for your kidneys, liver, colon, and blood. Prominent mention was made of this fact in each of the training programs presented in Part Two of this book.

The second step in building your solid foundation is to improve your body's wound-healing processes. After all, each intense workout inflicts tremendous stresses on your muscles and other tissues. The third step—accomplished right along with the second step—is to maximize your body's adaptive responses to the stresses of training. In these ways, your herbal-based foundation-building efforts gently and efficiently coax your body into a far more strategic position for maintaining improved growth, recovery, and repair for the months of hard training you are about to enter.

Here is a blend of herbs used for foundational training:

- Blood and liver: red clover, burdock, rhubarb, goldenseal, milk thistle, licorice, and dandelion
- Kidney: cornsilk, couchgrass, hydrangea, uva ursa, and althea root
- Colon: psyllium husk and flax seed

IMPROVING YOUR BODY'S ADAPTATION PROCESSES

Russian sports scientists, coaches, and athletes—even their elite cosmonauts—have known for years that your body has to be able to adapt to the rigors of high-intensity training if maximum gains in strength, recovery ability, and muscle growth are to be had. There is no magic formula or carefully guarded state secret about it. The one substance of choice over all other substances on the face of planet Earth the Russians use to accomplish this important mission is Siberian ginseng—eleutherococcus senticosus, or ED for short. They use it every day of their lives. So should you.

BUILDING MUSCLE MASS

When practiced individually, neither training nor eating can ensure that your muscles will grow to their full potential in size or strength. In the earlier part of this century, before drugs of any sort were ever invented, doctors and laymen alike knew that certain substances from Mother Nature's bountiful medicine chest provided mild, steady, long-term effectiveness in promoting tissue growth. The combination of botanicals in a well-designed herbal mass-building formula provides your body with both anabolism-enhancing and catabolism-limiting capabilities to make better use of your training efforts and nutritional intake in producing the maximum gains in muscle mass humanly possible.

Here's a blend of herbs that can be assistive, along with proper training and nutrition:

Sarsaparilla root (Smilax officianalis)
Wild yam root (Dioscorea villosa)
Saw palmetto fruit (Serenoa serrulata)
Siberian ginseng (Eleutherococcus senticosus)
Damiana leaf (Turnera Diffusa)
Avina sativa (oat)
Licorice root (Glycyrrhiza glabra)
Fenugreek seed (Trigonella foenum-graecum)

IMPROVING YOUR STRENGTH AND POWER

Like mass training, strength-training science has come of age and in the process has come full circle. We have finally come to realize the wisdom of the ancients in their reliance on Earth's bountiful plant life for sustaining, healing, and strengthening properties. Our modern advantage, however, is that we have borrowed age-old wisdom from the four corners of Earth and combined these strength-generating ingredients with our scientific knowledge of training science and nutrition.

This blend of herbs can improve your strength when combined with proper training and nutrition:

Ginkgo (Ginkgo biloba)
Yerba maté (Ilex paraguayensis)
Blue vervain (Verbena officianalis)
Wood betony (Betonica officianalis)
Avena sativa (oat)

IMPROVING YOUR
BODY'S RESTORATIVE PROCESSES

The advantage of youth is that you recover from the stresses of intense training or competition much faster. The faster you can restore your body, the more often you can train harder. That, of course, relates to better gains over a shorter period of time. The botanical ingredients contained in a well-conceived restorative formula are designed to restore this benefit of youth or, if you're already young, to amplify the benefits of youth by gently coaxing your body to restore itself faster and more fully. In addition, many of the ill effects of the natural process of aging can be either eliminated completely or radically slowed. Then, and only then, can you construct your training cycle in such a way that you can train harder more often for years to come.

Your body's restorative process can be assisted by the following blend of herbs along with proper training and nutrition:

Horsetail grass (Equisetum arvense)
Saw palmetto fruit (Serenoa serrulata)
Fenugreek seed (Trigonella foenum-graecum)
Teasel root (Dipsacus asper)
Fleece flower root (Polygonum multiflorum)
Ginkgo (Ginkgo biloba)
Capsicum fruit

OTHER HERBS OF INTEREST TO BODYBUILDERS

Scores of botanical preparations in addition to those mentioned above are or have been used for sports and bodybuilding purposes. Some of the more common ones are outlined in Figure 30-1. Others are briefly discussed in the following chapter.

FIGURE 30-1
Herbs and Their Historical and Bodybuilding Uses

Herb	Antistress	Immune response	Cardiovascular	Environ. toxins	Antiaging	Digestion	Sleep	Pain	Fat loss	Muscle	Energy	Recovery/repair	Female problems
PLANTAIN TREE								*				*	
YARROW		*			*			*				*	*
ALFALFA			*						*				
CHICKWEED		*						*	*			*	
COMFREY									*			*	
VERVAIN									*			*	*
EVENING PRIMROSE		*	*		*			*	*				*
ONION	*												
GARLIC	*												
GINGER													
CAYENNE	*	*	*			*						*	
BLACK COHOSH	*							*				*	*
SKULLCAP	*		*				*	*					
GENTIAN						*	*						
CHAMOMILE	*	*				*	*					*	
CELERY SEED								*	*				
WHITE WILLOW BARK								*	*				
CHAENOMELES LAGENARIA								*	*				
ELEUTHEROCOCCUS SENTICOSUS (SIBERIAN GINSENG)												*	
LICORICE										*			
XU DUAN										*			
HE-SHOU-WU					*								
JUJUBE										*			
KOLA NUT										*			
YERBA MATE										*			
ASTRAGALOS MEMBRANACEUS			*							*		*	
PRICKLY ASH						*						*	
SAINT-JOHN'S-WORT	*												*
BLUE COHOSH													*
CHASTEBERRY													*
CODONOPSIS											*		
REHMANNIA GLUTINOSA					*								
HAWTHORN BERRIES	*		*		*						*		
PASSIONFLOWER	*		*				*						
VALERIAN	*		*				*	*					*
CATNIP	*	*				*							
HOPS	*						*						
MILKWEED					*								
SARSAPARILLA			*			*			*			*	
BURDOCK			*			*						*	
RED CLOVER			*						*			*	
GOTU KOLA			*								*	*	
BERBERIS			*			*		*				*	
GOLDENSEAL	*	*	*			*						*	*
YELLOW DOCK		*	*			*						*	
ECHINACEA		*	*										
ORIENTAL GINSENG	*	*		*			*				*	*	*
ALOE VERA		*		*		*		*			*	*	
GINKGO TREE			*										
DANDELION ROOT				*	*	*					*	*	
CHAPARRAL		*		*	*								

*Ratings based on research and logical inference from theory and practice.

31

ANTIOXIDANTS: MOTHER NATURE'S ULTIMATE ERGOGEN

In your pursuit of excellence, you engage in high-volume, high-intensity training. The stresses on your body cause tissue hypoxia, and a performance-limiting array of metabolic wastes and blood-borne free radicals begin to accumulate. Fatigue and overtraining sets in.

Vince Lombardi said it best: "Fatigue makes cowards of us all." More precisely, postexercise fatigue can devastate your recovery capabilities. Postexercise fatigue limits everyone's ability to come back again, to train harder and more often for better gains.

Soviet dominance in the sports arena is legendary. That same dominance has, if the 1992 Olympic Games are any barometer, been carried on with the newly formed Commonwealth of Independent States (C.I.S.). For decades, the Russians' clear advantage in most sports has been a source of puzzlement to western coaches and athletes alike. How can they dominate the rest of the world in so many different sports? Do they have some sort of secret method or elixir that catapults their athletes beyond the abilities of their competitors?

Their sports scientists have known for years that postworkout fatigue and muscle soreness, and therefore overtraining, are caused by three major factors: tissue hypoxia (lack of oxygen to the working muscles), an accumulation of waste products such as lactic acid in both the liver and in the muscles, and cumulative microtrauma (a buildup of small but widespread tears in your muscle cells from training stress over weeks and months of time).

The greater the fatigue or overtraining, the lower your performance level will be. Decreasing your training load will not make you a better bodybuilder, and it won't allow you to achieve your true potential in mass. It's critical that you improve your recovery ability so you can handle greater training stresses better and more often.

While western sports specialists have concentrated on efforts to stimulate the body, C.I.S. teams of sports specialists focused on the more important problem of how the body recovers more quickly and more fully. By recovering more quickly, you can work out harder more often without overtraining or undue fatigue. That adds up to vastly improved performance. Interested?

THE PERPETUAL BATTLE AGAINST FREE RADICALS

You can take an immense step in the right direction now. That is, you can join in the ongoing fight—minute by minute—against the ravages of free radicals. You cannot win the war against fatigue and overtraining all the time, any more than you can win the war against old age. But you can win many, many of the battles. This approach to training for peak performance makes common sense.

Conditions of normal metabolism, radiation, exercise, ozone exposure, carcinogens, and other environmental toxins cause oxygen molecules inside our bodies to break down. Losing one of its electrons to another molecule during such processes causes the oxygen molecule to become highly reactive, capable of combining with other molecules in its quest for another electron to take the place of the one lost. In this volatile state, it becomes known as a free radical.

When the renegade molecule finds an electron mate, it bonds with it, causing it to have an extra electron. This new electron makes that molecule highly reactive, and a self-perpetuating vicious cycle begins. Cell membranes are destroyed, immune system integrity is compromised, and DNA—your cells' master regulators—is altered or destroyed.

The big question for bodybuilders is what to do about these little bitty devils scientists call free radicals. By far the most important prophylaxis against the ravages of free radicals is prevention. Some preventive measures are abstaining from smoking, strictly adhering to a carefully constructed—integrated—training program (including your diet), and avoiding pollutants and other toxic substances known to cause free radical formation.

There are also well-known scavengers of these free radicals, collectively known as antioxidants. Over the past few years, it has become scientific dogma that these antioxidants indeed make a difference in your ability to train and recover more quickly.

Dr. William Pryor, professor of biochemistry at Louisiana State University, says, "There's been a renaissance in free radical biology in the past decade. Within the next ten or so years, [our greater knowledge of how best to fight free radical damage] will promote a modest extension in life span—perhaps five to eight years."

Professor Pryor is not alone in this belief. Working in the USC-based Institute for Toxicology, Drs. Paul Hochstein and Kelvin Davies, together with their colleagues, have dedicated their total time and resources to understanding free radicals, the damage they cause, and how to combat them or prevent their formation. According to their research, your body's built-in repair mechanisms—certain enzymatic free radical–scavenging and salvage systems—aren't capable of handling the onslaught. The cumulative effect of free-radical damage over time may diminish the cell's ability to make these repairs. This may be what causes some of the physical degeneration of aging, explained Dr. Davies.

There is no doubt that the repair-limiting free radicals decrease an athlete's ability to recover from training as well. The following definitions are designed to further educate you on free radicals and how to fight them. There are also short descriptions of substances from Mother Nature's sports pharmacy which may prove to be powerful alternatives for you in your quest for bodybuilding excellence. Take them seriously.

FREE RADICALS

Free radicals are highly reactive molecules which target your tissue's protein bonds, the DNA in your cells' nuclei, and the important polyunsaturated fatty acids within your cells' membranes. Once initiated, a chain reaction begins that ultimately results in the total destruction of that cell. Scientists have determined that over sixty age-related maladies are a direct result of long-term damage resulting from free radical activity. There are seven different species of free radicals.

FIGURE 31-1

Species of Free Radicals and How to Combat Them

SPECIES OF FREE RADICALS	CORRESPONDING ANTIOXIDANTS
Superoxide anion radical	NDGA Vitamin C Glutathione (GSH) Maria thistle (assists GSH) Ginkgo biloba
Hydrogen peroxide	Glutathione (GSH) Maria thistle (assists GSH) Ginkgo biloba
Hydroxyl radical	NDGA Vitamin C Ginkgo biloba
Singlet oxygen	Vitamin A Vitamin E Glutathione (GSH) Maria thistle (assists GSH) Selenium and Bilberry (assists vitamin E) Ginkgo biloba
Polyunsaturated fatty acid radical	NDGA Vitamin A Vitamin E Selenium and bilberry (assists vitamin E) Maria thistle
Organic/fatty acid hydroperoxides	NDGA Glutathione (GSH) Maria thistle (assists GSH) Ginkgo biloba
Oxidized protein	Glutathione (GSH) Maria thistle (assists GSH) Ginkgo biloba

ANTIOXIDANTS

Antioxidants work both directly and indirectly against all or some of the seven known species of free radicals. They directly combat free radicals, potentiate other antioxidants, inhibit formation of free radicals, prevent the depletion of antioxidants, or prevent the depletion of other substances which potentiate the activity of antioxidants. The secret to successful antioxidant therapy is a combinational approach in which the antioxidants work synergistically in restoring normal function to all bodily tissues.

NDGA

NDGA (nor-di-hydro-guai-aretic acid) is the primary active constituent of the chaparral bush, which grows in the southwestern USA to over one thousand years old. It is widely known in the scientific community as a powerful antioxidant and has the official designation as a lipoxygenase inhibitor. Both research and folklore classify NDGA as effective in cellular respiration, analgesic activity, anti-inflammatory activity, and vasodepressant activity.

Bilberry

The active components of bilberries are the anthocyanosides. During World War II, bilberry jam became very popular among Allied Forces pilots because it promoted superior visual acuity, especially while flying at night. Both folklore and studies show that bilberry extract protects blood capillaries, protects the heart, shows excellent anti-inflammatory action, inhibits cholesterol-induced atherosclerosis, and inhibits serum platelet aggregation (clotting). Its chief action as an antioxidant is its powerful synergy with vitamin E.

Ginkgo Biloba

Native to China and Japan, the ginkgo tree lives over one thousand years. The active components of ginkgo leaves are quercetin and the flavoglycosides. Ginkgo extract is shown to reduce clots or thrombi formation in the veins and arteries, increase cellular energy by increasing cellular glucose and ATP, scavenge free radicals, prevent the formation of free radicals, reduce high blood pressure, promote peripheral blood flow (especially to the brain), and ameliorate inner-ear problems. Ginkgo also has been shown to improve alertness, short-term memory, and various cognitive disorders.

Maria Thistle

The active compound in Maria thistle is silymarin. It is known to be a potent hepatoprotector and antihepatotoxic agent (thereby restoring normal metabolic function to the liver), promote cellular regeneration via increased protein synthesis, aid in protecting the kidneys, and act as a powerful antioxidant principally through its sparing effects on glutathione (which also probably accounts for its potency in improving liver function).

Selenium, Glutathione, and Vitamins A, C, and E

The element selenium is an important constituent of the enzyme glutathione peroxidase. Vitamin E and selenium tend to enhance the effects of one another in that vitamin E works to prevent the formation of free radicals (peroxides) and glutathione peroxidase destroys those already present.

Selenium is an important part of the body's immune response system and blood-clotting mechanism. Vitamins A, C, and E are all powerful antioxidants. Natural vitamin E (d-alpha tocopherol succinate, as opposed to the synthetic version, dl alpha tocopherol acetate) is particularly effective in reducing exercise-induced lipid peroxide free radicals. Vitamin A (beta-carotene) appears particularly effective in preventing and treating pathologies involving singlet oxygen radicals triggered by intense sunlight. Vitamin C (ascorbate) is a real workhorse, both scavenging superoxide and hydroxyl radicals and potentiating the beneficial effects of many other substances in both the diet and certain nutritional supplements.

OXYGEN

It's life itself. To a bodybuilder, getting enough oxygen spells the difference between peak performance and also-ran status. The conventional method of delivering oxygen to your working muscles is breathing it. Period. Studies conducted over decades by C.I.S. sports scientists, and more recently in the U.S.A., show that when pure oxygen is taken into the stomach, the oxygen content of the blood, and therefore of the working muscles, is increased by 40 percent. The results are more effective repayment of the oxygen debt incurred during severe training, faster and more effective post-workout recovery, improved energy, improved tissue healing, faster waste elimination, and a decided upswing in performance and fitness levels.

Research has also shown that the oxygen content of the liver is increased by over 40 percent by ingesting oxygen combined with a specially formulated drink, as opposed to just 8 percent when oxygen is inhaled (Pilipenko, 1967; Gotovtsev et al., 1973; and others).

The "Oxygen Cocktail"

The concept of an oxygenated drink for athletes in need of rapid recovery was introduced to the world at the 1956 Olympic Games in Melbourne by the newly arriving Soviets (Yessis, 1990). The practice is reported to have originated with the Nazis in 1939, who used the technique to rejuvenate overworked factory personnel.

In the tradition of the Nazis' utilitarian approach, the Soviets' team of sports specialists focused on the problem of how the body recovers more quickly and more fully. By recovering more quickly, they reasoned, an athlete can work out harder more often.

Several methods of oxygenating the small and large intestines have been well researched (Ekkert and Gromova, 1986; Malone, 1987; Ugolev, Bagiian, and Ekkert, 1980). There is, for example, a substantial body of literature on the effects rectal oxygen insufflation has on oxygen diffusion through the mucosa of the colon (Klug, 1988).

In general, the findings as reported appear to fall into four broad categories of effect: improved transport of various nutrients (especially glucose); the beneficial effects of an oxygenated (as opposed to nitrogenous) intestinal atmosphere on the epithelium lining (and thus absorption of various nutrients); the reduction of endotoxin absorption (Shute, 1977); and the diffusion of oxygen through the mucosa of the colon into the vessels of the submucous coat and, in small but significant measure, into the general blood-stream (Klug, Knoch, and Muller, 1988).

Making more efficient use of inspired oxygen is another avenue of improving performance that has been reported in the literature. One technique that has received less than widespread attention is the use of various nutritional supplements and botanicals. One such aid, octacosanol, is contained in the commercial drink known as the Oxygen Cocktail.

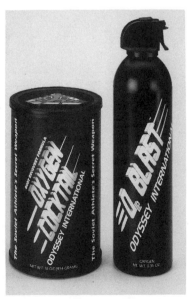

Octacosanol, the active component of the long-popular natural food supplement researched extensively by Dr. Thomas K. Cureton from the University of Illinois, wheat germ oil, has been shown to be an aid in improved stamina and endurance. Research shows that octacosanol reduces muscle cells' need for oxygen, meaning that you can go farther with a lower oxygen debt. It has also been shown to aid in the storage of muscle glycogen (stored sugar for energy). Curiously, according to one research study, it reduced reaction time.

While no non-Soviet research has been conducted recently specifically relating to the Oxygen Cocktail, there is substantial research evidence supporting the hypothesis that enteral delivery of oxygen results in a greater level of oxygen reaching the working muscles, resulting in an increase in work capacity and recovery ability. This improved oxygenation appears to be the result of one or more of the four avenues of effect noted above.

PART EIGHT

ADVANCED TECHNIQUES AND THEORIES

DEDICATED TO DAVID DEARTH

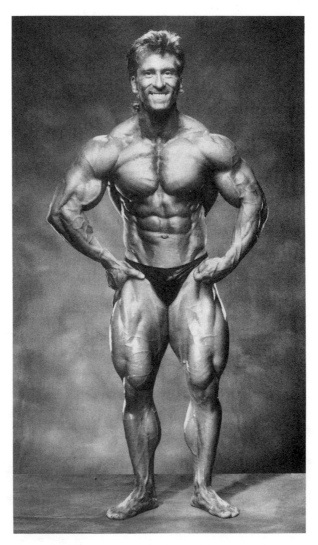

David Dearth

32

FORCED REPS

"Push, you wimp."

"Bear down!"

"Take it!"

Such noises are part and parcel of the everyday sounds in bodybuilding gyms everywhere. They're happy sounds, for they fill the air with the exuberance of striving for a goal with the joy of effort and, not so coincidentally, with the agony of defeat.

The failure that such sounds proclaim inspires one. You see, allowing yourself to be defeated by the heavy weight in your hands is not really failure at all. Your friend having to assist you on the last few reps does not really signal your demise. It simply means that you have learned a major lesson in achieving muscle building overload—you have finally learned the secret of taking your mind and body one step beyond mere sensation. You have learned how to coax your very being through the near-impenetrable barrier and into a twilight zone of painless effort, of positive failure, of incomprehensible growth potential.

Those of you who have experienced this advanced state of being know that I refer to a system of training dubbed forced reps. For those of you who haven't experienced it, you have my sympathy and my admonition to try. The time is now!

THE SCIENCE OF FORCED REPS

Rory Leidelmeyer, a great bodybuilder of the early eighties, related a story to me that very aptly describes the basic science behind forced reps. The story is a short one, so please bear with me.

A man decided to become a lumberjack and went into the woods to chop trees. All season he chopped away and his forearms grew from 12 inches to 15 inches in girth. The following year, he reentered the woods and came out again with 15-inch arms. Likewise the year after.

The point, said Leidelmeyer, is that the stress remained the same year in and year out. The lumberjack could not expect to get bigger arms merely by putting in more training time. The only way his arms could've grown beyond 15 inches is if he began using a bigger axe.

There are a lot of other ways of telling the same story. For example, all your life you've been walking on your legs. No additional walking is going to inspire them to further growth. No, you must begin to walk up stairs or walk with weights! Of course, an easier and more controllable alternative is to do squats.

The point is clear. Forced reps are a way of progressing one more rung up the ladder of training intensity. Forced reps are a way of making your muscles work harder than they have grown accustomed to and therefore continue growing.

The science behind forced reps, then, is the same science behind every other system of training you've ever experienced. Simply put, overload forces your muscles to adapt to ever-increasing stress. As one plateau is conquered, additional stress must be applied for continued adaptation to occur.

Partner-Assisted Exercise

Another name for forced reps is partner-assisted exercise. To the uninitiated or the inexperienced, having someone help you lift a weight seems somewhat self-defeating. "Why in blazes is he helping you lift?" is the erstwhile bodybuilder's query. "If you can't do it yourself, then it ain't doing you any good!" is the same dullard's admonition.

Tch, tch! I beg you to stop and think. As motor units shut down from fatigue (usually the fast-twitch fibers first) during a set, fresh fibers must bear the load. I believe that by rallying all of your inner reserves of strength and mental concentration, you assist in either lowering the excitation thresholds of hard-to-stimulate motor units, increase the level of millivoltage (stimulation) reaching the muscle, or both of the above.

With your partner assisting you through a tortuous three or four final reps, your mind and muscle have time to respond to this superstress. I believe the adaptive response you'll undergo is improved growth in size and strength. I believe it comes from the improved overload. The improved overload, in turn, stems from the greater time over which maximum overload is being applied.

One of the primary reasons why bodybuilders rarely do singles in training is they're not productive in improving size. Why? Not because the weight isn't heavy enough—rather, because the heavy weight isn't allowed to stress the muscle for a sufficient length of time!

Your partner helps you through three or four extra reps when you're using a heavy weight to increase the time that adaptive overload is being applied.

FORCED REPS WITH LIGHT WEIGHTS OR HEAVY WEIGHTS?

How much weight should you use when doing forced reps? There are many schools of thought on that one. Really, the answer is quite simple—it can easily be understood if you have any concept of the principles related in Parts One and Two.

Integrated training demands that you perform with heavy weights (myofibrillar elements in the muscle), light weights (for mitochondria in the muscle cells), fast movements (for the fast-twitch muscle fibers), slow movements (for the slow-twitch muscle fibers)—and everything in between!

Integrated training also demands the same kind of approach to your forced-reps training. The difference is that throughout all of your various sets (light, heavy, fast, or slow) you'll be using a weight that is about 5–10 percent heavier than you normally would use. For example, if you bench press with 300 pounds when you're performing sets of ten reps, you should add 30 pounds or so. Now, you'll only be able to perform six or seven reps and your partner will have to assist in the last three or four reps.

The same basic system can be applied to all of your sets and various exercises. Again, the only real difference between conventional set/rep systems and forced reps is that with forced reps you're using more weight than you can handle for the target number of reps in each set, and your partner has to assist. The same principles of training apply.

WHEN TO USE FORCED REPS

Should all bodybuilders use forced reps? Probably, but not as a sole means of applying overload and not all the time. Not when you're injured, overtrained, coming off an off-cycle, just beginning, or alone in the gym.

When beginners and bodybuilders returning to training after a layoff have accustomed themselves to the weights—a period generally lasting about 4–5 weeks at most—forced reps can be used effectively.

I have heard many bodybuilders and fitness experts tell beginners that forced reps should not be used by anyone other than the most experienced bodybuilders. Rubbish! Why not? Forced reps are a better way to overload and therefore can be used for greater gains by anyone. But because of the intensity involved, they should only be used once in a while. Many systems have been used over the years to incorporate forced reps into one's training. Here are a few of the most often used methods.

- One workout per week for each major muscle group
- Three workouts in a row followed by conventional training for the next three or four workouts
- Every other workout
- At the end of every steroid cycle (perhaps once popular, but nowadays considered nonsensical, unhealthy, and certainly against the law!)
- For a period of a week or so within the framework of a training cycle that goes from low- to high-intensity techniques over a period of 8–10 weeks total

All of these strategies are old technology at best and barely adequate by today's scientific standards. The bottom line is to use forced reps within the structure of the "ABC" integrated bodybuilding system (see Part Two) as follows: during "A" workouts only for muscles that Mother Nature intended to be used for heavy loads (e.g., your multipennate muscles such as delts or quads); during "B" workouts for lagging body parts especially, but any time you're doing sets of 12 reps; and never during "C" workouts.

33

CHEATING MOVEMENTS

The word *cheat* is used to describe someone who's trying to get away with something—someone who's looking for the easy way, typically at the expense of someone or something else. The same holds true when the word is applied to training science.

Erstwhile purists of the art and science of bodybuilding state that if you're cheating, you're trying to get something for nothing. They say that you'll end up getting nothing. But they're wrong.

In reality, the technique of cheating in bodybuilding can be done the right way or the wrong way, for the right reasons or the wrong ones. You can, during training sessions designed to emphasize your fast-twitch (white) muscle fibers, swing or heave the weight. That's one good reason for doing cheating movements. Two other reasons are not as good.

Some bodybuilders say that in cheating past a sticking point with a weight that ordinarily couldn't be lifted using strict form, they're getting adaptive overload during a portion of the muscle's range of motion that otherwise may never have received any. They also point to the fact that, since the weight being used is heavier, the overload is greater.

I reject both points of view as sheer poppycock. If you're engaged in good, scientific, integrated "ABC" bodybuilding (see Part Two), the only logical reason for selecting a cheating movement is for better white-fiber adaptation. However, this method of cheating should be done in such a way that the weight is heaved just far enough to get by your sticking point. For example, in doing curls, your sticking point will always be when the elbow is approaching a 90-degree angle.

If you cheat a weight all the way through the exercise movement, you run the risks of causing muscle, connective tissue, or joint microtrauma from ballistic stress or deriving too little adaptive overload. Swinging the weight all the way through a movement is only productive if you've mastered the technique of compensatory acceleration.

Compensating for a joint's improving leverage as movement continues by accelerating the bar has the net effect of improving the adaptive overload on the muscle. This is the same rationale used by the manufacturers of both accommodating resistance machines (such as Keiser air machines) and variable resistance machines (such as Nautilus machines).

However, these technologies compensate for improving leverage by controlling movement speed. They're both excellent. A far more natural way of compensating is to accelerate the bar. In so doing, you're getting adaptive overload throughout the entire range of motion and it's happening in a way that is not foreign to your body's motor memory. Mechanically controlled speed is not natural and is therefore foreign to your nervous system.

While accommodating and variable resistance technologies are good, compensatory acceleration is better. Remember, your white muscle fibers can only receive stimulation with explosive movements, so the cheating technique of compensatory acceleration is vital to maximum bodybuilding success.

34

TO BE GREAT, GET LAZY!

"Three in the afternoon. Fading fast. Gotta get psyched! Workout's at five! Coffee. Yeah! That's the ticket! Maybe if I take a walk or something! I'm so tired!"

If science has shown us anything about the ubiquitous midafternoon slump in energy, it's that you shouldn't fight it. It's a universal characteristic, it's normal, it's good, and it isn't necessarily due to poor eating habits, as is so often claimed. Go with the flow! Take a nap.

I know, I know! In our country, taking a nap—a midday siesta—isn't socially acceptable. Neither is it always feasible if you're working for a living. All over the world people close up shop for a couple of midday hours of snoozola. Not in the high-speed U.S.A. though. No, siree! It's as though taking a nap when your body's natural circadian rhythms beg for one would be considered laziness.

Too bad. If you're an athlete in heavy training—especially two-a-days or three-a-days, as most elite bodybuilders nowadays must perform—that nap can be mighty important. Not only will it revitalize you for a more intense noon or evening workout, but it'll provide an important growth hormone response for anabolism to occur, and it'll allow other recuperative processes to take place, making it possible to work out heavy more often.

Recovery. There's that word again. The Russians have spent a lot of time and rubles over the years studying the recovery process in elite athletes. In fact, most of their efforts in sports research has centered on recuperative techniques and substances. Let's look at but one factor in the recovery process—getting lazy.

- Take naps in the afternoon
- Take naps in the morning too if you can
- Keep your naps to about a half hour's duration. Longer than that, and you go into the deeper stages of sleep, causing you to feel groggy thereafter
- If you work during the day, find a nice shady tree or some secluded spot to grab a wink or two during lunch hour (take a late lunch if you can—around two in the afternoon would be ideal)
- Never eat a big lunch or drink alcohol during lunch, as these practices tend to exacerbate (not cause) the midday slump (bodybuilders eat small meals and avoid alcohol anyway)
- Don't sleep eight hours at night. That's too long. Opt instead for a six- or seven-hour sleeping schedule. You'll find that your midmorning and/or midday nap will be sufficient to bring you up to a total of eight hours per twenty-four-hour period.
- During the day, stay lazy. Avoid unnecessary activity, running around, taking long walks, or forcing yourself to stay awake when nature calls. Remember the lesson from the cattle industry—pen the cattle up so they can't range, and feed them plenty of protein throughout the day—and your muscle-growth efforts will be supportively served
- If you suffer from insomnia (about 10 percent of the population suffers from some form of sleep disorder), taking a nap may not be advisable. Instead, consult a sleep disorder specialist. Chronic daytime drowsiness is most often a function of how well—or how poorly—you sleep at night

The two most compelling reasons why elite athletes don't take naps or practice a more sedentary between-workout routine are your boss would fire you if you did and you feel guilty about your apparent laziness because of our social mores. If you can find a way around these two problems—and most athletes can if they really want to—your training and recovery efforts will surely improve.

Most sleep disorder scientists are in agreement that taking a midday nap can be normal, healthy, and contributory to improved alertness and creativity. Consider:

- Thomas Edison took naps
- Winston Churchill took naps
- Ronald Reagan (although he denies it) took naps
- In the final days of his reelection bid, Bush wanted to take naps

- Lee Haney takes naps, even if he has to find a closet to sleep in (true story!)
- Most kids—to support massive growth processes—take naps

Dr. Alan Lankford, director of the Atlanta Sleep Disorder Center, was recently quoted as saying, "people who, for whatever reason, need to take a nap in the afternoon, there's a payoff in increased alertness and better cognitive function, and they're likely to be more productive at work."

As I grow a bit older, I find that taking a nap comes more naturally. At a younger age, I remember wanting to take a nap, but I never did, for various reasons. Mostly because I was too busy, I guess. I didn't know of their potential for improving my training back then. Had I, I would've.

35

COMPUTERS CAN INTEGRATE
TRAINING TECHNOLOGIES BEST

No one can know everything there is to know about bodybuilding science. But a computer can come doggone close!

FOR THE ELITE BODYBUILDERS AMONG YOU

Hard-core ironheads dream a lot. Most elite athletes do. They dream about finding great new ways of getting the most out of their training efforts. They dream about finding some kind of magic elixir—short of drugs like steroids—that will help them along. And they dream about the future and what it may hold in the way of training technology.

Why do they dream? Why don't they just *do* it? You wouldn't ask that if you were inveterate in hard-core training! Training science is complicated—so many things to take into account.

Sure, I know I said training was as easy as ABC in Part One, but come on! Poetic license and all that. At any rate, those A, B, and C workouts—and all the multitudinous elements surrounding them—sure would be easier if there were a computer around, no?

FOR CASUAL BODYBUILDING AND FITNESS ENTHUSIASTS

Most personal trainers are pretty smart folks when it comes to training and nutrition. But in today's scientific world, there's too much to know. There's too much data to absorb and apply. If your personal trainer is so smart, how come he or she hasn't introduced you to integrated training and nutrition yet?

FOR PERSONAL TRAINERS

Most people seeking guidance from a professional fitness trainer are pretty smart folks. That's why they came to an expert like you. They know that in today's scientific world, there's too much information for one person to know and apply. If you're smart, you'll give your clients credit for their intelligence—and give them the sophisticated assistance they deserve and demand—by getting them hooked on integrated training and nutrition.

Your clients and athletes must eat right to lose fat, to develop lean muscle, and to remain healthy and responsive to their training. As a professional, you know that these goals are not easy to attain. That's why a professional group of certified trainers exists—to assist people in their quest for fitness or sports achievement.

I'm sure that you're familiar with the mythical concept of the balanced diet. People miss meals, they overeat, they snack on less-than-healthy food, and they live in and eat foods grown in a compromised environment. Couple these monumental problems with the fact that their rigorous training regimens literally cry out for maximum nutritional support.

Sports training experts have spent years trying to solve the utterly complex problem of creating a truly integrated approach to training, one that will provide maximally effective and personalized sports training, fitness, or fat-loss programs supported by scientific and easy-to-manage diet and nutritional supplementation schedules. All of them have done OK, but that's not good enough! You and your clients and athletes deserve more.

FOR EVERYONE WHO IS "OF IRON"

Brothers and sisters of iron! This is the age of computers!

Why have we been beating our heads against the proverbial brick wall when these powerful tools are there to help us? "Trouble is," you may argue, "if you put garbage into a computer, you'll get garbage coming out." I agree, and that's why so many people who have tried to use the computer in personalizing integrative training and nutrition have failed. Putting it bluntly, ISSA has succeeded. Here are some of the highlights of ISSA's computer support package.

1. The unique nutritional requirements associated with over one hundred common health conditions are accounted for
2. The latest scientific techniques of fat loss, promoting thermogenesis, fine-tuning metabolic adjustment to fat loss, and

improving your body's anabolic climate for more rapid muscle growth and recovery are all accounted for

3. Training periodicity—cycle training—is automatically calculated based on individual recuperative capabilities. Within your training periodicity schedule, microcyclic, mesocyclic, and macrocyclic needs are all accounted for

4. Nutritional supplement needs are outlined in detail, based on personal goals—both immediate and long-range in nature—and current nutritional status

5. Also, periodic followup computer programs and analyses are available in order that you may continually fine-tune your training to the nth degree

6. In addition to a personalized integrated training and nutrition plan, a printout of information on almost any health condition, dietary plan, or training protocol you can think of is available

I can assure you that there has never been such a comprehensive and scientifically supported approach to integrated training as ISSA's integrated training and nutrition support package. What's more, as the sciences of sports training, fitness, and fat-loss progress, you can rest assured that all relevant and useful information will find its way into our ISSA database.

FIGURE 35-1

An Example of a Profile Data Sheet for Use with the ISSA's Integrated Training and Nutritional Support Package

Client's Name: _____

Address: _____

_____ ZIP_____

Phone: (home) _____ (work) _____

Name and address of training facility and manager or owner: _____

_____

_____

Do you want a new training program?   Yes _____ No _____

Do you want a new diet?   Yes _____ No _____

YOUR TRAINING AND NUTRITION OBJECTIVE (circle one)

Fat Loss   Bodybuilding   Fitness   Aerobic Sports   Power Sports

Birth Date: _____ Sleep Time: _____ (in hours)

Height: _____ (in inches)   Weight: _____ (in pounds)

Sex: _____ (M or F)   Desired Weight: _____ (in pounds)

Daily Activity Factor: _____ (0 to 200%—See guide below)

  30% = Very light: sitting, studying, talking; little walking or other activities
     throughout the day

  55% = Light: typing, teaching, lab/shop work; some walking throughout the day

  65% = Moderate: walking, jogging, gardening type job with activities such as
     cycling, tennis, dancing, skiing, or weight training 1–2 hours per day

100% = Heavy: heavy manual labor such as digging, tree felling, climbing, with
     activities such as football, soccer, or bodybuilding 2–4 hours per day

130% = Exceptionally heavy: a combination of moderate and heavy activity eight or
     more hours per day

Number of Days to Achieve Goal: _____ (6 weeks minimum)

Smoke Tobacco: _____ (cigarettes per day)

Ingest Alcohol: _____ (beers or drinks per day)

Do You (or Your Spouse) Cook at Home Regularly?   Yes _____ No _____

Old and Recent Injuries: _____

_____

Other Medical Problems Not Listed Above: _____

_____

Foods You Can't or Won't Eat: _____

_____

Work Tasks: _____

Your Somatotype: _____

(Endomorphs tend to be fat; ectomorphs tend to be tall and thin; mesomorphs tend
to be heavy-boned and muscular)

TRAINING EXPERIENCE (read below and then circle one):

Beginner   Intermediate   Advanced

Beginners = Those just getting into training and dieting who work out three times weekly

Intermediates = Those who have worked out at least one year, are familiar with weight training exercises, and exercise 3–5 times weekly

Advanced = Bodybuilders, athletes, and fitness-oriented people who have been training seriously for a substantial period of time, are thoroughly familiar with training equipment and sound nutritional practice, and who train five or more times weekly

BODY MEASUREMENTS:

GIRTH MEASUREMENTS (IN INCHES)

Chest girth _____ Hip girth _____

Upper arm girth _____ Thigh girth _____

Forearm girth _____ Calf girth _____

Waist girth _____ Wrist girth _____

SKINFOLDS (IN MILLIMETERS)

Biceps _____ Suprailiac _____

Subscapula _____ Abdominal _____

Triceps _____ Thigh _____

HEALTH AND FITNESS PROFILE (If Available)

Resting heart rate _____   Blood pressure _____   Percent body fat _____
_____

Note: If you do not know your percent body fat, do you want a body-fat test performed?

YOUR MEDICAL HISTORY

Have you experienced any of the following?

Y	N	Heart attack, coronary bypass, or other coronary surgery?
Y	N	Chest discomfort (especially with exertion)?
Y	N	High blood pressure?
Y	N	Extra, skipped, or rapid heartbeats/palpitations?
Y	N	Heart murmurs, clicks, or unusual cardiac findings?
Y	N	Rheumatic fever?
Y	N	Ankle swelling?
Y	N	Peripheral vascular disease?
Y	N	Phlebitis, emboli?
Y	N	Unusual shortness of breath?
Y	N	Light headedness or fainting?
Y	N	Pulmonary disease (e.g., asthma, emphysema, and bronchitis)?
Y	N	Abnormal blood lipids (cholesterol, triglycerides)?
Y	N	Stroke?
Y	N	Recent illness, hospitalization, or surgical procedure within the past four months?
Y	N	Medications of any kind? (if yes, list all on back)
Y	N	Diabetes or other metabolic disorders?
Y	N	Are you pregnant now?
Y	N	Is there any reason your physician would object to your dieting?
Y	N	Is there a history of heart disease in your family?
Y	N	Is there any reason your physician would object to your exercising?

36

SAUNA

Most bodybuilders don't have to worry about working up a sweat. They sweat profusely every time they exercise, as the process of calorie burning generates heat and the body responds by cooling it down with perspiration.

Sweating is one of your body's healthiest reactions. For optimal health and greatly improved adaptive ability, you should be especially aware of the benefits you can accrue from taking a sauna. Not any sauna, however. The one I have in mind generates a different form of heat called infrared radiant heat.

Studies conducted by the Health Mate Company indicate that profuse sweating in an infrared sauna room produces many beneficial reactions for athletes. Studies showed that far infrared heat creates low-level thermal radiation (only 100°–120° Fahrenheit as opposed to the 210° Fahrenheit heat of conventional saunas) that penetrates 1½" into the body, stimulating sweating without the feeling of suffocation and the discomfort of high temperatures of standard saunas. It sets up a vibratory resonance between your own body's infrared emissions and those of the sauna. Heat, they concluded, is not the important factor. Instead, the vibratory stimulation deep under the skin appeared to be.

Heat, however, has been shown to be an extremely important therapy. Sweating in a sauna room is one of the oldest folk remedies in the world. "Give me a chance to create fever, and I will cure any disease," said Parmenides two thousand years ago. Ancient Greeks and Romans had their hot baths, and Native Americans built sweat lodges for both health enhancement and treating illness.

Sweating by overheating the body has these effects:

- Produces a pronounced thermogenic response (burns calories), thereby assisting in speedier fat loss
- Speeds up metabolic processes of vital organs and endocrine glands
- Places demands upon cardiovascular system, making the heart pump harder and producing a drop in diastolic blood pressure
- Creates a fever reaction which kills potentially dangerous viruses and bacteria and increases the number of leucocytes in the blood, thereby strengthening the immune system—important for fighting colds, flu, and cancer and bolstering resistance to infections
- Excretes toxins from the body, including cadmium, lead, zinc, nickel, sodium, sulfuric acid, and cholesterol
- Stimulates vasodilation of peripheral vessels, which relieves pain and speeds healing of sprains, strains, bursitis, peripheral vascular diseases, arthritis, and muscle pain stemming from intense training
- Promotes relaxation, thereby lending a feeling of well-being
- Promotes release of growth hormone from the anterior pituitary gland, which in turn promotes a pronounced anabolic effect in the body

Nobel Prize–winner Dr. A. Lwoff, a French virologist, believes that high temperature during infection helps combat the growth of virus. "Therefore, fever should not be brought down with drugs," he said. Two medical doctors, Werner Zable and Josef Issels, have this to say about fever: "Artificially induced fever has the greatest potential in the treatment of many diseases, including cancer."

Dr. Ernst, a German physical education professor, has found that there are no cancer patients among marathon runners. He conducted a study of marathoners who log about 20 miles a day. Analyzing their sweat, he found it contained cadmium, lead, zinc, and nickel. Dr. Ernst concluded that these athletes excrete these potential cancer-causing elements from their bodies by perspiring. He and other scientists conclude that it is necessary to sweat profusely at least once a day to maintain good health.

Ward Dean, M.D., a U.S. Army flight surgeon who has researched the physiological effects of sweating in a sauna, finds that it can be as effective as regular exercise in conditioning the cardiovascular system and burning calories. Sweating in a sauna is a good workout for people unable to exercise, such as disabled people in wheelchairs or immobilized athletes recovering from injuries, according to Dr. Dean.

Dr. Paavo Airola, well-known authority on holistic health, says that sweating in a sauna stimulates the body's own healing systems. "The healing of many chronic and acute conditions, such as colds, infections, rheumatic diseases, and cancer, is accelerated by the body's own curative forces. The body is thoroughly cleansed and rejuvenated inside and outside . . . Many toxins, accumulated in the system as a result of metabolic wastes and sluggish elimination, are thrown out of the body with perspiration. The sauna increases the eliminative, detoxifying, and cleansing capacity of the skin by the stimulating action on the sweat glands."

As for me, I like the sauna simply because of its relaxing, soothing effect. I find that by taking a 20-minute sauna—and engaging in some visualization training while doing so—after intense training sessions, my recovery time is improved. According to research reports, the improved recovery most likely stems from the growth hormone response accompanying the stress of artificially induced fever.

In any event, it doesn't hurt, and it most certainly has the potential of doing a lot of good. Try it regularly for a while. You just may grow to both like it and depend upon it.

37

NEW TRAINING TECHNIQUES
AND TECHNOLOGIES

LUMBAR TRAUMA

In the normal lifting posture, the lower back is unnaturally hyper-flexed. This rounding of the lower back is often exacerbated by the fact that, during the lift, your legs are bent at the knees, causing a gradual deterioration of flexibility in your hamstrings. Since the hamstrings attach to the pelvis, they pull downward when too tight, causing a further rounding of the lumbar spine, even during the day away from the weights.

Over time—over months of training—the characteristic slump of the lower back coupled with the rearward tilt of the pelvis caused by tight hamstrings exert damaging stress upon your vertebral discs. Once these discs are damaged—and they will be—no chiropractor in the world can fix them. Then it's time for surgery, often an excruciating ordeal.

Is There a Solution?

What's a person to do? Quit training? Put up with the ill effects? Neither. There is an answer. It's so simple that it may make you want to cry over all the years you've been inflicting unnecessary trauma to your back. It's called a training belt—but not in the traditional sense of the word.

Why Wear a Training Belt?

The early weightlifters in Olympic competition used to do a standing military press—pushing the barbell overhead to arm's length. This maneuver required bending backward radically (hyperextension), exposing the lumbar spine to tremendous stress. They devised a belt that was supportive in the back to help alleviate this debilitating lumbar stress. A weightlifting belt is four inches wide in the back and only two inches wide in the front.

Powerlifters were a bit more scientific than their weightlifting cousins. They realized that by pressing the belly hard against the front of the spine, instead of trying to support it only from the rear, they could actually get far more protection. They reasoned that if their supportive belt were wide all the way around, they'd get support from both sides. They were only partly right.

THE LORA

Dr. Mike Yessis, Professor Emeritus at California State, Fullerton, adopted some research from Russian sports scientists and, more recently, from the U.S. Army and applied it to what our powerlifters in this country already knew about supporting the back. Dr. Yessis, this country's foremost Soviet-watcher for many years (he published a quarterly journal called the *Soviet Sports Review*, which later became the official journal of the International Sports Sciences Association, renamed, *The Fitness and Sports Review*), devised a belt after a primitive Soviet version. It completely eliminates lumbar trauma.

I collaborated with Dr. Yessis in developing the concept. Today the belt is known as the LORA (acronym for Lumbar Orthopedic Repositioning Appliance) in chiropractic circles and simply the Belly Belt in the world of sports and fitness training.

The Belly Belt stabilizes the lumbar spine into a fused group of aligned vertebrae. It prevents the viscera from crunching together, so nerve damage from lifting or squatting with a rounded back and constant jarring from running, plyometric training, or other forms of low-back stress are all practically eliminated. Everything is held together in perfect, precise position.

For many of you, the Belly Belt will add years to your bodybuilding careers. But for all of you, it'll add a dimension of safety and health to your spine during any predisposing movements or activities that you've all been in need of for a long, long time.

Research clearly shows that the Belly Belt is markedly superior to any of the weightlifting and training belts out there. Even office workers, housewives, factory workers, and athletes in all sports and ability levels can benefit from wearing the Belly Belt.

It's not restricted in its usefulness to training!

SAFETY SQUATS

Despite the fact that they have been much maligned by physicians who rarely have the opportunity to observe healthy people (they usually only see sick people), squats are the single most effective leg exercise ever conceived. This is true whether your training goals are those of a bodybuilder, power athlete, endurance athlete, or fitness freak.

In all honesty, however, and in deference to the good doctors who eschew squats, they have to be done very carefully. To work best—with the utmost safety and effectiveness—squats must be done with an upright torso, with knees not extending beyond your feet in order to protect the integrity of the tissues comprising your knee joint. You should go to a depth necessary to stimulate maximum quadriceps contraction but not so deep that hyperflexion of your lumbar spine exposes you to serious back injury (i.e., thighs approximately parallel to the floor).

Powerlifters, of course, turn to the more effective technique of spreading the stress to the hips, hams, back, and quads when it comes time to enter contests. But even the most scientific powerlifters train with the upright bodybuilding style during the off-season.

All too often, bodybuilders with knee problems or bad backs have felt doomed to remain squatless in training. Nowadays, there's a training device called the safety squat bar (more often than not, it's called the Hatfield Bar because of my outspoken belief in it, the fact that they call me Dr. Squat, or both) which can give you a new lease on effective leg training.

Regular Squats

Conventional straight-bar squats (called Olympic or Bodybuilding squats) have several inherent weaknesses or dangers:

1. The chance of leaning forward or rounding your back under heavy loads is always a problem
2. Falling off-balance forward or backward also jeopardizes your safety during heavy squatting
3. Your shoulder girdle, shoulders, wrists, and elbows often take a beating holding the straight bar firmly in position
4. Missing a squat attempt is something which happens to all of us from time to time, often with dire consequences
5. Discomfort to the back of the neck (typically at the seventh cervical vertebra) where the bar sits is a problem we all shrug off as part of the game

6. Individual anatomical peculiarities often make it extremely difficult—if not impossible—to assume the most efficient stance in order to derive maximum benefit from squats

7. Not being able to squat because of the lack of competent spotters has been one of my personal gripes

8. Perhaps the most dangerous part of squatting is the need to take several steps backward to set up and then return to the rack after squatting. This factor alone accounts for over 75 percent of all squatting-related injuries

All of us put up with these problems and get on with the business of learning good technique, taking proper precautions, and doing what we know is best for us. We squat no matter what because it has always been thought of as best to do so. That we've gotten by and made progress with conventional squats is due in no small measure to our belief that squats work best, and we make them an important part of our program.

The Safety Squat Bar

Reducing or eliminating these problems inherent with conventional squatting will allow you to realize faster gains, less stress and strain on your back, knees, and other joints, fewer potentially devastating misses under heavy iron, and in general a far more enjoyable workout. The exquisite isolation the Safety Squat Bar provides for your quads will be a truly unique experience, I assure you.

Let's go over the good points of the Safety Squat Bar one by one.

1. Your hands are not holding the bar. This allows you to grasp the handles on the power rack. Because of the heavy loads involved in squatting when returning to the upright position, there is a tendency to round your back and place unnecessary stress on your lower back. This is avoided by exerting pressure against the power rack handles and thus maintaining a perfectly straight back throughout the entire squatting motion. Using your hands to spot yourself prevents you from falling forward or backward.

2. Squatting with a straight bar, you're forced to use a load that you can handle in the weakest position. This results in using an inadequate amount of weight in the strongest position of the squatting motion.

This problem is solved by use of the hands in the Safety Squat Bar. When the sticking point is reached, the hands can be used to help you through it. This unique feature allows you to work with heavier weights in the ranges of movement where you are strongest

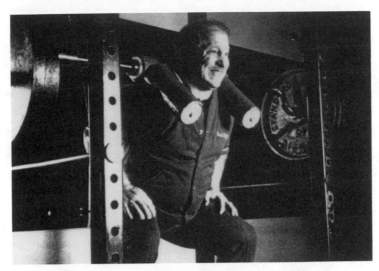

The Author Using the Safety Squat Bar

and gives you help when you are weakest. You are exerting closer to your maximum effort through the entire range of motion.

3. The padded yoke of the Safety Squat Bar virtually eliminates neck and shoulder girdle discomfort. The fact that you needn't use your hands to hold the bar on your shoulders eliminates wrist, shoulder, and elbow discomfort.

4. By using your hands to regulate body position, your posture under the bar can be adapted to suit your own anatomical peculiarities so that you can literally tailor your squatting style to afford maximum overload and consequently more efficient quad development.

5. Conventional squatting places the weight behind you, fully four inches behind your body's midline. That caused you to lean forward for balance. The Safety Squat Bar distributes the weight directly in line with your body's midline and completely eliminates the need to lean forward.

6. Finally, because you are holding onto handles built onto the squat rack, you do not back up before squatting, and you are not obliged to walk back into the rack after squatting. This element alone has the potential of eliminating up to three quarters of all squatting-related injuries.

Back problems and knee problems preventing you from training may never get solved completely. But you can squat more safely, more effectively, and quite probably with bigger weights than ever before. That amounts to better progress toward your bodybuilding goals.

PART NINE

PROBLEM AREAS
FOR BODYBUILDERS

DEDICATED TO VINCE COMERFORD

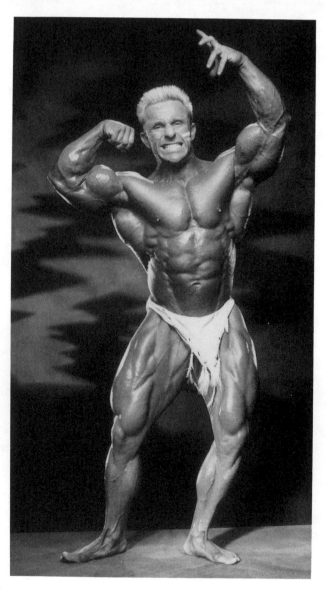

Vince Comerford

38

OVERTRAINING AND AVOIDING INJURY

OVERTRAINING

No exercise or training program proceeds completely free of difficulty. There are certain problems you're bound to encounter and, therefore, should be on the lookout for. Thorough knowledge of a potential problem is half the solution to it. If you know what to watch for, you're less likely to take the wrong path to begin with. It's discouraging to lose your forward momentum when you're already well into a serious training cycle, and an injury or a miscalculation in the amount of training you need to do can hurt you in more ways than one.

Young, strong, enthusiastic bodybuilders tend to overdo it once in a while. They want to train hard and fulfill their potential. They want to be the best they can be. Sometimes they don't know when to stop—when enough is enough—or they're just not willing to admit it, so dedicated are they to bodybuilding perfection. Well, that's great attitude but excess in anything can lead to distress. Too much of anything is no good for you, and that most definitely applies to the sort of intense loads borne by young bodybuilders trying to get into contest shape.

Overtraining doesn't always mean that you have trained too much. Perhaps you have trained for too long at the same level or you've overdone it with one or two exercises (e.g., too much weight, too frequently).

Conditioning yourself to respond in an optimal manner to every training session can be extremely rewarding—for a while. As you continue to live up to your own expectations, you hit a stale period, a state of poor performance, and skid into a slump. If three or four workouts in a row seem to be subpar you may be in a state of overtraining. You may have let other factors, along with your leveling-out of limit strength, influence the way you feel, react, and train.

While the main culprit causing overtraining is overuse, often there is no one identifiable factor. Overtraining can sometimes be attributed to several factors that converge at the same time.

You must be able to respond well to stress, not just physically, but mentally and emotionally. Therefore, there are other, nontraining-related elements that affect your conditioning, some in ways that you don't even perceive. Problems in the following areas could have an effect on your training.

- Academic/studies
- Financial status
- Family
- Sexuality
- Personality conflicts
- Schedule conflicts
- Poor training facilities
- Monotony in training or lifestyle
- Poor diet or sleep habits
- Inadequate coaching
- Lack of encouragement
- Time-consuming or strenuous job that interferes with your workouts
- Drugs
- Poor coaching or personality conflicts with coach
- Inflicting too-severe exercise stress upon your body—this is by far the *most* significant cause of overtraining

It used to be believed that there were two different types of physical overtraining, Addisonic overtraining and Basedowic overtraining. Nowadays, however, it is believed that the symptoms for each of these two types are what gave rise to the names and that both stem from a common cause, cumulative microtrauma. This is just a fancy name for getting a whole bunch of tiny (microscopic in size) tears in your muscles and connective tissues through high-frequency severe or improper training.

Addisonic overtraining is named after Addison's Disease, in

which the adrenal and pituitary glands malfunction. Some of the symptoms of this form of overtraining resemble those of the disease. This form of overtraining usually affects older or advanced athletes and includes a slightly overtired feeling but no increase in sleep needs, no weight loss, unusually low resting pulse rate, normal metabolic rate, higher blood pressure, but normal temperature and no psychological changes.

Like Addisonic overtraining, the name of Basedowic overtraining is derived from a disease (Basedow's disease) in which the thyroid function is too high. Symptoms of Basedowic overtraining include tiring easily, reduced appetite and weight loss, needing more sleep, a fast resting pulse rate, higher temperature and blood pressure, slower reaction time, and inability to perform skill movements. This type of overtraining is more commonly seen in strength athletes and explosive athletes such as sprinters, jumpers, and lifters. It also occurs in young athletes, less advanced athletes, and easily excitable ones.

Avoiding Overtraining

1. Develop a schedule that doesn't stress you. Too much in one area tends to hurt another
2. Develop a rational training program
3. Conform your workouts to cycle training principles
4. Vary your training methods
5. Sleep 8–10 hours a night
6. Follow sound nutrition practices
7. Make the athlete/coach connection and work together
8. Take one or two naps a day. A 20-minute nap is all it takes to rejuvenate and energize you
9. Find a sports-medicine clinic or practitioner who can help you monitor blood pressure and other symptoms of overtraining
10. Let logic—not ego—rule your training
11. After workouts, whirlpool affected muscles, then massage them vigorously for a minute or so. Use the "buddy" system for the vigorous massage

INJURY-FREE TRAINING

Every time you climb under a bar crammed with pig-iron plates, you risk the ultimate nightmare of all powerlifters—injury. An injury can do more than put a crimp in your training program or sideline you for a few weeks. It can severely limit or end your lifting career.

It's very important to devote time and attention to safe training practices and methods of conditioning that will keep you injury-free.

Your muscles and joints undergo an amazing amount of stress in even the simplest of sports and athletic movements. You can imagine the stresses they undergo while powerlifting. Therefore, no unnecessary chances should be taken.

Strong muscles and connective tissue can prevent injury. Further factors can also ensure a state of overall fitness that protects your body from the problems every athlete risks.

Guard against muscle weakness or imbalance. If you build one muscle more than another you risk injuring the weaker muscle. For instance, if you're a runner and want sprint speed, you'll work on your quadriceps. If you build great strength in the quadriceps without also building strength in your hamstrings, you have a muscle imbalance and leave yourself open to a hamstring pull. In the same manner, powerlifters often develop lower-back muscle problems because they neglect their abdominal muscles, which are crucial to back support.

Flexibility counts. When you strengthen or enlarge muscles you also tend to increase their tone, and that sometimes limits flexibility. To keep your muscles from getting too tight, you must have an ongoing flexibility program as part of your training. If you develop a muscle without also stretching for flexibility and strengthening your muscles while they are in the stretched position, you leave yourself open to injury. If you simply stretch without strengthening, you can often leave yourself open to injury as well.

Sports scientists have identified many other common causes of sports injuries. Sometimes poor body mechanics, spinal imbalance, poor nutrition, dehydration, drug use, or problems related to these areas can lead to injuries. But two special areas of potential injury must be looked at more closely.

Congenital Weakness

Your spine is a key factor in body mechanics. Its shape and resilience to stress are important. If you have too much curvature you could strain your back muscles. Also, malformed vertebrae can lead to muscle injury.

Some people are born with these kinds of structural problems, and that is what is meant by congenital weakness. Such weaknesses are liable to appear anywhere in the body, not just the spine. Often, a coach, health instructor, or doctor can help you identify these problems and then work out a program for you to stretch or strengthen the necessary muscles so as to lessen the possibility of injury.

The same kind of problems exist with knock-knees and pronated (inward-drifting) feet. Corrective devices have been developed to treat these conditions.

Pushing Too Hard, Too Fast

Lack of progress or susceptibility to injury means something is wrong. If this happens, you must take a close look at your training. You should never advance so quickly in your powerlifting routines that you experience high levels of pain. Also, if you train too long and/or too often, your muscles won't have a chance to adapt.

Most of the coaches of elite athletes will tell you that the single biggest problem with their athletes is not that they don't train enough, but that they train too much. All progress must be gradual. Your conditioning efforts are not like a silver bullet—they won't give you immediate success at your sport, and they can hamper your progress if you push too hard too soon. Take your time, be scientific and thorough, and—above all—stick to the cycle training program.

As long as you consistently follow an integrated training program, working out hard, but wisely, adding flexibility exercises where necessary, following sound nutritional guidelines, and getting sufficient rest, you'll achieve your strength goals much faster and become better able to keep yourself in top condition. The better condition you're in, the easier it is to recover from an injury or to avoid one in the first place.

Remember to dedicate yourself to the health of your body as much as to the performance of your sport.

39

BODYBUILDING BURNOUT

Fatigue can cause that dreaded scourge of athletes of all persuasions—burnout, overtraining, staleness, plateauing. Whatever name you call it, this general syndrome is of the sort that makes second-place finishers of us all.

A lot of mechanisms are believed to be responsible for long-term as well as short-term fatigue. By cursorily reviewing the mechanisms of short-term fatigue, we can gain a more complete perspective of the dynamics of long-term fatigue, or burnout. You will see that short-term fatigue can involve any or all of the various mechanisms involved in movement, from the thought process to the final contraction of the muscle. See Figure 39-1.

Back in 1978 exercise scientists H. Gibson and R. T. H. Edwards divided short-term fatigue into two groups: central fatigue and peripheral fatigue. The causes of central fatigue include diminished motivation, impaired transmission of nerve impulses down the spinal cord, and impaired recruitment of motor neurons. The causes of peripheral fatigue, on the other hand, involve impaired function of the peripheral nerves serving the individual muscles, impaired transmission of electrical impulse at the neuromuscular junction, and impaired processes of stimulation within the muscle cell (including metabolite changes resulting in depletion of ATP and thereby the function of the contractile machinery of the cell).

It's clear that central fatigue only happens among the uncommitted. None of those around here, right? Let's concentrate on a more useful understanding of peripheral fatigue. Those same scientists subdivided peripheral fatigue into two groups: high-frequency fatigue and low-frequency fatigue.

FIGURE 39-1

Possible Fatigue Mechanisms*

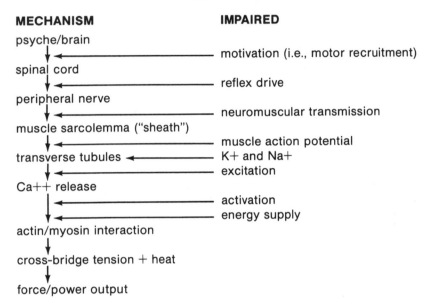

MECHANISM

IMPAIRED

psyche/brain

motivation (i.e., motor recruitment)

spinal cord

reflex drive

peripheral nerve

neuromuscular transmission

muscle sarcolemma ("sheath")

muscle action potential

transverse tubules — K+ and Na+

excitation

Ca++ release

activation

energy supply

actin/myosin interaction

cross-bridge tension + heat

force/power output

*Adapted from H. Gibson and R.T.H. Edwards, "Muscular Exercise and Fatigue," *Sports Medicine*, March/April, 1985.

FIGURE 39-2

Comparison Between Force Output and Twitches Per Second Between High-Frequency Fatigue and Low-Frequency Fatigue*

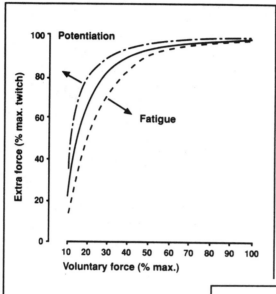

High-Frequency Fatigue

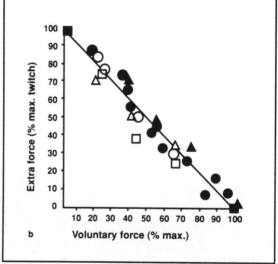

Low-Frequency Fatigue

In high-frequency fatigue, there's a direct relationship between force output and the number of twitches per second. In low-frequency fatigue, however, there's a shift to the right in the curve, indicating a fall in the ratio of force generated by low-frequency stimulation as compared to high-frequency fatigue.

*Adapted from H. Gibson and R.T.H. Edwards, "Muscular Exercise and Fatigue," *Sports Medicine*, March/April, 1985.

High-Frequency Fatigue
(Electromechanical Fatigue)

In sports where you sustain rapid movement patterns for over 60 seconds, force output losses typically result from the failure of action potentials (the ability of the membrane to conduct electrical impulses) along the surface membrane (sarcolemma) of the muscle cell. The sarcolemma transmits electrical impulses into the tiny openings on the muscle cell's surface (called t-tubules) and on to the individual actin/myosin filaments deep within the muscle cell. Failure of the action potentials is believed to be due to a buildup of potassium both inside the t-tubules and between the actin/myosin filaments, not a result of lactic acid buildup or too little oxygen.

High-frequency fatigue (electromechanical failure) typically occurs most readily in cold muscles, although maximal and repetitive movement over about 60 seconds' duration is also believed to cause such nervous-system fatigue. It probably has little bearing on short- or long-term fatigue of the type seen among bodybuilders.

Low-Frequency Fatigue
(Mechanico-Metabolic Fatigue)

In this type of fatigue, low-frequency force output is limited despite adequate electrical stimulation. Everyone knows that it's the buildup of lactic acid that causes this sort of fatigue, right?

Not necessarily. Back in 1981, Ciba Corporation funded research showing that short-term fatigue can be experimentally induced among individuals with metabolic defects which influence energy pathways and lactic acid accumulation. What then, is the most important mechanism causing fatigue? Cellular damage!

Whoa! Conjures up all sorts of wondrous theories, doesn't it? It is believed that low-frequency fatigue (especially involving eccentric muscle contraction as opposed to concentric) results from tearing and rending those very cellular structures which carry the electromechanical impulses to such a degree that, not unlike a torn or frayed electrical wire, the electrical impulses are considerably weakened. If you'll look at Figure 39-3, you'll clearly see that force output decreases faster following eccentric contraction.

FIGURE 39-3

The Difference in Low-Frequency Fatigue Between Concentrically and Eccentrically Contracted Muscles*

Concentric contractions

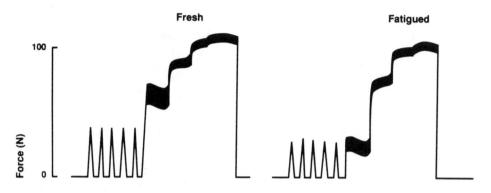

Eccentric contractions

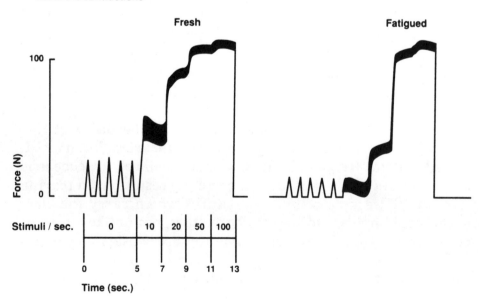

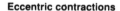

Note that greater low-frequency fatigue occurs after eccentric contractions, an indication that cellular damage caused the fatigue.

---

*Adapted from H. Gibson and R.T.H. Edwards, "Muscular Exercise and Fatigue," *Sports Medicine*, March/April, 1985.

LONG-TERM FATIGUE

Here we are to the burnout stage.

The microtrauma resulting from eccentric contraction (and, to a lesser degree, with concentric contraction) begins to accumulate because you're not taking proper restorative measures between workouts or you're engaging too heavily in eccentric work, or both. The cumulative microtrauma disrupts the electromechanical impulses which drive the contraction process. Those impulses never get to the actin and myosin in sufficient intensity (twitches per second) to generate maximum force.

This is what the British scientists refer to as the catastrophe theory of fatigue. Drs. Gibson and Edwards explained that, in aerobic exercise, the marginally deficient rate of ATP supply resulting from such electrochemical deficiency may indeed go unexplained. This being the case, cumulative microtrauma is never tended to and restoration is never complete, a situation which may indeed result in an overtrained state over weeks of time.

Among anaerobic athletes, it's a bit different. Gibson and Edwards continued to explain that, after an isometric contraction, for instance, the recovery of both ATP and excitatory capabilities of the muscles is rapidly restored. If high-frequency fatigue is stimulated, again recovery is instantaneous (ruling out metabolic fatigue and supporting the lowered excitation explanation).

According to Gibson and Edwards, what's left as the most tenable explanation for fatigue is the catastrophe theory. But they never really looked at the long-term effects of continually eliciting countless minuscule catastrophes inside the muscles, day after day, workout after workout, for months on end.

Let's do that now.

BURNOUT AND OVERTRAINING AMONG BODYBUILDERS

Listen up! There are two ways to cope with cumulative microtrauma. You can avoid it, or you can treat it. You avoid it not by avoiding lifting or by avoiding a small amount of (normal) cellular destruction, but instead by not letting microtrauma accumulate. You do this the same way you treat cumulative microtrauma.

- Sensible, scientific weight training and light resistance systems of training which employ a carefully devised periodicity or cycle method

- Sensible, scientific application of the many therapeutic modalities at your disposal (especially whirlpool, heat, ice, massage, and neuromuscular re-education)
- Sensible, scientific nutritional practice (especially maintaining an adequate amino acid pool to effect protein turnover, adequate energy foods to replace those depleted during intense training, and a minimum of five meals daily)
- Sensible, scientific nutritional supplementation (especially the branched-chain aminos, glutamine, adequate protein intake multiple times daily, vitamin and mineral intake, and other state-of-the-art supplements and herbs designed to aid tissue recovery and healing)
- Good technique in your lifting and skills, especially avoiding excessive eccentric contractions (negatives) and uncontrolled ballistic movements (controlled ballistics are reserved for special training during various periods of your training cycle for maximum stimulation of the fast-twitch muscles, but not excessively)
- Getting plenty of rest both between workouts and at night (try to get at least 8 hours per night, plus at least one or two short 20-minute catnaps during the day)
- Taking advantage of various psychological techniques which promote restoration (especially meditation, visualization training, hypnotherapy, or self-hypnosis techniques)

It all boils down to a simple plan—to do things the best way that science can provide. The above list ought to at least get you thinking along some reasonable pathway in that regard.

Remember that there is no decidedly wrong way to train. If you are a raw beginner just getting into sports or bodybuilding in a serious way, anything you do, provided it doesn't kill you, will probably help, but only for a while. If you get the iron bug and begin training at least daily, you're bound to overtrain eventually. If you're an inveterate lifter, you've probably been operating in at least a minimal state of overtraining for your entire career (that is, unless the points outlined above have been adhered to religiously).

Good, better, best is how things go in the gym. Which do you prefer? If you're committed (there's that word again!), there's only one way to go.

40

A THUMBNAIL SKETCH
OF THE FACTORS INVOLVED
IN RECOVERY

Right up front, let me tell you how I feel about recovery. It is the single most important factor in promoting bodybuilding success. In fact, it's so important in all sports that the Soviets spent a huge majority of their research efforts as well as their sports budgets' rubles in understanding and promoting it.

There are four key questions all bodybuilders ask.

1. What is a bodybuilder's or athlete's most important goal in his/her quest for improved performance capabilities?

- The ability to recover from intense training fully and quickly

2. What are the factors involved in improved recovery?

- Improved blood circulation during and following intense training for removing catabolic wastes and delivery of nutrients and oxygen
- Protein turnover—sloughing off destroyed muscle cells and bringing aminos (especially the branched-chain aminos leucine, isoleucine, and valine) in to facilitate anabolic processes of new growth and stress adaptation—and fighting the unnecessary destruction of cells through the use of anticatabolic agents such as L-glutamine
- Energy replacement must take place before anabolic processes can begin (blood sugar left over from preworkout meal is used for glycogen storage inside muscle cells)
- Supercompensation processes including improved stress

tolerance (connective tissue), strength (muscle tissue), and circulation (capillarization)

- Postexercise clearance of adhesions stemming from destroyed tissue
- Free radical scavenging (exercise creates massive influx of free radicals into the bloodstream)
- Improved adaptogenic ability for return to homeostasis
- Improved sleep quality (with REM sleep comes a significant growth hormone response, which is highly anabolic)

3. Which of those factors can be augmented or improved upon?

- All of them. An integrated approach must be used. The best approach to training always involves integration of all key technologies

4. What are the supplements and other technologies that can help in each of the processes of improving recovery ability?

- Blood circulation: vasodilator (e.g., cayenne or niacin); viscosity reducer (e.g., aspirin); therapeutic modalities (e.g., heat, ice, whirlpool, sauna)
- Protein turnover: BCAAs and L-glutamine; immune system booster (e.g., mumie); B-complex (especially B_6 and B_{12}); dibencozide (coenyzme B_{12})
- Energy replacement: short, medium, and long-chain carbos; glycoinulinides
- Supercompensation: mucopolysaccharides (connective tissue) such as purified chondroitin sulfates; twenty-two aminos with all cofactors (muscle tissue); GH releasers
- Adhesion preventive: proteolytic enzymes, therapies (e.g., deep fiber massage, ultrasound)
- Free radical scavengers: NDGA; vitamins A, C, and E; glutathione; selenium; green tea; ginkgo biloba; and many other substances
- Adaptogenic agents: eleutherococcus senticosus, reindeer antlers, mumie
- Improved sleep quality: serotonin activator (e.g., tryptophan)
- Improved immune system competence: vitamin E, mumie

It seems apparent that many of the above-listed substances and practices are worthy of inclusion in your training regimen. Perhaps, after you've used them for a few months, your question of whether you can improve your ability to recover without having to resort to drug abuse will be answered.

41

YOUR TOLERANCE TO EXERCISE

Arthur Jones, the King of Nautilus Fitness Machines, is a thinking man. More than once this acknowledged marketing genius has held me spellbound, laying waste to training notions I previously held dear.

After years of insistence that one set to failure was the only way to train, Jones turned his back on this singular concept that made him famous in some circles and infamous in others. Even after his retraction, his former disciples nonetheless clung to the archaic dogma that gave rise to one of this century's most influential gym marketing policies.

Arthur (finally) noticed that some people tend to thrive on far less exercise than normal, while others seemed to be incapable of making gains no matter how hard and long they trained. He wondered why. He termed this one's "tolerance" to training stress. Let's explore this concept from the perspective of scientific reason.

THE NORMAL CURVE

If all the bodybuilders in the world were dumped into a pile after going through a sort of sifting machine that graded them according to their exercise tolerance, we can assume that the pile they made would approximate a normal distribution. (See Figure 41-1.)

Scientists have studied this distribution for years and have catalogued its properties rather completely. One such property is its ubiquitous nature—we see it in almost all walks of life. Intelligence. Testosterone levels. Pain tolerance. Height. Weight. And so forth.

FIGURE 41-1

Normal Distribution and How Bodybuilders Compare in Their Tolerance to Exercise

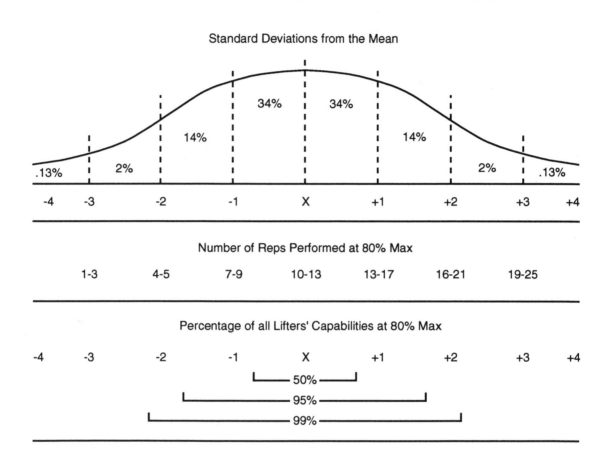

Sometimes the pile is skewed one way or the other. Sometimes there are two or more humps in the pile, a phenomenon referred to as a multimodal distribution. The actual shape of the pile is most often determined by the interplay of many factors that tend to affect the trait being observed.

Since virtually no significant studies have appeared which treat tolerance to exercise as the focal variable, we have only our powers of reason to guide us in determining what kind of shape the pile of bodybuilders would take. There are too many variables that can affect your exercise tolerance, including

- Red vs. white fiber ratio
- Tolerance to pain
- Perceived exertion

- Incentive level
- Strength-to-weight ratio
- Time of last meal (energy)
- Type of foods eaten at least meal (glycemic index)
- Metabolic rate
- Use of ergogenic techniques or substances
- Musculoskeletal leverage factors
- Motor-unit recruitment capabilities
- Skill level at exercise being performed
- Equipment quality
- Environmental factors (e.g., heat, cold)
- Size of muscle being exercised
- Exercise intensity

All these factors, and perhaps several more as yet undreamed of, will affect your ability to perform to your true tolerance level.

In the absence of any concrete guides available from the glistening towers of academia, all we can do at the moment is assume that the pile (created by dumping all the bodybuilders as one might dump a bucket of sand onto the ground) will be very symmetrical, approximating the normal distribution shown in the illustration on the opposite page.

TOLERANCE TO EXERCISE

Keeping in mind that many variables affect your exercise tolerance, let's look at a sample exercise, bench pressing. When my bench press was at maximum (about 550 pounds) I generally stayed around 70–80 percent of max during the last phase of my peaking cycle. I was able to do about six reps with 500 pounds (approximately 80 percent of max).

Curious over Arthur Jones's prognostications regarding how lifters differ in their abilities in this regard, I began charting other lifters' reps at 80 percent max. I found that guys who were so-called fast gainers were only able to do 4–6 reps at 80 percent, while lifters who seemingly never made great gains were able to rep out at around 15–20 reps with 80 percent of their max. Apparently, so-called fast gainers have rather poor anaerobic strength endurance. This is explainable in part by the fact that they're probably mostly white muscle fiber, which has fast-twitch/low-oxidative capabilities. Conversely, slow gainers are probably mostly red muscle fiber (slow twitch/high oxidative) and therefore may possess greater ability for rapid during-set recovery.

Arthur Jones, it seemed, was dead right.

The problem is, however, that each muscle group's tolerance to exercise probably differs. Each exercise you do for each body part can—and often does—elicit an entirely different response in output at 80 percent max. Determining your exercise tolerance on any sort of comprehensive level seems, at best, a pipe dream.

Hold on! Remember the normal curve. We're talking about averages here. Getting a handle on your exercise tolerance level—albeit a tenuous handle—is better than having no grip on it at all, so let's back up and start again.

Individual Differences

For simplicity's sake, let's divide your body into the traditionally identified body parts, then delineate some rough guidelines regarding what the tolerance levels are for each.

FIGURE 41-2

How Many Reps Can You Do?

Fill in the blanks.

BODY PART	TYPICAL EXERCISE	100% MAX (APPROX.)	80% MAX (APPROX.)	MAX REPS PERFORMED
Chest	Bench press	_____	_____	_____
Delts	Lateral raises	_____	_____	_____
Biceps	Curls	_____	_____	_____
Triceps	Pushdowns	_____	_____	_____
Lats	Pulldowns	_____	_____	_____
Upper back	Bent rows	_____	_____	_____
Hips/thighs	Squats	_____	_____	_____
Quads	Leg extension	_____	_____	_____
Hamstrings	Leg curls	_____	_____	_____
Abdominals	Crunchers	_____	_____	_____

Figure 41-2 gives you an idea of how to set up your own personal table, depending upon how you divide your body into parts and which exercises you prefer for each. The idea is to

1. Determine your one-rep maximum for each exercise (you need only approximate this number)
2. Load 80 percent on the bar and rep out with it for one all-out effort to see how many reps you can do
3. Apply this information to the illustration of the normal curve (Figure 41-1) to determine each body part's exercise tolerance

4. Critically evaluate whether your predicted exercise tolerance levels (as measured) stand up to what you know from experience to be true (e.g., low tolerance means easy gains; high tolerance means difficult gains) for that body part

FIGURE 41-3

Knowing Your Tolerance to Exercise

REPS PERFORMED	STANDARD DEVIATION FROM MEAN	TOLERANCE LEVEL	ABILITY TO MAKE GAINS
1–3	−3	Very, very low	Fast gainer
4–5	−2	Very low	
7–9	−1	Low	
10–13	Mean (average)	Average	Gainer
13–17	+1	High	
16–21	+2	Very high	
19–25	+3	Very, very high	Slow gainer

The Importance of Knowing Your Exercise Tolerance

Have a lagging body part? Most bodybuilders do. But what do you do about it? Most people will blitz the dickens out of that muscle, assuming that more is better. Not necessarily true! Maybe you're working the muscle beyond its tolerance point.

By critically evaluating your individual muscle's tolerance to exercise, you can more easily fine tune your training regimen to provide maximum gains in the shortest possible time. But don't forget the other factors that may affect your recovery rate. How have you accounted for each of these variables' effect on your progress? Have you raised or lowered your reps and sets accordingly? Have you increased or decreased the frequency of your workouts or training intensity commensurately? Have you taken into account the ratio of white versus red fiber and adjusted your exercise load and movement speed accordingly?

I cannot, at this time, predict with absolute certainty that any of this stuff will even make an iota of difference in your gains, although my strong suspicion is that it will. Perhaps it's time we started to get a bit more scientific—sophisticated—in how we approach our training. One thing is for sure: to become the best there is, was, or ever will be, you're going to have to get more scientific.

42

SYMMETRY

Back in the Stone Age when I was a bodybuilder (yes, I was one once), I had a problem. My right lat was shapely, large, and well proportioned while my left lat was, well, just there. No shape, no eye appeal. It didn't have the same sweep or shape as my right one did.

What's worse, I couldn't rectify the imbalance no matter what I did. I didn't lose any sleep over the problem, mind you, but at contest time the problem became difficult to hide and was quite probably one of the reasons I wasn't able to beat Mike Katz back in the sixties when we competed for the Mr. Connecticut title. (For the record, while I came in second, I did beat him for the "Most Muscular" award.)

A lot of bodybuilders have problems with symmetry. One arm is bigger or more shapely than the other, the lat spread is unequal, or pectoral development is uneven. Those are three common sources of asymmetry, but there are others. Asymmetry problems aren't necessarily restricted to size differences occurring bilaterally. Shape differences are also sources of consternation to the perfection-conscious bodybuilder. The big question is, "Can anything be done about asymmetrical development?"

WHAT ARE YOUR OPTIONS?

As I see it, there are five options open to you if you're one of the unlucky ones who, upon conception, got a swift kick in the proverbial genes.

1. You can apply electrostimulation to the offending muscle
2. You can have deep fiber massage performed
3. You can apply a system of unilateral exercise
4. You can go to a neurologist or (less feasible) a chiropractor to determine whether your problem is rooted in nerve damage or impingement
5. You can hide it through creative choreography in your posing routine

Then again, you can simply forget about the problem. Let's review these options one by one to see whether you're a candidate for any restructuring efforts.

Electrostimulation

Actually, applying electricity to a muscle is a form of exercise. It's all the rage these days to refer to such a technique as passive exercise, but there's nothing passive about it, I assure you. It can prove to be a very stressful form of exercise.

Your individual muscle cells each have their own excitation threshold—the level at which they're stimulated to contract. Some can be easily stimulated with as little as a couple of millivolts of juice from your central nervous system. Others, especially the highly fatiguable, explosive white fibers, need as much as 15–20 millivolts of electrical current in order to stimulate them to respond contractively.

When your brain sends down its electrochemical message to muscles, it's like stepping on the accelerator pedal in your car. A little gas, the car goes slow. A lot of gas and it goes fast. That's the way your muscles work, too.

With a lagging muscle, it's important to get maximum excitatory stimulation in order to force previously unreached muscle fibers to contract. Doing so may be just the ticket you were looking for to get that muscle to grow to the proportions of the opposite side, and it can be done with a simple muscle stimulator device equipped with electrodes and a variable current selector switch.

It's not advisable for you to apply electrostimulation yourself. I recommend soliciting the assistance of a skilled technician. A half hour daily of electrostimulation on the offending muscle equates to a couple hours or more of intense training.

The trick is to get just the right amount of current to surpass the excitation threshold ordinarily generated during normal training. More colloquially, apply the progressive resistance principle.

Deep Fiber Massage

By now most bodybuilders have heard of deep fiber massage. Drs. Gary Glum and Joseph Horrigan, two chiropractors with offices in Los Angeles, developed this idea years ago. Ask any bodybuilder who's gone to see these guys for therapy and they'll rave about the newfound dimensions of individual body parts. Theoretically, by freeing the individual fibers which comprise a muscle (they stick together because of injury-prompted adhesions and scar tissue), it will assume a normal shape and size. Think of it as a liberation therapy—a release of bound-together muscle cells.

The docs call their technique neuromuscular reeducation. Bodybuilders call it fantastic. One very nice side benefit of the treatment is that it definitely improves strength. Freeing adhesions and scar tissue allows the affected cells to contract more fully, more forcefully, and with greater range.

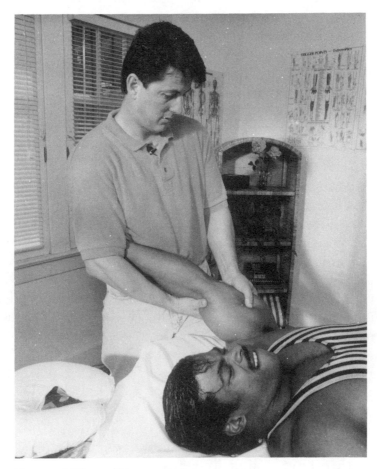

**Deep Fiber Massage
(Neuromuscular Reeducation)**

Of course, liberating the offending muscle group will no doubt prompt you to want all of your muscles similarly treated. Once done, it's anyone's guess whether the asymmetry will be rectified. One thing is for sure, though. It's worth a try.

Unilateral Exercise

Exercising the offending muscle and totally ignoring the good side is perhaps the most commonly applied remedy for asymmetrical development. In my opinion, it's too late by then—the asymmetry has appeared, and there's no point in ignoring your good side in favor of the "bad." That technique will simply create two bad sides instead of one.

However, one way of exercise may prove beneficial. Exercise your good side as you normally have in the past, but apply exercise to the offending side with a totally different form of stress. For example, if you're used to doing sets of ten reps or so (as most bodybuilders do), continue that form of stress on your good side, but do explosive sets of five or six reps on the bad. Also, try doing sets of 30–40 reps with slow, continuous tension movements to the bad side. Theoretically, as the cellular elements respond to this new form of stress, you may spark new growth there. It may be that your muscle has already adapted to the level and type of stress you have been applying and is in need of a new level and type of stimulation.

See a Doctor

I have seen many bodybuilders, athletes, and powerlifters with asymmetrical development resulting from nerve damage. Most typically the damage has occurred in the spine and has impinged or damaged the nerve that services the offending muscle.

The three most typical asymmetry problems—lats, arms, and chest—have nerves servicing them which emanate from the cervical spine. Your asymmetry may be nothing more than a nerve-adjustment problem, though that's unlikely. More commonly a disc is damaged.

Not being a physician, I hesitate to go beyond that meager description of a potential remedy. See a neurologist if you suspect nerve damage to be a potential problem.

Posing Routine Choreography

It seems prudent for you to get with a good choreographer and structure your posing routine in such a way that your good points are emphasized and your bad points are hidden. That's what I did when I was competing. Being somewhat naive to science back then, it seemed the logical answer for me. It worked, too.

But today, with bodybuilders nearing perfection, I doubt that taking this tack will prove effective enough to get you to Olympian stature. You're going to have to do more than hide a body part from the scrutiny of the vigilant judges. Try the other four options first. Then, if need be, hide. You may even want to get out of the sport.

For my money, asymmetry shouldn't be a problem anymore. If it is, maybe you should just try to forget competing. Even if you don't compete, you can still enjoy the sport of bodybuilding. It has much to offer.

43

GETTING A
COMPETITION TAN SAFELY

Competition bodybuilders' accepted onstage look is one which appears healthy, active, and finished. Part of the tradition of the sport is that these appearance factors include a tan. In years past, a tan was thought of as part and parcel of a healthy lifestyle.

But is it? Not necessarily, say dermatologists who study the effects that overexposure to the sun's rays has on our skin. Let's explore the problem in detail.

THE SUN'S RAYS

That portion of the sun's energy that is useful for tanning is only about 5 percent of the sun's total radiation. Visible light is about 40 percent and infrared about 37 percent of the total output. We cannot see nor feel ultraviolet light.

Ultraviolet light comes in two lengths, long and short. The short is called melanin-stimulating ultraviolet light, or UVB. The long is called oxidizing ultraviolet light, or UVA.

The melanin-stimulating rays (UVB) are one thousand times more powerful in causing sunburn than are the oxidizing rays (UVA). Outdoor sunshine contains ten times more strength in the stimulating rays than in the oxidizing rays; this is the reason sunburn can occur so quickly out-of-doors. Sunscreen lotions were developed to filter out the stimulating rays, yet leave the oxidizing rays. The problem with sunscreen lotions is that they become invisible when applied. You can't tell how completely the skin is covered or how long the protection will last.

Fortunately, modern technology has finally produced indoor ultraviolet light made just for tanning. The guesswork required in outdoor tanning is a thing of the past.

WHAT CAUSES TANNING?

Specialized cells in the skin, called melanocytes, are photosensitive. Like pulling down a sunshade when the sun gets too bright, these melanocytes respond to the melanin-stimulating rays and release a granulelike substance called melanin into the upper cell layers of the skin. Melanin eventually becomes what we call a tan. Under a microscope, melanin appears much like little sand pebbles.

The melanin-stimulating rays (UVB) cause this release of new melanin. The oxidizing rays (UVA) have less ability to stimulate new melanin production. They only oxidize melanin once the melanin exists in the skin.

Melanin is produced deep in the skin. It then migrates to the uppermost layers of the skin, called keritinocytes. It usually takes two to four days before enough of the melanin granules arrive close enough to the surface to cause color change—what we call tanning. As more and more melanin accumulates, the tan improves. However, if the melanin were not oxidized, the color would be very pale.

FIGURE 43-1

Definition of Skin Types

SKIN TYPE I

Very fair, burn easily, tan with extreme difficulty, possibly freckle a great deal. Usually red hair, very blond, or blond with some red color.

SKIN TYPE II

Fair complexion. Eventually tan with extra work. Burn easily when outdoors. Freckling moderate or not at all.

SKIN TYPE III

Sometimes burn, but always tan. Even when out of the sun for some time, there is still some color to the skin. Usually darker hair, except those blonds who tan exceptionally—sometimes attributed to a Scandinavian heritage.

SKIN TYPE IV

Never burn, always tan well. Usually dark hair and brown eyes. Always have some hue to the skin.

For all Caucasians, whether fair or dark, melanin in and of itself is not dark. It is commonly a yellow/brown or a red/brown, not a dark brown. Melanin must be oxidized, so your skin can change from its normal, very weak, pale, red/brown or yellow/brown color to the dark, golden brown color that we prize and adore as a tan.

People with dark complexions produce some melanin continuously. Should such individuals use the oxidizing rays (UVA), the melanin they possess would darken quickly, given sufficient intensity of the oxidizing rays. This would be particularly true for the face and also quite true for the chest and back. However, it may not be true for the legs, particularly in men and especially if they had an outdoor tan recently. Nevertheless, oxidation of melanin occurs very rapidly. For example, if a piece of tape were placed somewhere on the upper body of that person with a dark complexion, there could be a visible tan line where the tape had been after just one session, if the intensity of the rays was sufficient.

Those with fair complexions would see no such results at first. Since they hereditarily have almost no melanin in the skin, they must wait for the melanin-stimulating rays to affect the release of new melanin. The newly produced melanin must then migrate to the upper cell layers of the skin before color change could be seen.

ACQUIRING THE DARKEST POSSIBLE TAN SAFELY

Some areas of the body have more layers of cells and can retain more melanin. For example, the skin of the legs is considerably thicker than the skin of the nose or ears. Therefore, a tan of the legs may appear darker, since more melanin can be stored, and will retain its color longer. The skin of the nose and ears is thin, having fewer cell layers. Thus, these parts of the body will never tan as dark as other parts. The skin of the nose and ears will burn easily and lose color more quickly.

Normal body functioning causes the skin to shed those upper cell layers. With that shedding goes the accumulated melanin, and gradually the tan disappears. Actually, it will take three months or longer for all parts of the body to lose their tan completely. The face loses color first because there are fewer cell layers in which to store melanin. The legs lose their tan last.

In order to obtain a great tan, the melanin granules must be oxidized—changed from their pale color to a deep, golden brown. This is the primary job of the oxidizing rays. If the oxidizing rays are administered with sufficient intensity, the skin darkens. They have little ability to stimulate new melanin production but are very effective in changing the color of melanin once the melanin exists.

Tanning is just a question of intensity. When outdoors, we accumulate ray intensity by staying out longer and by being outside when the intensity is greatest, at midday rather than morning or evening.

Indoor tanning intensity is accomplished in other ways.

1. The wattage of the lamp used (just as home lighting has 100-watt, 200-watt bulbs, etc., so fluorescent lamps have different wattage)
2. Distance of the lamp from the body
3. Reflection and concentration of the light
4. The nature of the white coating inside a fluorescent lamp (there are slight variations among manufacturers)
5. The type of glass used in making the fluorescent lamp
6. Heat control
7. The type of control in delivering electricity to the lamp—performed by "ballasts"
8. The number of lamps used for a given space

These factors become important, particularly for the oxidizing rays. The amount of UVA required to effect the oxidation of melanin is enormous relative to the amount of the stimulating rays needed to effect the release of new melanin. Sunbeds use UVA lamps of medium wattage and bring the lamps as close to the skin as possible, all in an effort to maximize intensity.

Enjoy your tan. Having a nice tan has always been "in" and considered a symbol of health and vitality. Carried to extremes, however, tanning can be both unhealthy and cause premature signs of aging. Tan wisely and in moderation.

PART TEN

PSYCHOLOGICAL STRATEGIES FOR SUCCESS

DEDICATED TO AARON BAKER

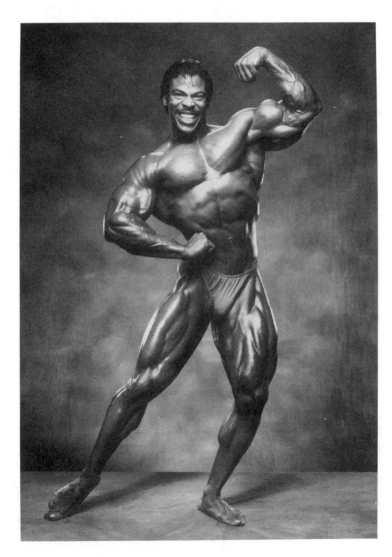

Aaron Baker

44

CONDITIONING YOUR MIND

Beyond pumping iron there is another kind of preparation for body-building competition, a preparation just as important and one that involves subtle factors concerning your attitude and mental approach to training and competition. You can achieve great things with your body if you learn how to use your mind. Learning to harness the power of your mind can advance your physical training a giant step further. It can also make the difference between winning and losing in competition.

Mind power and success through mind conditioning only comes with a sustained and sincere effort. You can't make a wish, hope that it comes true, and forget about working on it. The mind reacts much the same way the body does. If you train and condition it regularly, it responds with great efficiency and effectiveness. On the other hand, if you assume, as so many bodybuilders do, that it's good enough the way it is, your chances of achieving your maximum potential are greatly diminished. If you had foolishly assumed that attitude about your body, you would never have entered the gym to train in the first place.

Some of the key ingredients to an effective mind conditioning program are motivation, incentive, visualization, and, most important of all, belief. You've got to believe. You've got to believe in yourself, in your talents and capabilities, in your goals and all you hope to achieve, and in your methods for achieving them.

The key to understanding what your mind holds in store for you is a simple realization. Realize that within you is all the power you need to succeed both in training and in competition. Within you is all the potential for success. Within you is the brainpower of an infinitely superior person, physically, spiritually, and mentally.

Once you reach this realization—that your mind holds a vast wealth of knowledge, information, control, power, ability, and potential—you can start to tap into it. You can delve into your own secret depths and find out what you're really made of.

MOTIVATION AND DISCIPLINE

Motivation is the state of mind that generates positive feelings about achieving a purpose. Some people are motivated by financial rewards, others by primitive urges for physical pleasure. For you, the most highly motivating element in your life must become your dream of acquiring unsurpassed, mind-blowing power and mass.

But to be motivated isn't enough. You also need discipline. Discipline is what keeps you consistently scientific in your actions as you strive to achieve your goal.

Here is a simple step-by-step method to getting what you want.

Step 1

Define your ultimate goals clearly and write them down. This means being specific about what you want. What kind of improvements are you looking for? Do you want simply to increase your overall strength or your lean body mass, or reduce your body-fat percentage? Is your goal to compete in the NPC Championships? The Olympia? Then concentrate specifically on the actual aspects you wish to improve, and write them down. You'll be surprised at how much clearer your objectives become when you simply put them in words. When you have to select the exact words to define what you want, you tend to develop a superclear image of your goal.

Step 2

Devise a series of short-term goals that will ultimately lead you to realizing your main goals. It's easier to attain a short-term goal that's within your reach than to try and make great leaps in progress all at once. When you try to do too much at once and fail, you tend to get discouraged. Instead, knock off a number of short-term goals one at a time. Focus exclusively on the short-term goal you wish to achieve most of all; don't even think about the next short-term goal or the long run. Each one of your short-term goals should be a stepping stone, not an end in itself—that's why they have to be accomplished one at a time. As you complete them, you will find that you are all the more motivated to continue striving for your long-term goal—your trek to greatness.

Step 3

Create your strategy for success. This is your game plan, your integrated training program. On the same sheet where you wrote your long-term goal and listed the short-term goals that will get you there, break down your daily activities into the best means to get you where you're going. This means routines, exercises, sets, reps, intensity, practice, rest periods, diet, naps, posing practice, and so on. Follow your own plan to success. Prepare a daily schedule that takes you in the direction you want to go, and recognize right from the start that you are a unique individual who requires a program that's necessarily different from anyone else's. Keep your goal sheet current and review it day by day.

A good place to start is with the "daily clocks" presented earlier in this book. These daily clocks are designed to allow you to take advantage of all the various technologies science has to offer and, at the same time, let you thoroughly personalize your goal-oriented training.

Step 4

Visualize yourself succeeding. No one would attempt to build a house without using a set of blueprints. Likewise, you must plan your success strategy and actually see yourself, in your mind's eye, accomplishing your goals. Your inner feelings, your thoughts, your daydreams must all be filled with images of your ultimate success. Twice a day—once after training and once before bedtime—read your goal sheet out loud. Close your eyes and with crystal clarity see yourself becoming exactly what you want to be. But see yourself actually accomplishing your goals of acquiring great muscular size and proportioning, not just wistfully thinking about how nice it would be to look that way.

Step 5

Align your mind, body, and spirit with achievement. By affirming your commitment to your stated goals and actually visualizing and verbalizing your commitment, you will find that your mind, body, spirit, and emotional self all become one. The power of this union will send an emotional supercharge to your body by stimulating secretion of your body's emotion-producing biochemicals.

The alignment is accomplished by actually verbalizing your commitment while visualizing it. For example, say, "I am committed to becoming the most massive and cut bodybuilder in history." Repeat your commitment statement before, during, and after your success visualization every day.

Step 6

Give yourself a reward for your accomplishments. After you've achieved a subgoal or your ultimate goal, reward yourself in a significant fashion. I don't mean just having an ice-cream cone after a contest peaking cycle—that's not substantial enough to anchor the significance of your achievement firmly in your mind and soul. Personally dwell upon your achievement and your success. Congratulate yourself and savor the feelings of pride and confidence in having taken direct action to make yourself bigger and stronger.

The key to mental conditioning is to make your new thoughts and new approach a habit. The more regular your new habit becomes, the more quickly old and destructive habits fade away. The only way to continue making progress is to regularly reinforce your new, goal-directed integrated training.

It usually takes about three weeks to implement this revised way of thinking. During that time you're likely to feel tempted to return to old patterns and habits, feeling that the old way was easier and good enough. Don't do it!

The more you resist old habits, the stronger you'll become until you develop an iron will to succeed and you no longer even think about returning to old habits. Going back to your old mental habits would be akin to leaving the gym forever.

Remember to create a goal, visualize it as real, and work regularly to successfully attain firm footing on each of the stepping stones that will take you to it. When you get there, you'll know.

PASSION

Let's back up for a minute before we review the steps toward goal achievement. What got you into bodybuilding? Was it seeing a bodybuilding show? Was it the incredibly huge and muscular kid next door or your older brother or sister who bodybuilds? Whatever it was, it no doubt fostered in you a deep, abiding sense of passion for bodybuilding. All champions begin with an abiding passion for what they do. With such passion, motivation almost always comes naturally.

Passion is a hard word to define. It's a burning desire to exceed all bounds, to totally dominate all situations. Passion is not doing what it takes to win—it's doing what it takes to exceed. It most certainly is not force of skill or muscle. Rather, it's the explosive, calamitous force of will.

Passion is all-consuming. That is what it takes to become a champion, and that is what it'll take for you to achieve your ultimate bodybuilding goals. If you haven't acquired passion, seek it first. Find it. Do not begin without it, for without it you will be severely limited in your quest for greatness.

INCENTIVE: THE MOTHER OF MOTIVATION

Motivation and passion begin and end with incentive. You have to know what you want and why you want it, and achieving it may be reward in and of itself. This is called intrinsic reward. Extrinsic rewards are such things as money, trophies, or prizes. In both intrinsic and extrinsic cases, the rewards serve as incentive to continue.

In bodybuilding, this may mean that achieving a specific improvement provides the incentive for going after it. More strength, stamina, cuts, or sheer muscle mass are various incentives. But they may also be a part of larger incentives such as being liked and admired, being a winner or achiever, enjoying success, shaping a personal identity, or gaining peer acceptance.

Recognize incentive as a powerful motivating force, not as something potentially destructive, evil, trivial, or shameful.

STEPS TO GOAL ATTAINMENT

1. Set realistic short-term goals.

2. Short-term goals should lead you to a long-term goal. Allow for occasional setbacks along the way, but regard them as learning experiences, thereby turning those setbacks into something positive.

3. Set a training schedule and stick to it. Again, the best place to find such a training program is from among the integrated training programs described right here in this book.

4. Make pain and fatigue work for you, as signs that your all-out effort is helping you attain your goals.

5. Constantly challenge yourself in your training.

6. Devise your own personal definition of success. Success is what you say it is, not what someone else says.

7. Believe in yourself and foster positive aggression in your training.

8. Build a strong ego, but a restrained one.

45

YOUR EMOTIONAL STATE

Your mind and your emotions are tightly tied together. It's up to you to find a balance between them and exert absolute control over them.

Your emotional state plays a large role in your overall training. The way you're feeling inside has repercussions on your behavior and performance on the outside. Many different factors go into the makeup of a solid emotional base. Some of these factors are:

- Personal life
- Sexual life
- Family life
- Job
- Daily schedule
- Diet
- Financial matters
- Health concerns
- Most importantly, self-esteem

Your own self-esteem contributes greatly to the level of your sports performance. Self-esteem can vary greatly within the time confines of a single training session, and it can mean the difference between winning and losing in a competition setting. One minute you may hate yourself over an error you've committed on the posing platform or in the gym, and a few moments later you could reverse that feeling completely by performing exceptionally.

This sort of event can—and often does—lead to superlative performance throughout the remainder of your training session in the gym or in your onstage performance. In either case, your mental appraisal of yourself—your self-esteem—counts for a great deal in your performance.

This sort of scenario may be common, but it is not desirable. It would be far better if your self-esteem going into the gym or competition was such that only superlative performance throughout was possible. Day after day, month after month, building only the possibility of success into your training by careful, integrated application of science will tend to maintain peak mental attitude and feelings of self-esteem.

Success begets success.

FEAR AND SELF-ESTEEM

Fear of Failure

Fear, depression, anxiety, or overarousal can all lead to subpar training or competition performance. For every winner, there are many losers. Often the distinguishing features between the two are attitude, positive thinking, and the absence of inhibiting fear.

Fear of the competition, for instance, can put you in a defeatist frame of mind even before the competition begins. If you're so psyched out that you consider your opponent unbeatable, then you have defeated yourself. Your goal is to foster belief in yourself, train hard to achieve the means to victory, then realize you have made your belief work for you.

All your success comes first out of belief in yourself. In fact, belief and success go hand in hand. Once you rid yourself of fear, you begin to see yourself as potentially better than your opponent. That's the key to winning! In a state of fear, you will never see yourself as potentially better than your opponent.

It's obvious, then, that your state of mind determines to a large extent whether or not you ever see victory.

Fear of Injury

Fear of injury is another inhibiting factor. Doubtless you've heard of the oft-injured athlete who is forever on the disabled list. Sometimes, when this athlete returns to active play, he or she tends to be slightly gun-shy and might even alter his or her style of play to protect against injury. Ironically, playing to protect yourself against injury often leads to it, because you're pulling up, not following through with movements, and contracting your muscles irregularly.

The same sort of protective training occurs in bodybuilding.

The effects of a torn rotator cuff, a pulled hamstring, or whatever injury you may have suffered all tend to linger long after the injury is healed sufficiently to be trained again. Being careful is prudent, but being unreasonably careful will only keep you from your goal.

Fear of Success

Picture this scenario. Your best buddy is your training partner. He means a lot to you, and you don't want to embarrass him by showing him up with your superior physique, strength, or pain tolerance. Where does this lead? Believe me, this sort of fear is not all that uncommon.

Being pals is one thing, but a real pal will recognize (although perhaps not acknowledge or accept as permanent) your superior abilities. Turn your friendship with your training partner into a healthy, constructive, *friendly* competitive situation.

If you feel that your training partner is holding you back, don't train with him anymore. If you're an aspiring elite bodybuilder, your training program isn't going to match his anyway. Being buddy-buddy to the extent of following identical training programs rep-per-rep, exercise-per-exercise, day after day is downright stupid.

Other situations involving unreasonable fear of succeeding include not wishing to attain your ultimate goal for fear of no longer having anything to strive for, not wishing to be forced to accept the sociopsychological responsibilities associated with being the champion, and not wanting to totally commit to doing everything necessary in order to become a champion.

The first step in eliminating these sorts of fears is to realize that they exist. Then, it's a simple matter of intellectual reasoning as to why such fears exist and how utterly silly such fears really are. A skilled sports hypnotherapist or sports psychologist may be able to assist you in eliminating these potentially debilitating roadblocks to success.

CONCENTRATION

Success in sports performance can be likened to practicing Zen. The concentration is so complete that there is no consciousness of concentration. The player must be one with his sport in order to execute it to his optimal ability.

You have no doubt been in a situation where your entire attention was so rapt and absorbed in one thought that you completely blocked out all others. This was probably due to your high concen-

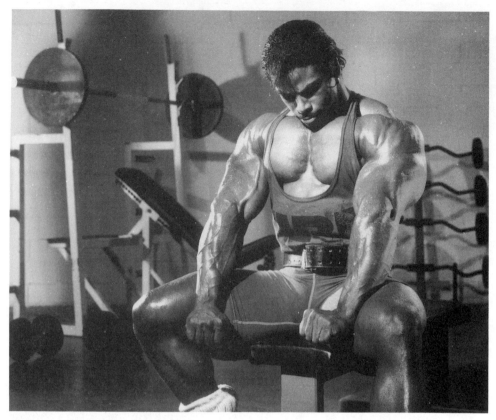

Concentrating to Win!

tration level on some thought of great importance to you. This kind of focus can be a confidence builder.

The more you focus on what you're working to achieve, the fewer distractions enter your awareness. This lifts you out of the state of mind that can't see success. Once you begin to see success, you consider yourself potentially better than the competition. Little by little, you concentrate more and more, until you're unaware of anything in your way. You see your way clearly to victory and success. This is total concentration.

This kind of total concentration comes to those who develop total self-confidence. You must have high self-esteem and high motivation and be consistent in your training program. You must develop your mind to the point that total concentration is merely a learned response, one you never consciously think about anymore.

Apply this sort of laser focus rep-per-rep and set-per-set in your workouts. Apply it in your daily integrated training program. Just as success begets success, imperfect practice makes your performance imperfect.

46

DEPRESSION

All of us get depressed from time to time. But at what point should the garden-variety sadness all of us suffer occasionally be regarded as a problem? Perhaps more importantly, is depression a tear or misplaced stitch in the fabric comprising one's personality, or is it a legitimate, physically-based illness that may be treatable?

Bodybuilders (with their well-known egos) may, on first reflection, seem less susceptible to the potentially mind-crippling ravages of self-doubt, melancholy, and despondency than your average pencilneck—you know, the old "C'mon, life! Hit me with your best shot!" attitude that all tough-minded athletes seem to possess. This kind of mental armor assists them in maintaining focus for the duration of their ascendancy to sports honor—maybe even until the heights of Olympia are conquered.

That armor, fellow iron freaks, is naught but a tenuously fastened exoskeleton protecting an infinitely fragile id. The eddy and swirls of gloom, prccipitated by events only God fully comprehends, inevitably seep in.

Depression states vary by name, symptom, and origin. In recent years, especially in the past year, scientists have made mighty strides in uncovering many of the causes and a growing number of treatments and cures for depression. One factor has consistently emerged in the research literature on depression—it's an illness.

That means that it can be treated and controlled. The day a cure is forthcoming for some of the more serious forms of depression seems just over the horizon. Less serious forms of depression appear now to be entirely curable.

WHAT IS DEPRESSION?

Think of depression as a hollow in an otherwise smooth surface. Sort of like the Grand Canyon, with some gradual drops and some precipitous ones. Think of depression as akin to being lower than a snake's belly or, more deeply poetic, lower than the proverbial whale dung on the bottom of the deepest ocean.

Depression is typically thought of in those terms. Extreme feelings of sadness, despondency, dejection, emptiness, lack of worth or purpose—often growing past the bounds of reason and reality, on to the point of suicide—are all symptoms of this illness. It would be a mistake for you to confuse these symptoms with the full definition of depression. To do so would perpetuate the same misconception of years past that depression is a disease of the mind. It is not. It is a disease that affects the mind. To fully define this common malady, you must also identify the root causes of depression.

Before you get bored with this stuff, let me direct your focus to my intent in writing about depression. I see depression far more frequently among competitive bodybuilders than any other class of athlete. There are some good reasons for this seemingly paradoxical observation.

WHAT CAUSES DEPRESSION?

Most people who suffer from depression aren't depressed all the time. Usually they go in and out, sometimes precipitously and sometimes gradually. Sometimes they sink low, low, lower, and sometimes they don't. Understanding the psychological and biochemical correlates to these variable mood swings will give you a clearer idea of the many treatments available for depression.

In the past, scientists recognized that exercise—particularly aerobic exercise—often seemed to be a powerful antidote for depression. These explanations included:

1. Exercise distracts sufferers from their suffering because it's enjoyable
2. Exercisers reap social reinforcement for their efforts
3. Depressed people see a measure of improvement in their physical condition, which gives them a lift in mood
4. Depressed people benefit from exercise because they are doing something for themselves and by themselves, thereby giving them a sense of power and control
5. Exercise improves circulation of blood to the brain, thus getting more oxygen there

6. Exercise causes the production of morphinelike endorphins and enkephalins which lift the mood as might other drugs
7. Neurotransmitters associated with the depressed state (or states of well-being) are stimulated or blocked (e.g., norepinepherine and other amine neurotransmitters)

These explanations of why exercise seemed to help gave no clue as to what caused the depressed state in the first place, however. It would be fallacious to argue that the lack of physical conditioning predisposes one to depression. Also, exercise only seemed to work part of the time, and only with certain individuals, in reducing or controlling depressive states.

A love affair gone bad, job-related stress, the death of a loved one, overwork, social isolation, all seem to be causative factors in plummeting a person headlong into a depressive state. But are such external events capable of being the prime causative?

Scientists now recognize that mood disorders are a result of complex interactions between a variety of biochemicals, including neurotransmitters, hormones, and many dietary cofactors such as the amino acid L-tryptophan and vitamins C, B_{12}, and B_6. To make matters more complex, there is a decided hereditary component to depression. Locked inside some strand of DNA (or a combination of loci on different chromosomes), a genetic code predisposes that person to an easier triggering of whatever mood shifts and/or bodily functions initiate the depressed state.

It's well known by now that sadness, happiness, anger, and other such states of mind are accompanied by vast biochemical changes inside the brain. Some of these biochemical changes are becoming better understood thanks to psychiatry's breakthrough discoveries of late. In some individuals, the biochemical changes associated with stress, grief, or other such external events become runaway, assumably due to genetic predisposition, drug abuse, infection or disease, nervous system disorder, allergy (especially cerebral allergies), or inadequate dietary intake or sunlight. Drugs, exercise, psychotherapy, electroconvulsive therapy, and even intense light therapy and other treatments all have the net effect of controlling the runaway biochemical response.

DIAGNOSING DEPRESSION

According to the American Psychiatric Association, depression is diagnosed when at least four of the following symptoms persist for two weeks or more.

- A marked increase or decrease in appetite accompanied by significant weight changes
- Insomnia or excessive sleepiness
- Hyperactivity or hypoactivity
- Loss of interest in sex and/or other activities typically regarded as pleasurable
- Reduced concentration, thinking ability, and recurrent thoughts of death and/or suicide
- Feelings of worthlessness, guilt, or self-reproach.

Guilt feelings or feelings of inadequacy may not be overtly apparent. That is, the person experiencing them may hide such feelings from others. However, attendant behavior most often becomes apparent to others. These behavioral changes frequently include

- Withdrawal from normal relationships
- Overreacting to the normal irritations of daily life
- Frequent crying spells
- Constipation, headaches, gastric upset, sexual dysfunction, anorexia, insomnia, early morning waking, and other unusual symptoms

Severely depressive patients frequently

- Hear voices accusing them of unpardonable sins
- See visions of dead friends or relatives
- Feel that someone is watching them
- Suffer from delusions of sinfulness, worthlessness, or incurable diseases

These symptoms range from mild to severe and are certainly nothing to take lightly at any level of intensity. It's advisable for depressed individuals—during a more lucid moment—to seek professional assistance. You can't fight the fight alone.

BODYBUILDERS AND DEPRESSION

It's both axiomatic and paradoxical that bodybuilders preparing for competition are malnourished to the point of sickness. Their strange and ritualistic eating behaviors, borne by naught but whim and propagated in myth alone, are believed to be just and proper precompetition necessity.

When are you going to learn? Months of muscle building, attitude adjustment, fat reducing, nutritional planning, and supplementation constitute proper preparatory technique. Crash dieting is *not* an acceptable component of scientific contest preparation.

The mythic beliefs about what constitutes good nutrition, attitude, and behavior among some bodybuilders can—and does—create a biochemical atmosphere conducive to the onset of a depressive state. Consider the following:

- Overindulgence in raw or lightly cooked egg whites can cause depression. Raw egg whites contain a protein that binds to biotin, making that important vitamin unavailable to the body

- Crash diets often severely limit the amount of vitamin B_6 (pyridoxine) available to the body. Since B_6 is a metabolite of tryptophan, and tryptophan is shunted into making more B_6, little is left for the manufacture of serotonin, a neurotransmitter which, in times of low supply, is implicated in depressive states

- Crash diets also often severely limit vitamins C and B_{12} (cyanocobalamin), deficiencies of which can cause depression

- Sad but true, many obsessive bodybuilders still cling to their abusive practices of shotgunning different drugs into their systems. Many of these drugs—especially those which alter estrogen and other hormonal levels—interact to produce depression. Examples are amphetamines, human chorionic gonadotropin (HCG), and L-DOPA. Combinations of estrogen blockers, steroids, amphetamines, and other drugs also cause variable and unpredictable interactions, some of which can involve depression.

When such bodily abuse is combined with the stresses of training and, ultimately, the tragically common happenstance of not winning the contest (there can be only one winner), you have a somatic and psychic potpourri of circumstance which are all-too conducive to depression.

WHAT ARE THE ALTERNATIVES?

As with most illnesses, depression can be prevented. Sure, there are treatments. There are, in some instances, outright cures. But by far the best alternative is to avoid depression in the first place.

1. Ensure that your diet is well balanced
2. Ensure that your diet is fortified with good-quality vitamins and minerals
3. Avoid the abusive drugs commonly used in some bodybuilding circles

4. Foster a lifestyle that is fun-filled and rewarding

5. Avoid unnecessary mental and physical stresses that so often accompany today's frenetic pace

6. Having job problems? Love partner problems? Financial problems? Solve them! One (often unspoken) way to solve such problems is to simply get rid of the source

7. When you begin to notice symptoms in yourself or in someone close to you, do something about them. That will usually involve seeking professional help. Nipping such problems in the bud is the best way to avoid future problems. A full-blown case of depression is one problem you certainly don't need.

FIGURE 46-1

States of Depression, Symptoms, and Treatments

PSYCHOSIS

A mental disorder of either a physical or emotional source, psychosis is marked by delusion, hallucination, illusion, depression, or excitement of major proportions and in which the individual is incapable of functioning within the scope of reality. The disorder is typically bipolar in nature; that is, sometimes manic (excessive excitement, overactivity, a marked reduction in one's need for sleep, and an inability to concentrate) and sometimes depressive (apathetic, excessive sadness, loneliness, guilt, and unrealistically low self-worth).

PRIMARY CAUSE(S)

Genetic predisposition
Severe stress
Drug abuse
Disease (nervous system disorder, cancer, infection)

TREATMENT(S)

Electroconvulsive therapy (in older patients)
Lithium carbonate (primarily in manic phase, but also shows effectiveness as an antidepressant)
Carbamazepine (manic phase)
Valproic acid (manic phase)
Psychotherapy:
    Cognitive therapy (helps change negative thinking patterns)
    Interpersonal therapy (helps in interpersonal relationships)
Psychoanalysis
Aerobic exercise (sometimes anaerobic as well)
Combinational approach (drugs, psychotherapy, and psychoanalysis most often prove more effective than drugs, psychotherapy, or psychoanalysis alone)

TYPICAL PROGNOSIS

Thirty percent respond well to treatment(s) but do not get completely well.

SEVERE (CLINICAL) DEPRESSION

Typically unipolar in nature (compared to the bipolarity of psychosis), clinical or severe depression is characterized by inability to sleep or eat, extreme feelings of sadness, lack of self-worth, dejection, and emptiness. This form of depression can range from a slight inability to concentrate and lack of motivation to severe changes in bodily functions. This type of depressive disorder was for years referred to as melancholia. In combination with manic-depressive disorders, it affects nearly 30 million people in the U.S.A. alone.

PRIMARY CAUSE(S)

Genetic predisposition
Stress
Traumatic event(s)
Drug abuse
Hormonal imbalance (can be induced or genetic)
Poor diet
Disease (nervous system disorders, cancer, infection)

TREATMENT(S)

Tricyclic antidepressants (disturbed sleep patterns, apathy, appetite loss)
Prozac (increases brain levels of serotonin)
Anafranil (increases brain levels of serotonin)
Wellbutrin (mood elevator)
Diet therapy
Psychotherapy
Psychoanalysis
Aerobic exercise (sometimes anaerobic as well)
Combinational approach

TYPICAL PROGNOSIS

Thirty percent respond well to treatment(s) but do not get completely well.

ATYPICAL DEPRESSION

This form of depression is marked by the same mood and self-worth reductions as clinical depression. However, it is characterized by a person eating more (not less) and sleeping more (not less). It is current thinking that this atypical behavior stems from factors related to specific hormonal imbalances.

PRIMARY CAUSE(S)

Same as Clinical Depression, with the emphasis on hormonal imbalances

TREATMENT(S)

Monoamine oxidase inhibitors (MAO metabolizes tyramine in the gut; MAOI prevents this breakdown, thereby leaving tyramine intact to allow release of norepinepherine)
Diet therapy
Psychotherapy
Psychoanalysis
Aerobic exercise (sometimes anaerobic as well)
Combinational approach

TYPICAL PROGNOSIS

Thirty percent respond well to treatment(s) but do not get completely well.

SEASONAL AFFECTIVE DISORDER (SAD)

This state of depression is common in the Arctic and Antarctic regions. With the gradual disappearance of sunlight, despair sets in and lasts until the sun returns six months later.

PRIMARY CAUSE(S)

Lack of sunlight (believed related to body's inability to synthesize vitamin D)
Poor diet

TREATMENT(S)

Light therapy (sitting in front of intense light)
Antidepressants
Take a vacation to a sunny beach
Diet/vitamin therapy
Combinational approach

TYPICAL PROGNOSIS

Energy and high spirits return with sunlight and/or good diet

DYSTHEMIA

Dysthemia has been likened to a low-grade infection that simply takes time to go away. It is a chronic, though milder, form of depression that can last for months or even years. You just don't feel good. This feeling of malaise is dispiriting and affects nearly 10 million Americans.

PRIMARY CAUSE(S)

Continued poor diet
Continued inactivity
Continued stressful lifestyle
Traumatic event(s)
Drug abuse
Disease (infection, hormonal imbalances, dysfunctional bodily process(es))
Cumulative consequence of above factors

TREATMENT(S)

Diet therapy
Antidepressants
Exercise (aerobic or anaerobic seems to help)
Lifestyle change and/or change in domicile
Stop abusing drugs
Psychotherapy
Psychoanalysis

TYPICAL PROGNOSIS

While some forms of this depressive state take longer to treat than others, most appear curable. All appear controllable with a tailored program of ongoing therapy.

REACTIVE DEPRESSION

Normal (reactive) depression is a healthy response to a specific event. The event can be emotionally based (divorce, job loss, neglect, unrealistic expectations, midlife crisis, loss of parent or loved one) or biologically based (premenstrual syndrome, postpartum depression, sickness, injury).

PRIMARY CAUSE(S)

The unwanted/unavoidable event

TREATMENT(S)

Time

TYPICAL PROGNOSIS

Time cures all.

PART ELEVEN

CONTEST PREPARATION

DEDICATED TO TONY PEARSON

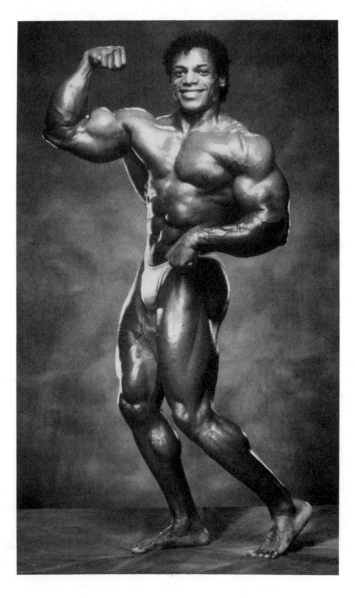

Tony Pearson

47

PRECONTEST PREPARATION

"We're all individuals with different needs" is a phrase you'll hear repeated ad nauseam. For the most part, it's a cop-out. Most bodybuilders think they know what's best for them. I have found that, upon being prodded for some semblance of scientific rationale, they really don't know. True as it may be that all of us are unique, the similarities between competing bodybuilders far outweigh the differences.

Need more beef in the upper chest region? That's a difference you may regard as unique. OK. Train your upper chest with a vengeance. Kind of weak in the biceps department? Blitz 'em. Tend to put on a bit of fat because your metabolic rate is a bit slow? Well, then, eat and supplement a bit more fastidiously in the off-season.

But don't—I repeat—*don't*—resort to Herculean efforts involving severe caloric restriction and endless aerobics during the precontest phase of your training. If science has taught us anything, it's that bodybuilding must be a lifestyle commitment. It must not be merely a precontest commitment.

All of us are indeed unique. Build your training regimen to reflect your unique qualities and weaknesses. In the meantime, recognize that your physiology—your anatomy and your biochemistry—is quite the same overall as the others against whom you intend to compete. On that note, it makes scientific sense to construct a training shell which will be modified to reflect your uniqueness.

Outlined in this chapter is that universal shell. Assuming that you've laid a solid bodybuilding foundation over years of time already, it takes sixteen weeks to really get contest-ready. This is the only system I've ever seen that makes total sense. Other systems are good—they work. Some systems of training are better than others, but there is only one best system. Here it is. Go with it!

SIXTEEN WEEKS OUT

Assessment time. Take a look in the mirror. Have your coach or a qualified judge look you over. Be critical. Where are your weaknesses? Your strengths? Rearrange your training regimen to maximize your efforts at alleviating weaknesses in proportioning now. Later, it'll be too late to worry about weaknesses. At contest time, it's not your strengths that will put you on the winner's podium—it'll be your lack of weaknesses. Remember that!

It is a universal requirement for all bodybuilders to come in as massive, proportioned, and cut as possible. Universal laws of science dictate how this is best accomplished. (Note: I said "best." I didn't say "good" or "better.") Since you're already taking care of your proportioning through selective arrangement of your exercises, and since you've been reasonably fastidious (as you should have been) at keeping down the excess baggage (fat) during the off-season, let's concentrate on getting bigger muscles without putting on fat during this early cycle.

You put on muscle, my friend, by ensuring that every subcellular element of every muscle in your anatomy is forced to adapt. Compensatory adaptation can only take place if the stress you impose is of sufficient frequency, intensity, and duration. Since each subcellular element requires a different form of stress (frequency, intensity, and duration), you must use a holistic approach to your training—heavy weights, light weights; fast movements, slow movements; high reps, low reps; and everything in between!

One more thing. How does a muscle grow? By feeding it! If any one of your muscles is not adequately capillarized, you can't get enough nutrient-laden blood there, nor can you remove the wastes generated by muscle work. Slow, continuous tension movements performed at high reps (forty or more) are essential during this phase of training in order to ensure that capillarization occurs. This will support your mass training efforts, and it will also lay a foundation for the following training cycle which emphasizes recovery ability.

It's critical to note that the vascularization process takes about two months to complete. You will notice little or no progress during that time in your ability to perform high reps. All of a sudden, it happens! You will suddenly be able to do around 80 reps with the same weight that, days before, you could only do 40–50 reps with. These new capillaries don't open until they're fully developed. Now you can grow because you have an ample supply line to your muscles to support that growth.

Be patient, and trust science.

NINE WEEKS OUT

About nine or ten weeks prior to your competition or target date, you should do a cleanse of your gastrointestinal tract. In this way, your entire system will gear itself up for the grueling weeks of contest training or rigorous mass training ahead. Part Seven contains some of the methods of accomplishing this.

Now it's time to up the intensity. Stay with some heavy stuff for limit strength and mass increase, but be sure that your high-intensity microcycles (body part per body part) are more frequent. That'll mean you have to begin concentrating more on recovery. Try increasing intensity without tending to your recuperative capabilities, and you will surely overtrain.

FIGURE 47-1

Coordinating Your Precontest Training Intensity, Caloric Intake, and Body Weight

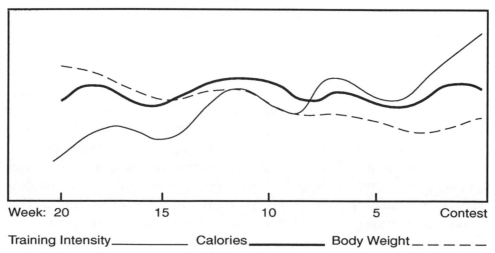

Week: 20   15   10   5   Contest

Training Intensity_____ Calories_____ Body Weight _ _ _ _ _

You're still improving on your mass and strength so that, as your recovery abilities improve, you can lift even heavier weights more frequently. What does that spell? Even more mass. It also spells an improved metabolic rate for fat control. Remember, bigger muscles burn more calories than smaller muscles.

The net result of this form of training is that your body weight will stay relatively stable but your ratio of fat to muscle will change. You'll be getting harder and harder.

FOUR WEEKS OUT

Whoa! Time's a' wastin'! You're as big right now as you're going to be. Now, as you look in the mirror, you'll say, "Dude, you're already ready!" You look better than you have ever looked—vascular, ripped, and massive.

But wait! No striations. Holding a bit of water. Here and there—if you're really critical with yourself—there are tiny pockets of fat visible. Usually they show up on your lower butt at the hamstring tie-in area and around the rear portion of your obliques. That spells only one thing—you *aren't* ready!

Your job during these last few weeks is to improve your anaerobic threshold training. Perhaps a bit of aerobic training will be called for as well, so long as it's not overdone. Too much aerobic training tends to waste muscle tissue and mobilize the triglycerides for that long-term energy aerobic training requires.

But please don't forget that beautiful mass that you've worked so hard to acquire! You've got to keep training with heavy weights, and you've got to keep pushing the intensity to the absolute limits of your pain threshold. With an amped-up metabolism and some moderate aerobics, you'll burn more calories, even while you're resting and sleeping, so be careful! Those big muscles aren't regarded by Mother Nature as important to your survival, and she'll cannibalize them for fuel way before she'll dip into your dwindling fat stores. What does that mean? You've got to keep the calories coming in—plenty of protein, and plenty of carbs. Keep the dietary fat down to around 5 percent of your total caloric intake, because the only way you can metabolize that fat is through muscle wasting aerobic training.

THE LAST SEVEN DAYS

How many times have all of us seen it happen—a week out you look great. You panic: "Maybe I can do more! Maybe Joe Blow *is* better than me! Maybe if I just take this, or do that, I'll get even better." This is called self-doubt. You show up holding water, drawn out to the max, lighter than you intended, and (predictably) you lose. A day after the contest, you look great again.

When are you going to learn? Even the big guys—the superstars of bodybuilding—are guilty of this scenario once in a while. Even they can make mistakes sometimes. Sure, they're great, but our honest belief is that there's still plenty of room for improvement. Someday, you'll see a normal height guy walk out onto the stage weighing in at 300 pounds and ripped to shreds. It's possible, but only through integrative science.

Your sodium/potassium ratio is critical in these last few days. Careful manipulation of the mechanisms responsible for extracellular water levels is a must. But get this straight right now—you cannot get rid of a significant amount of fat in the last four or five days, and you can't get bigger muscles either. That has to have already happened over weeks of time, so don't try. Keep the caloric intake where it should be—normal! All you have to do during the last days prior to the contest is ensure that your extracellular fluid is managed properly. All the other work is already done.

An age-old technique that's tried and true works every time—for everyone. It's called glycogen supercompensation, or carbo-loading. Then, and only then, will you hit it exactly on schedule and look your best at the prejudging.

Get this, and get it good! If you want to play with the big boys, you're going to have to be willing to pay the price. You aren't going to beat any serious competitors in the elite ranks of bodybuilding with one-a-days. Even two-a-days is going to be barely adequate. You need to couple smart training with all of the other things that go into making a champion.

In short, you've got to want it.

48

CARBOHYDRATE SUPERCOMPENSATION ("CARBO-LOADING") STRATEGIES FOR LOOKING YOUR BEST AT PREJUDGING

Your muscles use carbohydrates as their main source of energy. The carbohydrates in your diet are converted into glycogen and stored in your muscles and liver. When you are at rest, your body burns carbohydrates and fats at an equal rate, but as you increase your training intensity, carbohydrates become the more important source of fuel for your muscles. At very high training intensities, carbohydrates become the sole energy provider.

Several decades ago, Swedish scientists used this knowledge to devise a method of packing greater than normal amounts of glycogen inside endurance athletes' muscles. It allowed them to run for longer periods without hitting the wall. More recently, bodybuilders found that the practice of carbo-loading gave their visible muscles a fuller, more striated, and denser appearance.

There are basically three ways to load carbohydrates. It's up to you and your coach to find the one most suitable for you. Together with integrated training, carbo-loading makes it possible for you to pack 40 to 60 percent more glycogen than normal into your muscle cells, providing a far better onstage appearance.

CARBO-LOADING METHOD 1

The first method is the most simple to follow. Three days before a competition, consume only low-glycemic-index carbohydrates. Eliminate your intake of refined sugars (refer to the glycemic index presented in Chapter 22). Keep your calorie sources at a ratio of 1:2:3 for fats, protein, and carbohydrates, respectively, for each of your 5–6 daily meals. Maintain a very high training intensity, keeping your workouts less than 30 minutes in duration. Throughout the three days, be sure to use your supplements as directed.

CARBO-LOADING METHOD 2

The second method is a bit more exacting. Beginning one week before your contest, train to exhaustion for four days in order to deplete your existing glycogen stores. Your food ratio remains 1:2:3 (one part fats, two parts protein, and three parts carbohydrates) during this carbohydrate depletion phase. Continue eating 5–6 meals daily. Then, during the three days prior to competition, load up on carbohydrates with a glycemic index of below 50 (refer to the glycemic index chart in Chapter 22). During this final precontest period, you should alter your intake of fats, protein, and carbohydrates to a ratio of 1:2:5 with little or no fats and protein prior to the prejudging round on contest day. Throughout the seven days, be sure to use your supplements as directed.

CARBO-LOADING METHOD 3

The final carbo-loading system is the most rigorous. Beginning six days before your contest, reduce your carbohydrate consumption to about 20 percent of your daily caloric intake for three days, maintaining very high training intensity. With a caloric ratio of 1:3:1 for fats, protein, and carbohydrates during the carbohydrate depletion phase, it's possible that you will feel fatigued and weak and possibly lose potassium and muscle tissue. To avoid this, you must ensure that you're taking in ample calories. Do *not* starve yourself. Continue to eat 5–6 meals daily.

During the carbohydrate loading phase, increase your intake of low-glycemic-index carbohydrates to 70–80 percent (refer to the glycemic index chart in Chapter 22). Your ratio of fats, protein, and carbohydrates is now about 1:2:8. This carbo-loading phase should last three days with reduced training during the first two days and none on the last day before competition. During the carbohydrate loading phase you should rest a lot and keep your workouts very high in intensity and only 30 minutes in duration. Throughout the seven days, be sure to use your supplements as directed.

Although any carbohydrate source can help refill glycogen stores, lower-glycemic-index carbohydrates are best. Why? Since these carbohydrates tend to enter your bloodstream slowly, they are able to maintain a steady release of insulin that activates the enzyme glycogen synthetase, which is essential for glycogen storage. Carbohydrates with a high glycemic index—those which raise your blood sugar rapidly—cause wild fluctuations in your insulin level, and your carbo-loading efforts will not be as effective.

For each gram of glycogen stored inside your muscle cells, about 3–4 grams of water are stored along with it. This is what gives your visible muscles a dense, full, striated appearance. For this reason, reducing water consumption during the carbo-loading phase is ill-advised. You should ingest at least 8 ounces of water with each meal, and more depending upon your overall lean body mass.

Scientists recommend that carbohydrate loading be practiced no more than three times a year. More, they believe, will decrease its effectiveness. Under normal off-season and precontest training conditions, a 1-2-3 diet (one part fats, two parts protein, and three parts carbohydrates), consumed 5–6 times daily, will ensure that sufficient glycogen is stored to fuel even the most rigorous body-building schedule.

PART TWELVE

MYTHIC CONCEPTS IN BODYBUILDING

DEDICATED TO TROY ZUCCOLOTTO

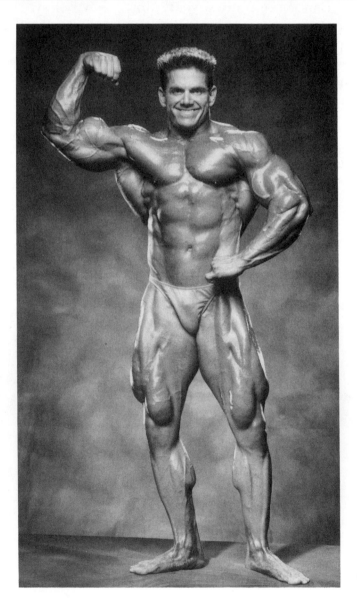

Troy Zuccolotto

49

MYTHS ABOUT DRUGS, NUTRITION, AND TRAINING

INTRODUCTION

Ironheads often become crusaders for their lifestyle, much in the tradition of the misguided Christians of the dark ages, the Nazis of the darkest ages, and even current-day cultists. In their characteristic zeal, they embrace beliefs that seem at the time of acceptance to be logical and just—or, at least, worth the risk.

Later on, realizing that their belief structure has been based on half-truths, lies, misinterpretations of legitimate research findings, out-of-context quotes, and a host of other tenuous infrastructural lattices, they are forced into a situation not unlike the crusaders, the Nazis, and the Scientologists. They hunker down and defend the beliefs they've held dear for so long with an abiding vengeance. You see, their very souls had gone into believing. For them to abandon that which was once held dear for something as trivial as truth would lay waste to their very souls and beings.

Consider this common phenomenon in psychology. A man buys a Chevy. He saved for a long time to buy that car and tried his best to get the most for his money. He tried hard to buy a vehicle that his peers would hold him in high regard for purchasing—a vehicle befitting his social position. Someone comes along and proves to him that, had he bought a Ford, he'd have gotten more for less.

Bang! The mind closes tight and hunkers down into a defensive position. All references to Fords (or any other vehicle) are burned or avoided like the plague. This man had invested too much to admit that he had erred. He doesn't even want to be reminded of it! Despite the fact that he is patently aware of his mistake, he is obliged, by all he holds dear, to defend his position to the death if necessary.

Such is the human condition, and such is the state of the art and science of bodybuilding, fitness, and sports training. These activities lend themselves to the crusading spirit. They represent a lifestyle which, upon its acceptance, sets the believer apart from all others on the face of planet Earth.

There's a new day dawning on us. New-age science has spawned breathtaking advances enabling us to make muscle gains like never before. It all started with the electron microscope, then came magnetic resonance imaging, genetic engineering, and a veritable cascade of technological breakthroughs of such a profound nature that 95 percent of the entire history of man's inventiveness would be cited in the scientific annals of a single quarter century.

Looking to science for your important training questions, and the simpler ones as well, you will be swept away on a journey you won't believe—on into the innermost regions of space, inside the cells themselves, into the individual organelles comprising the cells, and the genetic codes to which they individually owe their existence. You are minutely advancing toward a profound understanding of the very essence of life itself.

Poof! Gone are the mythic beliefs. Open your minds to modern science! You owe it to yourself to make the gains you have heretofore only dreamed about.

I propose herein to systematically shatter some of the mythic beliefs of irondom. If you're still not convinced, hopefully you will at least stand back and think. The alternatives to the myths—the *truths*— are only briefly presented herein. The complete pictures are to be found elsewhere. Be aware that this is not *my* science. I did not invent it, nor did I singlehandedly interpret it. I merely serve as your humble archivist.

MYTHIC CONCEPTS ABOUT DRUGS

Myth One: Anabolic Steroids are Dangerous

The fact is, the folks who misuse or abuse them are. Guns aren't evil either; the misuse of them is.

Myth Two: Without Steroids, I Can't Make the Same Gains

Have you tried applying integrative science yet? Don't knock it until you've tried it! It may take more discipline and time, but it most certainly can be done.

Myth Three:
All the Top Bodybuilding Stars Have Learned How to Circumvent Detection in the Drug Tests

The fact is that some have, but most who have tried got caught. As testing procedures become more discriminatory, the misuse and abuse of steroids and other banned drugs are on a decided decline in all sports. In the World Wrestling Federation (as in the ill-fated World Bodybuilding Federation), testing has already been taken to the highest level of discriminatory detection ever through the efforts of Dr. Mauro DiPasquale of Canada.

Myth Four:
Testosterone Is a Great Substitute for Steroids

Testosterone is highly androgenic. It is not highly anabolic. When it's abused as a substitute for anabolic steroids, it bloats the abuser (among other dangerous side effects), with little or no lasting strength gains forthcoming.

Myth Five: There Aren't Any Other Anabolic Agents on the Horizon That Can Compare to Steroids in Effectiveness

There are, but they too are dangerous and are illegal or banned by sports governing bodies. There are some nutritional and nonnutritional substances which are safe, legal, and at least marginally effective. Give them a try within a scientifically formulated training regimen. You will be pleasantly surprised.

Myth Six: Smoking Dope or Snorting Coke Can Help Me in My Training Efforts

These drugs are dangerous, quite addicting (physically and psychologically), and, especially in the long run, thoroughly bad for training because they take away your drive and cause many unwanted side effects.

Myth Seven: Uppers Will Help Me with My Training and Fat-Loss Efforts

Only in the short-run. In the long-run, they will cause both physical and psychological dependency to the extent that they become more desirable than scientific training or dieting. At that point, you lose.

Myth Eight: As Long as There Are Bodybuilders Who Want to Win, There Is Going to Be a Drug Problem in the Sport of Bodybuilding

If we can instill a new moral ethic among our youth, drug abuse in sports will over a generation or two become regarded as an ancient and archaic attempt on the part of desperate athletes to excel. Parents, clergy, coaches, scientists, doctors—and the kids themselves— all working together can make this happen.

MYTHIC CONCEPTS IN THE TRAINING SCIENCES

Myth Nine: With the Proper Choice of Exercises, I Will Be Able to Control the Shape of Each One of My Muscles

The good Lord, in His infinite wisdom, gave you genes that will determine your individual muscles' shape. Your job is to make them big or strong. You can, however, shape your body. You can also shape a body part comprised of several muscles.

Myth Ten: The Nautilus Principle of One Set to Failure Is More Effective Than Any Other Method for Bodybuilders and Fitness Enthusiasts Alike

It is not effective for serious bodybuilders, and it is marginally effective in casual fitness training. Its originator, Arthur Jones, publicly turned his back on this (principally marketing-oriented) myth. There are many great ways to train. This is not one of them.

Myth Eleven: The Top Pros Know How to Train, and They Know Why They Do What They Do

Some have a good idea. Most, however, do not and became great primarily as a result of a gift from God (genetic predisposition) and hard (not necessarily smart) work. You'll no doubt get some good advice from the pros, but you'll be better off seeking competent advice from trained experts, of which there are precious few.

Myth Twelve: If I Train Longer and Harder Than Anyone Else, I Stand a Good Chance of Becoming Better Than They

Almost never. You'll overtrain yourself every time you try. Smart work—not hard or long work—is the only way to go.

Myth Thirteen: In Order to Get Maximum Development in My Muscles, I Have to Attack Them from Different Angles— with Several Different Exercise Movements

When you make a muscle contract against resistance, do so in such a way that the targeted muscle contracts hard enough to force an adaptive response. It is not necessary to get cute with many different exercises, because the training effect is generalized throughout the entire muscle, never only in one spot or border of that muscle.

Myth Fourteen: Answers to All My Training Questions on Bodybuilding, Fitness, and Sports Training Can Be Obtained from Exercise Physiologists or Sports-Medicine Doctors

Most of the time this is not true, unless they have hands-on experience in training themselves. Answers to most training problems have come from the trenches, and few have come from the ivory towers of academia.

Myth Fifteen: Heavy Weights (Low Reps) Make You Bigger, and Lighter Weights (High Reps) Get You Cut

The truth is, there's a better way. Get your muscles big through a holistic approach (heavy weights, light weights, fast movements, slow movements, high reps, low reps, and everything in between). Get your cuts from careful, scientific dieting and supplementing.

Myth Sixteen: I Can't Make It to the Top Because I Have a Full-Time Job, a Family, and Other Obligations That Keep Me from Training

Excuses all! Get up early and train. Bring a brown bag full of good food with you to work so you can eat five or six times a day. Grab a few sets during your scheduled lunch hour. Work out at least once in the evening (you may wish to get in two short workouts instead). The answer is dedication, discipline, and frugal use of available time.

Myth Seventeen: Those Electrostimulators, Bullworkers, Stretchie-Cords, and Other Gadgets on the Market Have No Place in a Bodybuilder's Training Regimen.

Au contraire! All such devices work fine. The secret is to use them regularly. Frankly, weight training is the best alternative, but that's not to say the other stuff doesn't work. In fact, under certain conditions, such items may be more appropriate than a weight workout.

Myth Eighteen:
Squats Give You a Broad Butt, Leg Extensions Are Good for Cutting Up the Quads, Hammer Curls and Variations Thereof Will Elongate the Biceps

Your genes will determine the shape of your muscles once you've hypertrophied them through weight training. Careful scientific training and nutrition—not necessarily the inclusion or exclusion of a particular exercise—will determine the extent of hypertrophy, but never the shape, of a muscle.

MYTHIC CONCEPTS IN NUTRITION

Myth Nineteen:
I Can Get as Big as I Am Physically Capable of Getting by Eating Three Square Meals Per Day

It takes five or six meals a day, each with an array of food groups and each with an appropriate balance of fats, carbohydrates, and protein to ensure maximum growth. Let's not forget training, either.

Myth Twenty: The Scientists Who Established the RDAs Had Bodybuilders and Other Athletes in Mind When They Made Their Recommendations

The FDA is concerned with feeding the masses. They have never given any thought whatsoever to elite athletes. Maybe that'll change once the masses get involved in fitness.

Myth Twenty-One: If You Can't Find It in the Research Literature, Forget It—It's No Good

This is the prevalent thinking among legitimate scientists. They say, "Where are your data?" as if its absence signifies illegitimacy. The truth is, a vast majority of training wisdom emanates from the trenches and sometimes, if we're lucky, gets tested years later by these scientists.

Myth Twenty-Two: If You Can Find It in the Research Literature, Embrace It as the Truth

Much of the research done thus far in the general area of fitness and sports training has contributed to the body of knowledge without contributing one iota to sports or fitness in an applied sense. Further, much (particularly the nutrition literature) was performed for one semester using college freshmen (hardly a representative sample of fitness or sports people), rendering findings pretty much externally invalid. There is, however, much good research, and it's wise to use it.

Myth Twenty-Three: All Those Pills, Potions, and Powders Being Ramrodded Down the Throats of Unwary Consumers with Promises of Bigger Muscles Are Just Plain Garbage and Don't Work

It is true that science has not produced the magic bullet that steroids were. That's not to say that some of the substances on the market nowadays aren't effective. Some are, but you have to use them for a long time; they're very expensive; you have to ask, "Does the cost justify the small gains they produce?" and there may not be sufficient data to support the claims made by the manufacturer. Usually such claims are outrageous and ill-founded. Sometimes, however, if you look past the hype and bombast, you'll find a pretty good (and worthwhile) supplement.

Myth Twenty-Four: More Is Better

Better is better.

Myth Twenty-Five: Dieticians, Medical Doctors, Chiropractors, and Nutritionists Are Your Best Bet for Good, Sound Nutritional Advice to Support Your Training Efforts

Most are highly conservative in their nutritional approaches to fitness and sports excellence. Most are concerned with the health of the relatively sedentary masses because that's where their training is and that's where the money is. Nonetheless, you're going to get better information from them than from an uneducated gym rat. Better that you go to a sports or fitness-oriented physiologist with extensive experience in the trenches as well as an academic background.

Myth Twenty-Six: I Don't Have the Time, Money, or Patience to Eat Right

Reread the response to Myth Sixteen.

Myth Twenty-Seven: I'll Be Healthier If I Stay Away from Fats, Sodium, and Sugar

There's nothing wrong with fats and sugar, just don't eat too much of them. Do, however, eat *some*. They are healthy, necessary, and good. As for sodium, seek medical advice before eliminating it from your diet. Sodium serves many important functions in the body and happens to be our chief source of iodine these days (too little fish is eaten nowadays).

Myth Twenty-Eight: Assuming I Need 3,000 Calories a Day (for Example) and Must Eat Five Meals Per Day, Then All I Have to Do Is Eat 600 Calories Per Meal

This method is fine for general fitness and is certainly better than eating three or fewer meals per day, but it's not enough if peak performance is your goal. Before each meal, ask yourself, "What am I going to be doing for the next three hours of my life?" Then, apportion your caloric intake accordingly. Never eat for what you just did—only for what you're going to do.

POSTSCRIPT

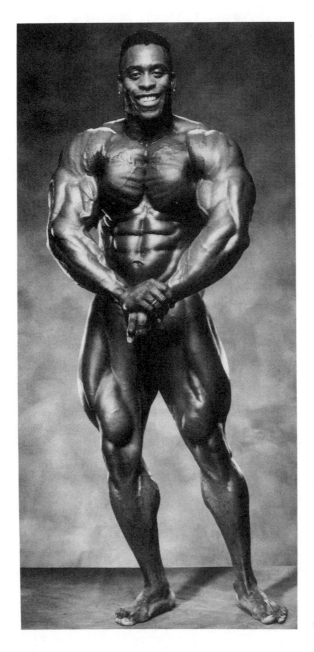

Johnnie Morant

A BROTHER'S SAGA

The mighty men of Iceland sing
    against the wind and winter's sting.
Viking blood and Viking ale
    have conquered worlds in truth and tale,
But never a man of ice and winter
    doth lift the Manhood Stone like Hinter.

Doth lift the Manhood Stone like Hinter.

Blue lagoons and lava caves;
    geysers blow, volcanos rage.
Such a place is Hinter's host;
    "the Gates of Hell" it's called by most.
But never a man loved home like Hinter;
    he reveled in the cold, dark winter.

He reveled in the cold, dark winter.

Now cometh to this Viking land
    a man called Squat, with steel in hand.
Of Norsemen's blood by mother's mother,
    he braved the cold to seek his brother.
And never a man from Norse begot
    doth lift the heavy steel like Squat.

Doth lift the heavy steel like Squat.

Then cometh he to Hinter's lair
    where fires glow on women fair
And geysers blow from Hell's fires burning
    a drink men drink called Black Death, churning.
Though steel and stone are worlds apart,
    still Hinter shook the hand of Squat.

Still Hinter shook the hand of Squat.

Why come you here to seek your kin?
    The days grow short and winter's in.
My brother's here—I feel his soul.
    I'll find him though the nights turn cold.
But first let's drink some Viking beer!
    My brother lives; I have no fear.

My brother lives; I have no fear.

So drank these mighty men of old,
    the Black Death steaming and Viking Gold.
So drank till nightfall came and went,
    till six months passed and stories spent,
But never a word was ever spoken
    of stone and steel, or strength feats broken.

Of stone and steel, or strength feats broken.

The Clash of Giants contest nears.
    The crash of stone and steel one hears.
Hinter lifts the Manhood Stone
    while mighty Squat bears steel on bone,
But neither winces at the strain,
    and both men feel the other's pain.

And both men feel the other's pain.

And never a man of ice and winter
    doth lift the Manhood Stone like Hinter.
And never a man from Norse begot
    doth lift the heavy steel like Squat.
Now, come you to the place of Vikings
    to test your might on steel and stone.

To test your might on steel and stone.

From throughout Iceland giants lift
    to prove their worth and win the gift.
More steel, more stone to hand is taken,
    till one man fails, his honor shaken.
When stone is gone and steel bars bent,
    just two men stand, the others spent.

Just two men stand, the others spent.

Squat shares a kinship brothers may
    with mighty Hinter on this day,
For both have won the cherished gift
    of Vikings past who made the lift.
The gift of Brotherhood, 'tis told,
    is Viking blood, worth more than gold,

And *brotherhood's* worth more than gold.

                                  Dr. Squat

GLOSSARY

Abduction—Movement of a limb away from middle axis of the body, such as extending arms outward at shoulder height from a hanging-down position.

Abs—Slang for abdominal muscles.

Absolute strength—Developed through heavy weight training, typically involving above the 80–85 percent of maximum effort for each lift. Its three components are concentric, eccentric, and static strength. No ergogenic aids (e.g., drugs, therapies, or nutritional products) are used in training for absolute strength, whereas such ergogens are used to acquire limit strength.

  1. **Concentric strength** refers to the one-rep maximum for a movement
  2. **Eccentric** is the one-rep maximum lowering a weight under control (usually 40 percent more than concentric)
  3. **Static** is the maximum holding strength in a given position (20 percent more than concentric)

Accommodating resistance—A weight training machine which, through the use of air, fluid, or clutch plates in tandem with a flywheel, controls the speed with which you are able to move. By controlling speed, the exertion you are able to deliver is always at maximum throughout the entire range of motion of an exercise. This technology is very useful during rehabilitation, when injuries are present, and also in sports training for speed-strength. See *variable resistance* and *constant resistance*.

Acetyl coenzyme A (acetyl CoA)—A chief precursor of lipids. It is formed by an acetyl group attaching itself to coenzyme A (CoA) during the oxidation of amino acids, fatty acids, or pyruvate.

Acid-base balance—Refers to the condition in which the pH of the blood is kept at a constant level of 7.35 to 7.45. The acidity of blood is kept from becoming too acidic or alkaline through respiration, buffers, and work done by the kidney.

Acromegaly—A chronic pituitary gland disorder developing in adult life characterized by increased massiveness of the bones, organs, and other body parts and elongation and enlargement of the bones.

Actin—One of the fibrous protein constituents of the protein complex actomyosin. It is a protein which when combined with myosin forms actomyosin, the contractile constituent of muscle.

Actomyosin—The system involved in muscle contraction and relaxation which is composed of actin and myosin protein filaments.

Additives—Substances other than a foodstuff present in food as a result of production, processing, storage, or packaging. Examples: preservatives, coloring.

Adduction—Movement of a limb toward middle axis of the body, such as returning arms to the side from extended position at shoulders.

Adenosine triphosphate (ATP)—The body's energizer, an organic compound present in muscle fibers that is broken down through a variety of enzymatic processes. The resultant spark of energy released stimulates hundreds of microscopic filaments within each cell, triggering muscle contraction.

Adhesion—Fibrous tissue holding muscles or other parts together that have been altered or damaged through trauma.

Aerobic exercise—Activities in which oxygen from the blood is required to fuel the energy-producing mechanisms of muscle fibers. Examples are running, cycling, and skiing over distance. Aerobic means "with oxygen."

Aerobic strength—Strength of effort (i.e., force) in the face of massive oxygen debt, as incurred in long-distance training or competition. It has three general components:

1. **Cardiovascular endurance** relates to the efficiency in getting oxygenated and nutrient-rich blood to the working muscles and spent blood back to the heart

2. **Cardiorespiratory endurance** involves the efficiency of the loop where the blood goes from the heart to the lungs, gets rid of water and carbon dioxide, picks up oxygen, and returns to the heart for pumping out to the body

3. **Max VO$_2$ uptake** (maximum volume of oxygen taken up by the working muscles), expressed in milliliters of oxygen per kilogram of body weight per minute (ml/kg/min)

Agonist—A muscle directly involved in contraction and primarily responsible for movement of a body part. Also called a prime mover.

Albumin—A type of simple protein widely distributed throughout the tissues and fluids of plants and animals. Varieties of albumin are found in blood, milk, egg white, wheat, barley, and muscle.

Aldosterone—A mineralocorticoid which functions as the primary electrolyte-regulatory steroid hormone. It is secreted by the adrenal cortex.

Allergen—A substance that causes an allergy or hypersensitivity.

Amino acids—The building blocks of protein. There are twenty-four amino acids, which form countless numbers of different proteins. They all contain nitrogen, oxygen, carbon, and hydrogen.

Amino acids are either essential or nonessential. The "L" isomer of the amino acids has greater biological value; it is distinguished from the "molecular mirror image" isomer, which is called the "D" form. Thus, references to the individual amino acids often begin with the prefix "L."

Essential aminos must be derived from food. There are eight of them: L-isoleucine, L-leucine, L-lysine, L-methionine, L-phenylalanine, L-tryptophan, L-threonine, and L-valine. Two others, L-arginine and L-histidine, are essential for children.

Nonessential aminos are manufactured internally in the quantities the body requires. Their names are glycine, L-alanine, L-asparagine, L-aspartic acid, L-citrulline, L-cysteine, L-cystine, L-glutamic acid, L-glutamine, L-ornithine, L-proline, L-serine, taurine, and L-tyrosine.

Some of their roles are:

- **Glycine**—Vital for the manufacture of amino acids in the body and in the structure of red blood cells. Glucose and creatine phosphate (CP), two substances pivotal to energy production, require glycine in their synthesis process.
- **L-alanine**—An energy producer and regulator of blood sugar.
- **L-arginine**—An essential amino for prepubescent children, arginine is converted to ornithine in the adult body. It's usually used in supplement form by adults in combination with ornithine (another amino) for growth hormone stimulation, a practice of unproven efficacy.
- **L-asparagine**—An important factor in the metabolic processes of the nervous system.
- **L-aspartic acid**—Involved in the conversion of carbohydrates to muscle energy. A building block of immune system immunoglobulins and antibodies.
- **L-citrulline**—Helps detoxify ammonia, a byproduct of protein metabolism.
- **L-cysteine**—Performs detoxification duties in combination with L-aspartic acid and L-citrulline. Helps prevent damage from alcohol and cigarette smoke. Stimulates hair growth.
- **L-cystine**—A major partner in tissue antioxidant mechanisms. Contributes to improved healing, diminished pain from inflammation, and strong connective tissue.
- **L-glutamic acid**—An important metabolic factor in energy production, brain function, and the immune system. In combination with vitamin B_6, glutamic acid is converted to L-glutamine in the liver, scavenging ammonia in the process.
- **L-glutamine**—Lymphocytes and other white blood cells, front-line fighters in the immune system, are strongly dependent on glutamine. Glutamine also helps memory and concentration and aids in neutralizing the catabolic effects of cortisol, which is released upon strenuous exercise.
- **L-histidine**—Along with growth hormone and certain other amino acids, is vital to tissue growth. Important in the production of red and white blood cells.
- **L-isoleucine**—One of the three branched-chain aminos, so named because of their branching molecular configurations. The other two are leucine and valine. Together, they are indispensible for muscle growth and recovery. See Branched-Chain Amino Acids (BCAAs).
- **L-leucine**—See L-isoleucine.
- **L-lysine**—Low levels can slow down protein synthesis, affecting muscle and connective tissue. Has inhibitory affect against viruses and used in treatment of herpes simplex.
- **L-ornithine**—see L-arginine.

- **L-methionine**—Removes poisonous wastes from the liver and assists in the regeneration of liver and kidney tissue.
- **L-phenylalanine**—Enhances learning, memory, and alertness. A major element in the production of collagen, the main fibrous protein tissue in the body. Very useful for pain reduction in its modified D, L-phenylalanine form.
- **L-proline**—A major ingredient in the formation of connective tissue.
- **L-serine**—Important for the production of cellular energy and the formation of acetylcholine, a paramount brain chemical that aids memory and nervous-system function.
- **L-threonine**—One of the amino detoxifiers. Prevents fatty buildup in the liver. Important component of collagen.
- **L-tryptophan**—Stimulates secretion of serotonin, a brain chemical that has a calming effect on the body. Used in the treatment of insomnia, stress, and migraines.
- **L-tyrosine**—Important to the function of adrenal, pituitary, and thyroid glands. Elevates mood and is used in the treatment of anxiety, depression, and insomnia.
- **L-valine**—See L-isoleucine.

Amino acids are one of the three major sources of energy in the human body, the other two being fatty acids and monosaccharides such as glucose.

Amino acids are linked together in construction of the body's proteins. Most amino acids are incorporated into proteins that are either structural or regulatory in nature. Structural proteins, such as collagen and elastin, make up the muscles, tendons, ligaments, and bones. Regulatory proteins, called enzymes, control the function of all of the metabolic pathways within the cells of the body. Some enzymes are general in their activity and help break down food. Class-specific enzymes regulate larger-scale processes.

Ammonia scavengers—Combinations of certain amino acids and minerals that help remove ammonia from the blood. Ammonia is a toxic by-product of intense training (caused by the breakdown of amino acids for energy) and endurance events. It can accumulate to cause severe fatigue.

Anabolic steroid—A synthetic chemical that simulates the muscle-building properties of the male hormone testosterone.

Anabolism—The metabolic processes which build up body substances: that is, the synthesis of complex substances from simple ones. Example: muscle-building. Anabolism uses the available energy generated by catabolic processes to form the chemical bonds which unite the components of increasingly complex molecules. Anabolism is the opposite of catabolism.

Anaerobic exercise—Highly intense, short-term activities in which muscle fibers derive contractile energy from stored internal compounds without the use of oxygen from the blood. Examples: short bursts of all-out effort, such as sprinting or weightlifting. Anaerobic means "without oxygen."

Anaerobic strength—Maximum or near-maximum force output not requiring oxygen.

1. **Local muscular endurance** is exerting continuous submaximum force output over an extended period, the energy for which comes principally from the glycolytic pathway. The emphasis is on repetitive muscular capacity such as is required in boxing, wrestling, tug-of-war, and high-repetition training (more than fifty reps) without entering the aerobic

phase of muscular energetics and which involves the development of severe oxygen debt

2. Speed endurance involves maintaining maximum speed over times lower than 3–4 minutes (e.g., 100-, 400-, 800-meter dashes in track and field)

3. Strength endurance is exerting maximum muscular effort time after time with no appreciable decline in force output. Football linemen display this quality play after play for four quarters

Anorexia—A condition in which a person experiences a loss of appetite, distinguished from anorexia nervosa, a serious nervous condition in which the person, usually a young woman, experiences extreme aversion to food due to emotional reasons, resulting in life-threatening weight loss.

Antagonist—A muscle that counteracts the agonist, lengthening when the agonist muscle contracts.

Antioxidants—Certain nutrients, substances, and vitamins and minerals that protect against free radicals, highly unstable molecular fragments unleashed by strenuous exercise, chemicals, polluted air, and other factors, that can cause extensive damage to the body. Free radicals are involved in emphysema, wrinkled skin, cancer, blood clots, damage to cellular components and DNA, as well as muscle pains, cramps, and fatigue, and a host of other ailments and diseases normally associated with aging.

Free-radical scavengers (another term for antioxidants) include vitamins A, C, and E, selenium, zinc, many different botanical preparations such as pycnogenol and nordihydroguairetic acid (NDGA), glutathione, superoxide dimutase, and others.

ATP—The organic compound found in muscles which, upon being broken down enzymatically, yields energy for muscle contraction.

ATP/CP sports—Explosive strength sports with movements lasting a second or two at most. Examples: shot put, powerlifting, Olympic weightlifting, vertical jump.

Atrophy—Withering away, a decrease in size and functional ability of bodily tissues or organs.

Back-cycling—Cutting back on either number of sets, number of repetitions, or amount of weight used during an exercise session.

Barbell—Weight used for exercise, consisting of a rigid handle five to seven inches long with detachable metal discs at each end.

Beta-carotene—A carotenoid (pigment) found in yellow, orange, and deep green vegetables which provides a source of vitamin A when ingested. This substance has been found to have antioxidant and anticancer properties.

Biceps brachii—The prominent muscle on the front of the upper arm.

Bile—A thick, sticky fluid secreted by the liver via the bile duct into the small intestine where it aids in the emulsification of fats, increases peristalsis, and restores putrefaction.

Normally the ejection of bile only occurs during duodenal digestion. The normal adult secretes about 800 to 1,000 milliliters daily.

Bioflavonoids (vitamin P)—Water-soluble substances that appear in fruits and vegetables as companions to vitamin C. By name, they are citrin, rutin, hesperidin, flavone, and flavonols. They increase the strength of capillaries and regulate their permeability for the countless biochemical transfers that occur between blood and tissue. No RDA. Dietary sources: citrus fruit pulp, apricots, buckwheat, berries.

Biomechanics—The study of the mechanical aspects of physical movement, such as torque, drag, and posture, used to enhance athletic technique.

Biotin—A member of the B-complex vitamin family essential for metabolism of fat, protein, and vitamins C and B_{12}. It helps alleviate muscle pains, eczema, dermatitis. No RDA. Dietary sources: egg yolk, liver, whole rice, brewer's yeast.

Blood—The fluid which circulates through the heart, arteries, veins, and capillaries. It is composed of red blood cells, white blood cells, blood platelets, and an interstitial fluid called plasma. It derives its reddish color from the iron within the hemoglobin.

   Blood functions to provide nutrition and respiration for tissues located far from food and air supplies. It also transports waste from the tissues to the excretory organs. Blood provides chemical and thermal regulation to the body and helps prevent infection by transporting antibodies.

Blood glucose (blood sugar)—Refers to sugar in the form of glucose. The blood sugar level in humans is normally 60 to 100 milligrams per 100 milliliters of blood; it rises after a meal to as much as 150 milligrams per 100 milliliters of blood, but this may vary.

Blood pressure—A measurement of the force with which blood presses against the wall of a blood vessel. Blood pressure, as popularly used, is the pressure determined indirectly, existing in the large arteries at the height of the pulse wave.

   When a blood pressure reading is taken, the systolic over diastolic value is determined. Systolic pressure is primarily caused by the heartbeat or contraction. The diastolic pressure is taken when the heart is filling with blood between beats. Blood pressure values vary appreciably depending on age, sex, and ethnicity. A typical adult reading may be 120mm Hg over 80mm Hg, stated 120 over 80.

BMR (basal metabolic rate)—The speed at which the body burns calories while at complete rest.

Bodybuilding—The application of training sciences, particularly nutrition and weight training, to enhance musculature and physical appearance.

Body fat—The percentage of fat in the body. In bodybuilding, the lower the percentage, the more muscular the physique appears.

Boron—A nonmetallic earth element. It is required by some plants as a trace element and occurs as a hard crystalline solid or as brown powder. Boron forms compounds such as boric acid or borax. Taken as a supplement (3 mg/day), it shows decidedly favorable antiosteoporosis activity in middle-aged women. Despite its widespread use as a bodybuilding supplement, there is no evidence that it has anabolic properties among otherwise healthy bodybuilders.

Branched-chain amino acids (BCAA)—The amino acids L-leucine, L-isoleucine, and L-valine, which have a particular molecular structure that gives them their name, comprise 35 percent of muscle tissue. The BCAAs, particularly L-leucine, help increase work capacity by stimulating production of insulin, the hormone that opens muscle cells to glucose. BCAAs are burned as fuel at the end of long-distance events when the body recruits protein for as much as 20 percent of its energy needs.

Brewer's yeast—A nonleavening yeast used as a nutritional supplement for its rich content of vitamins (particularly B-complex), minerals, and amino acids.

Bromelain—A protein-splitting enzyme in pineapple juice used to reduce inflammation and edema and accelerate tissue repair. Pineapple eaten fresh is the best source.

Buffed—Slang for good muscle size and definition

Bulimia—The abnormal and unhealthful intake of large amounts of food. It is often followed by the use of laxatives and/or self-induced vomiting.

Bulking up—Gaining body weight by adding muscle, body fat, or both.

Bursitis—An inflammation of a bursa, the fluid sac located between joints for padding and lubrication.

Caffeine—A chemical in coffee, black tea, and cola drinks with an ability to stimulate the nervous system. In small amounts, it can create mental alertness. In larger amounts, it can cause nervousness, anxiety, and sleeplessness and is used medicinally as a diuretic and headache remedy.

Calcium—The most abundant mineral in the body, a vital factor for bones, teeth, muscle growth, muscle contraction, the regulation of nutrient passage in and out of cells, and nerve transmissions. RDA: 800–1,400 mg. Dose increases with age. Dietary sources: milk and dairy products, soybeans, sardines, salmon, peanuts, beans, green vegetables.

Carbohydrate—One of the three basic foodstuffs (proteins and fat are the others). Carbohydrates are a group of chemical substances including sugars, glycogen, starches, dextrins, and cellulose. They comprise the body's main source of raw material for energy. They contain only carbon, oxygen, and hydrogen. Usually the ratio of hydrogen to oxygen is 2:1. Carbohydrates can be classified as either a simple carbohydrate or a complex carbohydrate.

Digested carbohydrate enters the circulatory system in the form of monosaccharides, primarily glucose. Lesser amounts of fructose and galactose are also absorbed, but these are eventually converted to glucose in the liver. Before they can be absorbed into the bloodstream, polysaccharides and disaccharides must be broken down into monosaccharides by specific enzymes during the digestive process.

Carbohydrate loading—An eating and exercise technique used to build up ultra-high reserves of glycogen in muscle fibers for maximum endurance in long-distance athletic events. Benefits only events over 60 minutes long, where glycogen can become depleted to inhibit work capacity.

Cardiac muscle—One of the body's three types of muscle, found only in the heart.

Catabolism—The breaking-down aspect of metabolism, including all processes in which complex substances are progressively broken down into simpler ones. Example: the catabolism of protein in muscle tissue into component amino acids, such as occurs in intense training. Both anabolism and catabolism usually involve the release of energy and together constitute metabolism.

Cholesterol—A lipid, or fatty substance, normally present in most body tissue, especially the brain, nervous system, liver, and blood. Produced in the body to form hormones, vitamin D, and bile. Dietary cholesterol is obtained from meat, eggs, poultry, fish, milk, and other dairy products. Dietary cholesterol raises blood cholesterol, a factor in arterial disease, but the effect is less pronounced than that of saturated fat.

Choline—A B-complex vitamin associated with utilization of fats and cholesterol in the body. A constituent of lecithin, which helps prevent fats from building up in the liver and blood. Essential for health of myelin sheath, a principal component of nervous tissue, choline plays an important role in transmission of nerve impulses. No RDA. Dietary sources: lecithin, egg yolk, liver, wheat germ.

Chromium—Along with niacin, this essential micronutrient activates insulin for vital functions relating to blood sugar, muscle growth, and energy and helps control cholesterol. Chromium deficiency is widespread. Exercise and high consumption of sugar causes depletion. No RDA. Average adult intake should be 50–200 micrograms. Dietary sources: brewer's yeast, shellfish, chicken liver, oysters.

Circuit training—A system of weight training involving a series of 10–20 exercises for all body parts performed in sequence with short rest intervals between exercises. Used to develop both aerobic and anaerobic strength.

Collagen—The most abundant type of protein in the body. Forms tough connective tissue, the scaffolding holding a muscle in place which becomes the tendons that tie muscles to bones. Connective tissue literally keeps your body together—skin, bones, ligaments, cartilage, and organs.

Compensatory acceleration training—A weight-lifting technique used to develop explosive strength whereby you accelerate the bar as leverage improves through the movement.

Complete protein—Refers to protein which contains all essential amino acids in sufficient quantity and in the right ratio to maintain a positive nitrogen balance. The egg is the most complete protein food in nature.

Complex carbohydrates—Foods of plant origin consisting of three or more simple sugars bound together. Also known as polysaccharides. The starch in grains is an example. Compared to monosaccharides (refined carbohydrates such as table sugar and white flour products), complex carbs require a prolonged enzymatic process for digestion and thus provide a slow, even, and ideal flow of energy. This avoids fluctuations in glucose (blood sugar) levels which can affect energy. Complex carbs contain fiber and many nutrients.

Concentric contraction—Shortening of muscle due to muscle contraction.

Connective tissue—Tissue, primarily formed of collagen, that binds, supports, and provides a protective packing medium around organs and muscles.

Constant resistance—Weight-training technology wherein the weight you are lifting always remains the same regardless of changing leverage throughout a given exercise movement. The standing example of constant resistance training is lifting a dumbbell or a barbell. See *accommodating resistance* and *variable resistance*.

Contraction—The shortening of a muscle caused by the full contraction of individual muscle fibers.

Cooldown—The tapering-off period after completion of workout. Activities such as slow jogging, walking, and static stretching are recommended.

Copper—A mineral that helps convert the body's iron into hemoglobin for oxygen transportation through the bloodstream. Essential for utilization of vitamin C. No RDA. Dietary sources: legumes, whole wheat, prunes, liver, seafood.

Cortisone—A hormone isolated from the cortex of the adrenal gland and also prepared synthetically. It is believed to be both a precursor and metabolite of cortisol (hydrocortisone). Prior to this conversion to cortisol it is largely inactive. Cortisol, however, is highly catabolic.

Cortisone is important for its regulatory action in the metabolism of proteins, carbohydrates, fats, sodium, and potassium. It is used pharmacologically as an anti-inflammatory in various conditions, including allergies, collagen diseases, and adrenocortisol replacement therapy. Disadvantages may include temporary relief and also potential toxicity.

Creatine phosphate (CP)—An organic compound in muscle fibers that is fractured enzymatically for the production of ATP, the body's basic fuel that generates contractions.

Cross bridges—Projections of myosin molecules that link with actin filaments to create a grabbing, pulling effect, resulting in contraction.

Crunches—Abdominal exercises.

Cutting up—Reducing body fat and water retention to increase muscular definition.

Deadlift—One of three powerlifting events. Weight is lifted off floor to approximately waist height. Lifter must stand erect, shoulders back.

Deltoids—The large triangular muscles of the shoulder which raise the arm away from the body and are active in all shoulder movements.

Depletion—Exhaustion following a workout before the body has fully recuperated. Never train when feeling depleted.

dl-Phenylalanine—dl-Phenylalanine (DLPA) is a mixture consisting of equal parts of the d- and l-forms of phenylalanine. Phenylalanine is a naturally occurring amino acid, discovered in 1879, essential for optimal growth in infants and for nitrogen equilibrium in human adults. See *amino acids*.

DNA (deoxyribonucleic acid)—A complex protein present in the nuclei of cells. The chemical basis of heredity and carrier of genetic programming for the organism.

Double split training—Working out twice a day to allow for shorter, more intense workouts. See *variable split training*.

Dumbbell—Weight used for exercising, consisting of rigid handle about fourteen inches long with sometimes detachable metal discs at each end.

Easy set—Weight-training exercise far from maximum effort, as in a warm-up.

Eccentric contraction—Muscle lengthens while maintaining tension.

Ectomorph—A thin person with a lean physique and light musculature.

Eicosapentaenoic acid (EPA)—A fatty acid found in fish and fish oils believed to lower cholesterol, especially cholesterol bound to low-density lipoproteins (LDL).

Ejection fraction—The percentage of blood inside the heart's left ventricle that is pushed out into the body after contraction. The average training athlete, working at 80 percent maximum, ejects about 75 percent. This factor is positively affected by either anaerobic or aerobic training.

Electrolytes—Minerals such as sodium, potassium, chloride, calcium, and magnesium that provide conductivity functions for fluid passage (osmosis) through cellular membranes.

Electron microscope—A microscope that uses electrons instead of visible light to produce powerfully magnified images of objects smaller than the wavelengths of visible light. Electron microscopy has greatly advanced sports science by unfolding the subcellular dynamics of energy and contractile processes and how they are affected by specific types of training. This has allowed athletes to develop greater strength, endurance, or hypertrophy based on precise applications of training stress.

Endocrine—Refers to a secretion that flows directly into the bloodstream. The opposite of exocrine.

Endocrine glands—Organs that secrete hormones into the blood or lymph systems to regulate or influence general chemical changes in the body or the activities of other organs. Major glands are the thyroid, adrenal, pituitary, parathyroid, pancreas, ovaries, and testicles.

Endomorph—A heavyset person with a predominantly round and soft physique.

Endorphins—Brain chemicals that ease or suppress pain; dl-phenylalanine, an amino acid, intensifies and prolongs the effects of these natural painkillers.

Energy transfer systems efficiency—The ability of your body to generate ATP under aerobic or anaerobic conditions.

Enzymes—A type of chemical ferment-protein secreted by or contained within cells, which acts as a catalyst to induce chemical changes in other substances without being changed itself. Enzymes are specific and act only on specific substances, called substrates. They are present in the digestive fluids and in many of the tissues and are capable of producing in small amount the transformation on a large scale of various compounds. They are divided into six main groups: oxidoreductases, transferases, hydrolases, lyases, isomerases, and ligases.

Ergogenesis—Refers to a new beginning—a genesis—for athletes attempting to divorce themselves of steroid use by utilizing nutritional, psychological, training, and biomechanical technologies. Substances and practices that improve sports performance are called ergogenic aids.

Estrogen—The female hormone, a generic term for estrus-producing steroid compounds formed by the ovaries, placenta, testes, and adrenal cortex. These compounds can also be isolated from plants or produced synthetically.

Besides stimulation of secondary sexual characteristics, they exert systemic effects, such as growth and maturation of long bones. Estrogens are used therapeutically in any disorder attributable to estrogen deficiency, to prevent or stop lactation, to suppress ovulation, and to ameliorate carcinoma of the breast and of the prostate. Estrone and estradiol, both estrogens, induce the growth of female genital organs and stimulate the changes characteristic of the estrus cycle.

Exertional headaches—Pain triggered by a variety of exercise activities ranging from weightlifting to jogging and including sexual intercourse.

Fast-twitch fibers—White muscle cells that fire quickly and are utilized in strength-dependent anaerobic activities such as sprinting and powerlifting.

Fat—One of the three basic foodstuffs (along with carbohydrates and protein). The most concentrated source of energy in the diet, fat furnishes twice the calories of carbs or proteins. The components of fat are fatty acids, saturated or unsaturated. Saturated fatty acids are generally solid at room temperature and are derived primarily from animal sources. Unsaturated fatty acids, on the other hand, are usually liquid and come from vegetable, nut, or seed sources.

Fat deposits surround and protect organs such as the kidneys, heart, and liver. Fats are the primary substance of adipose tissue. A layer of fat beneath the skin, known as subcutaneous fat, insulates the body from environmental temperature changes, thereby preserving body heat.

Fatigue—State of decreased capacity for work due to previous workload.

Fat-soluble vitamins—Vitamin A, vitamin D, vitamin E, and vitamin K. They are vitamins which can be dissolved in fats or fatty tissue.

Fat (total)—The fat consumed from both saturated and unsaturated sources. High intake of total dietary fat increases risk of obesity, some types of cancer, and possibly gallbladder disease.

Fatty acid—One of the building blocks of fat. Used as fuel for muscle contractions. Fatty acids aid in oxygen transport through blood to all cells, tissues, and organs. They help maintain resilience and lubrication of all cells and combine with protein and cholesterol to form living membranes that hold body cells together. They break up cholesterol deposits on arterial walls, thereby preventing arteriosclerosis. Fatty acids are necessary for the function of the thyroid and adrenal glands.

Fiber (dietary)—The part of plant food that is not digested by the human body, such as the husk of whole grains and the skin of an apple. Healthy intestines and regular elimination require adequate fiber, generally provided by complex carbohydrates. A diet low in fiber is associated with constipation, intestinal disorders, varicose veins, obesity, and heart disease.

Fiber (muscle)—The long and stringlike muscle cells which contract to produce strength. They range from microscopic in size to one foot long. There are several hundred to several thousand individual groups (fasciculi) of fibers in each major muscle structure. These groups are something like pieces of string bound tightly together inside a protective sheath.

Flexion—A bending movement in contrast to extending, as in leg flexions.

Flush—Cleansing a muscle of metabolic toxins by increasing the blood supply to it through exertion.

Folic acid—A B-complex vitamin essential in formation of red blood cells and metabolism of protein. Important for proper brain function, mental and emotional health, appetite, and production of hydrochloric acid. Very often deficient in diets. RDA: 400 micrograms. Dietary sources: green leafy vegetables, liver, brewer's yeast.

Food allergies—Sensitivities to certain foods which can cause both mental and physical symptoms.

Forced repetitions—Assistance to perform additional repetitions of an exercise when muscles can no longer complete movement on their own.

Freestyle training—Training all body parts in one workout.

Gamma oryzanol—A substance extracted from rice bran oil which some athletes believe has nonsteroidal, growth-promoting properties when taken as a supplement. It allegedly helps increase lean body mass and strength, decreases fatty tissue, improves recovery from workouts, and reduces postworkout muscle soreness. Recently, in preliminary testing, the active ingredient, ferulic acid, was reported to exert an even more pronounced effect than gamma oryzanol. The jury is still out.

Glucagon—A hormone secreted by the alpha cells of the pancreas, which stimulates the breakdown of glycogen and the release of glucose by the liver, thereby causing an increase in blood sugar levels.

Glucagon works in direct opposition to insulin. Liver glucose is freed when the blood sugar level drops to around 70 milligrams per 100 milligrams of blood. Exercise and starvation both increase glucagon levels, as does the presence of amino acids in the blood after a high-protein meal. Glucagon produces smooth muscle relaxation when administered parenterally.

Glucose (blood sugar)—A simple sugar, the breakdown product of carbohydrates that becomes the raw material for energy production inside cells.

Glucose-lactate cycle (Cori cycle)—The metabolic partnership between muscles and liver to support active muscle work, refers to the sequence involving breakdown of carbohydrates, glycogen storage in liver, the passage of glucose into the bloodstream and its subsequent storage in muscle fibers as glycogen, the breakdown of glycogen during muscle activity, the production of lactic acid in this process, and the conversion of lactic acid to glycogen again.

Glucose polymers—A state-of-the-art low-glycemic carbohydrate supplement that delivers a steady source of energy for workouts and restoration. It is available as drinks, powders, and tablets.

Glucose tolerance—Refers to an individual's ability to metabolize glucose.

Gluteals—Abbreviation for gluteus maximus, medius, and minimus; the muscles of the buttocks.

Glycemic index—A rating system that indicates the different speed with which carbohydrates are processed into glucose by the body. In general, complex carbohydrates are broken down slower, providing a slow infusion of glucose for steady energy. Refined, simple carbohydrates usually are absorbed quickly, causing energy-disturbing fluctuations of glucose.

Glycogen—The common storage form of glucose in the liver and muscles, biochemically processed as part of the energy-producing cycle. Glycogen, a polysaccharide commonly called animal starch, is readily converted into glucose as the energy needs of the body require.

Glycolysis—The anaerobic enzymatic energy-yielding breakdown of glucose into pyruvic acid or lactic acid.

Glycolytic sports—Sports such as wrestling, boxing, 200-meter dash, and other long sprint or middistance sprints wherein the glycolytic pathway of muscle energy production (the breakdown of muscle sugar—glycogen—in order to produce more CP and ATP) is involved. See *glycogen, ATP,* and *CP.*

Golgi tendon organs—Nerve sensors (proprioceptors) located at the junction of muscles and tendons that pick up messages of excess stress on the muscle and cause the brain to shut off muscle contracture. The shut-off threshold and potential for strength can be enhanced through jerk training, where you carefully perform repeated submaximum jerks with weights.

Growth hormone (GH)—Somatotropin, any substance that stimulates growth, especially one secreted by the pituitary, which exerts a direct effect on protein, carbohydrate, and lipid metabolism and controls the rate of skeletal and visceral growth.

Hamstring—The big muscle along the back of your upper leg from the hip to the knee

Hard set—Performing a prescribed number of repetitions of an exercise using maximum effort.

Heart rate—The number of heart beats per minute.

Hemoglobin—A crystallizable, conjugated protein consisting of an iron-containing pigment called heme and a simple protein, globin. It is the pigment of red blood cells. Hemoglobin carries oxygen from the lungs to the tissues.

Hormones—Chemical substances which originate in an organ, gland, or body part and are conveyed by the blood to affect functions in other parts of the body.

Human Growth Hormone (hGH)—A hormone secreted by the anterior pituitary gland in response to various stressful stimuli such as heat, starvation, or intense physical stress (e.g., exercise) as well as by an innate pulsatile periodicity. The principal functions of hGH are to stimulate anabolism and to mobilize stored fat (triglycerides) for energy, thus sparing muscle glycogen.

Hyperglycemia—A condition of abnormally high concentration of glucose in the blood, especially with reference to fasting level. Hyperglycemia accompanies diabetes mellitus and other conditions, as well.

Hyperplasia (muscle splitting)—A controversial subject among sports scientists regarding the possibility of actually splitting muscle fibers, giving more strength from increased contractile potential and/or connective tissue.

Hypertrophy—Increase in gross muscle size as well as individual muscle cell size resulting from training (especially weight training); due to the adaptive process whereby the muscles add more mitochondria, sarcoplasm, myofibrils, and interstitial substances such as water, fat, or satellite cells in response to highly specific forms of stress.

Hypoglycemia—Literally means low blood glucose level. There are two general categories of this disorder: fasting (or spontaneous) and reactive.

In fasting hypoglycemia, serum glucose levels are low in the fasting state (for example, before breakfast). This form of hypoglycemia is relatively uncommon and is not what most people generally refer to when they claim to have hypoglycemic symptoms.

In reactive hypoglycemia, fasting glucose levels are normal. They become abnormally low only in reaction to the increased serum levels of glucose which follow the ingestion of a meal.

Hypnotherapy—An effective method to shed accumulated negativity and self-doubt that can limit confidence and performance potential.

Impulse-inertial training—A system originally designed for NASA space stations whereby a moving, weighted sled is used to effectively improve the ability to exert explosive, starting strength bursts.

Inertia—The tendency of an object to remain in its current state (in motion or at rest).

Inosine—A naturally occurring compound found in the body that contributes to strong heart muscle contraction and blood flow in the coronary arteries. As a supplement taken before and during workouts and competition, it stimulates enzyme activity in muscle cells for improved regeneration of ATP.

Inositol—A B-complex vitamin that combines with choline to form lecithin, protecting against the fatty hardening of arteries and cholesterol buildup. Important in the nutrition of brain cells. Promotes healthy hair. No RDA. Dietary sources: liver, brewer's yeast, dried lima beans, beef brains and heart, cantaloupe.

Insertion—The attachment of a muscle to the more movable or distal (farther from the center of the body) structure.

Insulin—A peptide hormone made of two polypeptide chains and secreted from the beta cells of the pancreas. The function of insulin is to increase the ability of certain organs, such as muscles and the liver, to utilize glucose and amino acids. Insulin also increases the total quantity of protein in the body by increasing the flow of amino acids into cells, accelerating messenger RNA translation, and increasing DNA transcription to form more RNA.

Insulin is essential for the proper metabolism and proper maintenance level of blood sugar. Secretion is primarily dependent upon the concentration of blood glucose, an increase of blood sugar bringing about an increase in the secretion of insulin. Inadequate secretion of insulin results in improper metabolism of carbohydrates and fats and brings on diabetes characterized by glucose accumulating in the blood and wastefully excreted in the urine. Various forms of insulin may be prepared and administered to temporarily treat a diabetic individual.

Insulinlike growth factors (IGF-I and IGF-II)—Liberated into the interstitial spaces surrounding muscle cells (especially Type IIb fibers) damaged by severe stress (especially eccentric contractions). Their collective function is to ensure bonding between the nearby satellite cells with the damaged fiber, thereby increasing that fiber's proneness to injury. Perhaps the single most contributory factor in muscle hypertrophy.

Intramuscular/intracellular friction—The natural friction between and within muscle fibers caused by contraction (especially eccentric contraction). Leads to some reduction in strength output. The greatest amount of friction occurs in eccentric movements, such as the lowering of weights, where the muscle lengthens against resistance. This can be very damaging to contractile components inside fibers, and to the fibers themselves (called microtrauma).

Iodine—An essential element for the function of the thyroid gland, which regulates metabolism and energy. RDA: 150 micrograms. Dietary sources: all seafood, kelp.

Iron—Combines with protein and copper to make hemoglobin, a pigment that colors the blood red, and carries oxygen through the bloodstream from the lungs to all bodily tissue. Also forms myoglobin, which transports oxygen in muscle tissue for use in fueling contractions. Deficiency is common in athletes. Without enough iron, you cannot train. Iron is easily lost through sweat, urine, feces, and menstrual flow. Runners in particular are suspected of inefficient absorption of dietary iron. RDA: 10 mg (men); 18 mg (women). Dietary sources: liver, oysters, lean meat, leafy green vegetables, whole grains, dried fruits, legumes.

Isokinetic exercise—Exercise with accommodating resistance. Nautilus and Cybex are two types of isokinetic machines, whereby amount of resistance is altered by equipment to match the force curve developed by the muscle.

Isometric contraction—A muscular contraction in which the muscle retains its length while increasing in tension, but no movement occurs. Also called static contraction.

Isotonic contraction—A concentric muscular contraction in which the load remains constant but the tension varies with the joint angle. Also called dynamic contraction.

Ketone—Produced as intermediate products of fat metabolism. They are normally created in limited amounts when fat is oxidized. However, in drastic conditions where carbohydrate supply is insufficient or unavailable for energy needs such as starvation or untreated diabetes, excessive amounts of fat are oxidized and ketone bodies accumulate. This condition is known as ketosis.

Kilocalorie—A unit of measurement used in metabolic studies, being the amount of heat required to raise the temperature of 1 kilogram of water 1° Celsius at a pressure of 1 atmosphere. It is one thousand times larger than the small calorie used in chemistry and physics. The term is used in nutrition to express the fuel or energy value of food.

Kinesiology—Study of muscles and their movements.

Knee wraps—Elastic strips used to wrap knees for better support when performing squats and deadlifts.

Krebs cycle (Citric acid cycle)—Refers to a complicated series of reactions by which fragments from any of the energy nutrients (proteins, carbohydrates, and fats) are completely broken down to carbon dioxide and water, releasing energy for the formation of adenosine triphosphate (ATP). It is the final common pathway for all nutrient metabolites involved in energy production and provides more than 90 percent of the body's energy.

L-carnitine—A natural substance found in muscle tissue that helps release stored body fat (triglycerides) into the bloodstream for use in cellular energy production. Taken as a supplement, this nutritional factor may increase energy levels for long-term aerobic activity.

Lactic acid—A by-product of glucose and glycogen metabolism in anaerobic muscle energetics. A minute accumulation causes muscular fatigue and pain, and retards contraction.

Lactic acid is carried by the blood to the liver, where it is reconverted to glucose and returned as blood glucose to the muscles. This elevation of blood lactic acid in sustained strenuous exercise, such as in marathon running, results in muscle fatigue and pain. Recovery follows when enough oxygen gets to the muscle; part of the lactic acid is oxidized and most of it is then built up once more into glycogen. The metabolic cooperation between contracting skeletal muscle and the liver to support active muscle work is called the Cori cycle.

Lactose—A disaccharide of milk which on hydrolysis yields glucose and galactose. Bacteria can convert it into lactic acid and butyric acid, as in the souring of milk. It is used in infant feeding formulas, in other foods, and as an osmotic laxative and diuretic. Lactose is not tolerated in many persons after weaning, owing to a reduced lactase activity.

Lats—Short for latissimus dorsi, the large muscles of the back that are the prime movers for adduction, extension, and hyperextension of the shoulder joints.

Lean body mass—All of you, except your fat. Includes bone, brain, organs, skin, nails, muscle, and all bodily tissues. Approximately 50–60 percent of lean body mass is water.

Lever—A rigid object (bone), hinged at one point (joint), to which forces (via muscle contraction or resistance) are applied at two other points. A lever transmits and modifies force or motion, and has three parts: a fulcrum, a force arm, and a resistance arm. There are three classes of levers, depending on the location of the three parts relative to each other.

Ligament—A strong, fibrous band of connective tissue that supports and strengthens a joint by linking bones or cartilage.

Limit strength—Absolute strength enhanced by hypnosis, electrotherapy, ergogenic substances of any form (including nutritional supplements or drugs), or other techniques. Such aids increase the potential for strength above normal capacity. Absolute strength is reached solely through training.

Lower abs—Slang for abdominal muscles below the navel.

Magnesium—A pivotal mineral important to protein synthesis, energy production, muscle contractions, and a strong heart muscle. Essential for metabolism of calcium, phosphorous, sodium, potassium, and vitamin C. Chronic muscle cramps is a typical sign of a shortage. RDA: 350 mg (men); 300 mg (women). Dietary sources: figs, lemons, grapefruit, yellow corn, almonds, nuts, seeds, dark green vegetables.

Manganese—A key enzyme activator. Also vital to the formation of thyroid and reproductive hormones, normal skeletal development, muscle reflexes, and the proper digestion and utilization of food. No RDA. Dietary sources: whole grains, egg yolks, nuts, seeds, and green vegetables.

Max—Maximum effort for one repetition of a weight-training exercise.

Max VO₂ uptake—Oxygen utilization as measured in milliliters of oxygen per kilogram of body weight per minute.

Mesomorph—A person whose physique features powerful musculature.

Metabolism—The total of all physical and chemical reactions in the body, including catabolism (breaking down) and anabolism (building up).

Metabolite—Any substance which forms as a by-product of the catabolism, growth, or anabolism of living tissue.

Military press—Pressing a barbell from the upper chest upward in a standing or sitting position.

Minerals—There are 96 times more minerals in the body than vitamins. As vitamins, they are necessary for life itself and combine with other basic components of food to form enzymes. Minerals are ingested through food and water. Many minerals are deficient in the diet because of mineral-poor agricultural soil, the result of intensive farming and long-term use of chemical fertilizers and pesticides.

Mitochondria—The rod-shaped organelles found in the cytoplasm of cells. They are the source of energy in the cell and are involved in protein synthesis and lipid metabolism.

Moment arm—The perpendicular distance from the line of pull of a muscle to the axis of rotation.

Moment of force—See *torque*.

Motor unit—The basic unit of movement: a motor nerve fiber and all of the muscle fibers it supplies. In the quadriceps muscle, one neuron can activate as many as one thousand fibers. In the eye, where great precision is required, one nerve cell may control only three fibers.

Motor unit recruitment—One of the factors affecting strength. Refers to your ability to get maximum stimulation through the nervous system to trigger the maximum amount of muscle contractions. This can be built up over time through heavy resistance and explosive strength training.

Muscle—Tissue consisting of fibers organized into bands or bundles that contract to perform bodily movement.

Muscle fiber—Synonymous with muscle cell. See *fiber*.

Muscle fiber arrangement—Long fibers are created for large movements and speed rather than strength. Short fibers are designed for strength with a lesser movement capability. Knowledge of fiber arrangement can help you train muscle groups in a scientific manner.

Muscle pull (strain)—Major or minor damage to muscles from excessive stretching or use. The key to avoiding muscle pulls is proper conditioning and strict adherence to a thorough program of warm-up and cooldown.

Muscle spasm—Sudden, involuntary contraction of muscle or muscle group.

Muscle spindle—The "computer" of muscle tissue, a modified fiber which responds reflexively to mental impulses and muscle movement such as stretching. Measures and delivers the quantity of muscle force needed to perform a given action.

Muscle tone—The degree of tension and vigor in a muscle.

Myofibril—The functional units within muscle fibers that cause contractions. The more you have, the greater your strength. Myofibrillarization—increasing myofibrils—is achieved with the use of heavy weight training.

Myofilaments—The elements of a muscle cell which comprise myofibrils that actually shorten (thereby providing contractile force) by sliding across one another via action of cross bridges. They are comprised of the proteins actin and myosin.

Myoglobin—An iron-containing protein responsible for oxygen transport and storage in muscle tissue, similar to hemoglobin in blood.

Myoneural junction—The connection of a neuron to a muscle fiber.

Myosin—The most abundant protein (68 percent) in muscle fiber. It is the main constituent of the thick contractile filaments which overlap with the thin actin filaments in the biochemical sequence that produces contractions.

Nautilus—Isokinetic-type exercise machine which attempts to match resistance with user's force.

Negative reps—An eccentric contraction. One or two partners assist in lifting a weight up to 20–40 percent heavier than an individual could normally lift. Once hoisted to the extended position, the weight is slowly lowered without help. This type of exercise is extremely damaging to connective tissue and, according to the "cataclysmic" theory of overtraining, is the elemental factor in overtraining and cumulative microtrauma.

Neuromuscular reeducation (NMR)—Therapy involving deep rolfing massage and neuronal stimulation to eliminate painful strength- and movement-limiting adhesions and scar tissues caused by trauma to body parts. Developed by Dr. Gary Glum, a Los Angeles chiropractor, and Joseph Horrigan, a soft-tissue expert also from Los Angeles.

Neurotransmitter—A biochemical that spans the gaps between nerve cells, transmitting an electrical impulse.

Nicotine—An alkaloid found in the tobacco plant. Nicotine first stimulates the central nervous system, then depresses it. It is absorbed easily through the mucous membranes and the skin and is highly toxic; symptoms include nausea, vomiting, twitching, and convulsions. Nicotine is used as an agricultural insecticide.

Nitrogen balance—An estimate of the difference between nitrogen intake and output in the body to measure protein sufficiency, derived by subtracting amount of urea nitrogen in a urine sample from an individual's total protein intake. If urea value is larger than protein intake, the nitrogen balance is negative, indicating that not enough protein was eaten to meet the body's nutritional needs. In this situation, muscle protein is sacrificed to provide additional protein to fund metabolic processes. Prolonged negative balance results in muscle wasting. Positive nitrogen balance is achieved by ingesting complete protein to meet the body's metabolic needs.

Non-locks—Performing a weight exercise without going through complete range of motion, e.g., a squat without coming to full lock-out position of knees.

Nonresistance training—Training without weights in which you put muscle strength against body weight to develop general and aerobic fitness. Includes mild running, calisthenics, jumping, skipping, swimming, and bicycling.

Nordihydroguaiaretic Acid (NDGA)—Used as an antioxidant in fats and oils. It occurs in resinous exudates of many plants, particularly the chaparral bush.

Obliques—Short for external and/or internal obliques, the muscles to either side of abdominals that rotate and flex the trunk.

Octacosanol—The active, energy-boosting component of wheat germ oil which is known to improve endurance, reaction time, and muscle glycogen storage. Taken as a supplement.

Olympic lifts—The two movements used in Olympic competitions: the snatch, and the clean and jerk.

Olympic set—High-quality, precision-made set of weights used for competition. The bar is approximately seven feet long. All moving parts have either brass bushings or bearings. Plates are machined for accurate weight.

Origin—The attachment of a muscle to the less movable or proximal (closer to the center of the body) structure.

Ornithine—Produced in the urea cycle by splitting off the urea from arginine and is itself converted into citrulline. On decomposition it gives rise to putrescine. It has been demonstrated to be of value as a growth-hormone stimulator when administered intravenously; there is no solid evidence that it stimulates growth hormone to a significant degree (enough to stimulate muscle growth) when taken orally.

Overload principle—Applying a greater load than normal to a muscle to increase its capability.

Overtraining—Excessive training, principally of the eccentric contraction phase of lifting weights or running. Can cause injuries, loss of body weight, insomnia, anorexia, depression, and chronic muscle soreness and retard workout recovery.

Overuse syndrome—Injury resulting from overtraining.

Oxidation—The chemical act of combining with oxygen or of removing hydrogen.

Oxidative sports—Sports such as long-distance running or cycling wherein oxygen must be present to allow movement to continue. See *ATP/CP sports* and *glycolytic sports*.

Oxygen debt—The oxygen consumed in recovery from exercise above the amount that would normally be consumed at rest. In intense endurance activities, oxygen debt refers to the amount of oxygen owed to the system to oxidize lactic acid buildup. One's tolerance for an accumulated debt is generally proportional to the level of fitness.

Parcourse training—A concept borrowed from outdoor parks and applied to the gym during sports-specific phase of foundation training for aerobic athletes. Involves the performance of aerobic activities—jogging, skipping rope, straddle jumping, bicycle ergometer—between exercises of a weight-training routine.

Partial reps—Performing an exercise without going through a complete range of motion either at the beginning or end of a rep.

Peak contraction—Exercising a muscle until it cramps by using shortened movements.

Pecs—Slang for the pectoral muscles of the chest.

Peptide—Any member of a class of compounds of low molecular weight which yield two or more amino acids on hydrolysis. Formed by loss of water from the NH_2 and COOH groups of adjacent amino acids, they are known as di-, tri-, and tetra-peptides, depending on the number of amino acids in the molecule. Peptides (polypeptides) form the constituent parts of proteins.

Peripheral heart action (PHA)—An excellent all-around muscle and fitness system of weight training whereby muscles are exercised in an alternating sequence of upper and lower body. This method keeps blood circulating constantly throughout the body, prevents undue fatigue in any given muscle, facilitates recovery, and provides holistic muscular development. It is mildly cardiovascular.

Phosphorus—Works with calcium to build up bones and teeth. Provides a key element in the production of ATP. RDA: 800 mg. Dietary sources: animal protein, whole grains.

Physiology—The study of the body's functions.

Plyometrics—A system of training whereby you use an implement (such as a medicine ball) or the ground as resistance to develop muscle-tissue elasticity and stretch-reflex threshold for quick explosive strength. Example: jumping off a bench to the ground, then quickly rebounding to another bench.

Postexercise muscle soreness—Microtrauma to connective tissue causes irritation to local nerve endings, triggering pain. Typically occurs from exertion or concentrated movement after a long period of disuse but even affects the most physically fit athletes after excessively stressful exercise.

Potassium—Teams with sodium to regulate the body's water balance and heart rhythms. Nerve and muscle function are disturbed when the two minerals are not balanced. Insufficient potassium can lead to fatigue, cramping, and muscle damage. Physical and mental stress, excessive sweating, alcohol, coffee, and a high intake of salt (sodium) and sugar deplete potassium. No RDA. Dietary sources: citrus, cantaloupe, green leafy vegetables, bananas.

Power—Strength plus speed. Power equals force multiplied by distance, divided by time.

Powerlifts—Three movements used in powerlifting competition: the squat, bench press, and deadlift.

Power training—System of weight training using low repetitions and explosive movements with heavy weights.

Preload—The stretching of a muscle prior to contracting it, thereby providing both a stretch reflex and a viscoelastic component, adding to the total force output.

Progressive resistance—The basic principle of weight training where weight is increased as muscles gain strength and endurance.

Proprioceptor—Sensory organs found in muscles, tendons, joints, and skin which sense and provide information about movement, body position, and environment.

Protease—A category of enzymes which attack specific bonds between amino acids and proteins. The proteases break amino acid bonds to split up the protein molecule into smaller pieces of lined amino acids.

Examples of proteases are renin and pepsin; these enzymes can be found in animals. Renin is used in the thickening of milk and is isolated from the stomach of the calf; pepsin is found in the gastric juices of humans and other animals where it breaks down proteins at specific places.

Protein—One of the three basic foodstuffs along with carbohydrates and fat. Protein is a complex substance present in all living organisms. It comprises 90 percent of the dry weight of blood, 80 percent of muscles, and 70 percent of the skin. Protein provides the connective and structural building blocks of tissue and the primary constituents of enzymes, hormones, and antibodies. The components of protein are amino acids. Dietary protein is derived from both animal and plant foods.

Protein is essential for growth, the building of new tissue, and the repair of injured or broken-down tissue. Proteins serve as enzymes, structural elements, hormones, and immunoglobulins and are involved in oxygen transport and other activities throughout the body and in photosynthesis. Protein can be oxidized in the body, liberating heat and energy at the rate of four calories per gram.

Protein efficiency ratio (PER)—A system of rating the quality of dietary protein by the number and proportions of the essential amino acids contained in it. Eggs rank highest; they contain all eight essential amino acids in a proportion regarded as the most readily assimilable and usable combination of naturally occurring amino acids. Eggs are the standard by which all other protein sources are rated for assimilability.

Pulmonary (ventilatory) capacity—The efficiency of gas exchange in the lungs.

Pumped—Slang term to describe the tightness in a muscle made large through exercise. The pumped sensation results from blood engorgement and lactate increase in the muscle.

Pumping iron—Slang for lifting weights, a phrase used since the 1950s.

Pyramid training—A training protocol incorporating an upward then downward progression in weight, rep per rep or set per set.

Pyruvic acid—The end product of the glycolytic pathway. This three-carbon metabolite is an important junction point for two reasons: it is the gateway to the final common energy-producing pathway, the Krebs cycle; and it provides acetyl coenzyme A (acetyl CoA), through which fatty acids, and in turn fat, are produced from glucose. Pyruvic acid converts to lactic acid as needed. Pyruvic acid increases in quantity in the blood and tissues in thiamine (vitamin B_1) deficiency. Thiamine is essential for its oxidation.

Quads—Short for quadriceps femoris, the thigh muscles that extend the leg.

Quality training—Training prior to bodybuilding competition where intervals between sets are reduced to enhance muscle mass and density and a low-calorie diet is followed to reduce body fat.

Ratio of fast-, intermediate-, and slow-twitch fibers—A fundamental strength factor relating to the distribution and specific capabilities of fibers within muscle tissue. Fast-twitch (predominantly white fiber) muscles are stronger and more suited for strength activities. Slow-twitch (red fiber) muscles are more enduring and are better suited for long-distance exercise. This ratio can be changed only slightly through training. You must train fast to be fast and train long to be enduring.

RDA (Recommended Daily Dietary Allowance)—Estimates established by the National Research Council for nutritional needs necessary for prevention of nutrient depletion in healthy people. RDA does not take into account altered requirements due to sickness, injury, physical or mental stress, or use of medications or drugs, nor does it compensate for the nutrient losses that occur during processing and preparation of food. RDA standards do not apply to athletes, who have extraordinary nutrient needs. RDAs are far too low for serious athletes and even for fitness enthusiasts who exercise regularly.

Reciprocal innervation—A phenomenon in which the opposing muscle group is stimulated to relax while the prime mover muscle is simultaneously stimulated to contract, thereby allowing movement to occur.

Recruitment—Activation of motor units. The greater the resistance encountered, the greater will be the recruitment necessary to overcome its inertia.

Recuperation—A physiological process involving full body and muscle recovery and subsequent muscle growth during a rest period between training sessions. Optimum increases in muscle growth occur only with complete recovery.

Repetition—One complete movement of an exercise. Also called *rep*.

Rep out—Repeating the same exercise movement until you are unable to continue.

Resistance—The amount of weight used in each set of an exercise.

Rest interval—Pause between sets of an exercise which allows muscles to recover partially before beginning next set.

Rest pause training—Training method in which you press out one difficult repetition, replace bar in stand, then perform another rep after a 10–20-second rest.

Ripped—Slang, meaning extreme muscularity.

RM—Acronym for repetitions maximum. For example, 5 RM stands for the maximum amount of weight you can perform for five repetitions.

'Roid—Slang for anabolic steroid.

Rotator cuff—A band of four muscles that hold the arm in the shoulder joint.

Sartorius—The largest muscle in the body, involved in the movement of the thigh at the hip joint.

Saturated fat—Dietary fat from primarily animal sources. Excessive consumption is the major dietary contributor to total blood cholesterol levels and is linked to increased risk for coronary heart disease.

Saturated fatty acid—An acid which by definition has no available bonds in its hydrocarbon chain; all bonds are filled or saturated with hydrogen atoms. The chain of a saturated fatty acid contains no double bond. Saturated fatty acids are more slowly metabolized by the body than are unsaturated fatty acids.

Saturated fatty acids include acetic acid, myristic acid, palmitic acid, and steric acid. These acids come primarily from animal sources, with the exception of coconut oil, and are usually solid at room temperature. In the case of vegetable shortening and margarine, oil products have undergone a process called hydrogenation in which the unsaturated oils are converted to a more solid form. Other principal sources of saturated fats are milk products and eggs.

Selenium—A major nutrient antioxidant along with vitamins A, C, and E. No RDA. Dietary sources: wheat germ, bran, tuna.

Set—Fixed number of repetitions of an exercise movement. Example: there may be ten repetitions in a set of curls.

Siberian ginseng (eleutherococcus senticosus)—A cousin of traditional Oriental ginsengs widely used among Russian athletes for boosting stamina and endurance, to speed workout recovery, and as a health tonic to normalize systemic functions and counter stress. A substance that enables athletes over time to adapt to increased training intensity.

Simple carbohydrates—Monosaccharides and disaccharides occurring naturally in fruits, vegetables, and dairy products. Some examples of simple carbohydrates are glucose, galactose, and fructose, all of which are monosaccharides; sucrose, lactose, and maltose, all of which are disaccharides.

Most simple carbohydrates elevate blood-sugar levels rapidly, providing instant energy which is quickly utilized and dissipated. Fructose is an exception. Additionally, refined sources of simple carbohydrates, such as candy, contribute only calories to the diet. These empty calories are often consumed in place of foods that would provide important nutrients in addition to the energy.

Skeletal muscle—Muscle that attaches to the skeletal system and causes body movement by a shortening or pulling action against its bony attachment.

Slow-twitch fibers—Red muscle cells that fire slowly and are designed for aerobic (enduring) activities such as distance running and cycling.

Smooth muscle—Involuntary muscle tissue found in the walls of almost every organ of the body.

Snatch—Olympic lift where weight is lifted from floor to overhead (with arms extended) in one movement.

Sodium—An essential mineral for proper growth and nerve and muscle-tissue function. A diet high in salt (40 percent of salt is sodium) causes a potassium imbalance and is associated with high blood pressure. No RDA. Dietary sources: salt, shellfish, celery, beets, artichokes.

Specificity—Principle which states that your body will adapt in highly specific ways in response to variable forms of stress which you impose upon it through training.

Speed-strength—A type of strength typically referred to as power. Power, however, is an inadequate synonym as it does not differentiate between the two important types of speed-strength.

1. Starting strength involves turning on a maximum number of muscle fibers instantly in any given movement. Ballistic athletes, such as sprinters, need this strength the most to fire each muscle simultaneously with each stride. A boxer does the same with each punch, a baseball pitcher each time he hurls

2. Explosive strength describes the firing of muscle fibers over a longer period of time after initial activation, for the purpose of pushing, pulling, or moving a weighted object. Examples: weightlifting, shotputting, and football

Spinal nerves—The 31 pairs of nerves radiating outward from the spinal cord which relay impulses to and from the skeletal muscles.

Sprain—Joint injury involving partial or total rupture of ligaments.

Squats—The king of all leg exercises. Heavy-weight squatting with an erect torso puts an overload stress on the quadriceps muscles of the upper leg for maximum strength building.

Stabilizer—A muscle that stabilizes (or fixes) a bone so that movement can occur efficiently at another bone articulating with the stabilized bone.

Starch—A polysaccharide made of glucose linked together. The body must convert starch into glucose, which can be utilized for immediate energy or converted to glycogen and stored in the liver for later energy needs. Starch exists throughout the vegetable kingdom, its chief commercial sources being the cereals and potatoes.

Steroids—Naturally occurring and synthetic chemicals that include some hormones, bile acids, and other substances. See *anabolic steroids*.

Straight sets—Groups of repetitions (sets) interrupted by only brief pauses (30–90 seconds).

Strength—The application of force in any endeavor, such as to a barbell, a ball, or to the ground underfoot. There are five broad categories of strength, each with its own special training requirements: absolute, limit, speed, anaerobic, and aerobic.

There are over thirty different factors that affect strength, divided into five broad categories:

1. **Structural/anatomical:** muscle-fiber arrangement, musculoskeletal leverage, ratio of fast- to slow-twitch fibers, tissue leverage, motion-limiting factors (scar tissue and adhesions), tissue elasticity, intramuscular/intracellular friction

2. **Physiological/biochemical:** stretch reflex, sensitivity of the Golgi tendon organ, hormonal function, energy-transfer–systems efficiency, extent of hyperplasia (muscle splitting), myofibrillar development, motor-unit recruitment

3. **Cardiovascular/cardiorespiratory:** stroke volume of heart, ejection fraction, pulmonary capacity, heart rate, max VO_2 uptake

4. **Psychoneural/learned responses:** psych (arousal level), pain tolerance, focus (concentration), social learning, skill coordination

5. **External/environmental:** equipment, weather and altitude, gravity, opposing and assistive forces

Strength training—Using resistance weight training to build maximum muscle force.

Stretch reflex—To prevent overextension and serious injury to muscles and tendons, muscles are equipped with specialized nerve cells (spindles) that apply the brakes when maximum elasticity is reached. Careful ballistic training augmented with plyometric drills can heighten the threshold of the stretch reflex mechanism and improve strength-generating ability.

Striations—Grooves or ridge marks of muscles' individual myofibrils visible through the skin, resulting from both hypertrophy training and extremely low subcutaneous fat deposits. The ultimate degree of muscle definition.

Stroke volume—The amount of blood forced into the circulatory system with each beat.

Sucrose—A sweet disaccharide that occurs naturally in most land plants and is the simple carbohydrate obtained from sugarcane, sugar beet, and other sources. It is hydrolyzed in the intestine by sucrase to glucose and fructose.

Sulfur—A mineral of major structural importance to proteins, enzymes, antibodies, skin, and hair. No RDA. Dietary sources: beans, beef, eggs.

Superset—Alternating back and forth between two exercises until the prescribed number of sets is completed. The two exercises generally involve a protagonist and antagonist (e.g., the biceps and triceps, or the chest and upper back); however, common usage of the term also can mean any two exercises alternated with one another.

Supplements—Concentrated forms of nutritional factors, such as vitamins, minerals, amino acids, and fatty acids, taken to augment the nutritional value of food.

Synergism—The combined effect of two or more parts of forces or agents which is greater than the sum of the individual effects. Example: the synergistic effect of a multiple vitamin and mineral formula compared to the benefits of one or two vitamins.

Tendon—A band or cord of strong, fibrous (collagenous) tissue that connects muscles to bone.

Testosterone—The principal male hormone that accelerates tissue growth. Anabolic steroids are synthetic chemicals that mimic the muscle-building effects of testosterone. Testosterone is an androgen, a sex hormone produced by all humans. It is important in the development of male gonads and sex characteristics. In females, testosterone is an intermediate product in the production of estradiols.

As a pharmaceutical drug, it is used to stimulate sex characteristics, to stimulate production of red blood cells, and to suppress estrogen production. Long-term use can lead to kidney stones, unnatural hair growth, voice changes, and decreased sperm count.

Tissue elasticity (Viscoelasticity)—Involved in all explosive sports, including shot put, boxing, the baseball and javelin throw, and powerlifting. After being stretched, all bodily tissues—including muscles and tendons—return to their original shape. The quicker they do, the more force that can be exerted.

Tissue (or interstitial) leverage—The degree of extra mechanical advantage gained by superheavyweight strength athletes by packing sheer mass from extra fat, liquid, and protein between and inside muscle fibers.

Torque—Moment of force; the turning or twisting effect of a force.

Training effect—Increase in functional capacity of muscles and other bodily tissues as a result of increased overload placed upon them.

Training technologies—Athletes can tap into eight broad categories of accepted methods to attain performance goals: weight training, light resistance training, medical support, therapeutic modalities (jacuzzi, massage, acupuncture), psychological support, biomechanics, diet, and nutritional supplements.

Training to failure—Continuing a set in weight training until inability to complete another rep without assistance.

Transcendental meditation (TM)—An effortless meditation technique scientifically shown to sweep away energy-sapping mental and physical stress and deep-rooted fatigue. Among athletes it improves energy, reaction time, workout recovery, mental alertness, and coordination.

Traps—Slang for trapezius muscles, the largest muscles of the back and neck that draw the head backward and rotate the scapula.

Triceps brachii—The muscle on the back of the upper arm, a prime mover for extending the elbow.

Trimming down—Gaining hard muscular appearance by losing body fat.

Triglyceride—A combination of glycerol with three fatty acids: stearic acid, oleic acid, and palmitic acid.

Troponin—A protein that reacts with calcium to set the contractile mechanism into action within muscle fibers.

Universal machine—One of several types of weight-lifting devices where weights are on a track or rails and are lifted by levers or pulleys.

Unsaturated fatty acids (UFA)—Important in lowering blood cholesterol and may thus help prevent heart disease. They are essential for normal glandular activity, healthy skin, mucous membranes, and many metabolic processes.

Unsaturated fatty acids (UFA) are fatty acids whose carbon chain contains one or more double or triple bonds and which are capable of absorbing more hydrogen. They include the group polyunsaturates, are generally liquid at room temperature and are derived from vegetables, nuts, seeds, or other sources. Examples of unsaturated fatty acids include corn oil, safflower oil, sunflower oil, and olive oil.

A small amount of highly unsaturated fatty acid is essential to animal nutrition. The body cannot desaturate a fat, such as vegetable shortening or margarine, sufficiently by its own metabolic processes to supply this essential need. Therefore, the dietary inclusion of unsaturated or polyunsaturated fats is vital.

The three essential fatty acids (those which the body is unable to manufacture) are linoleic acid, linolenic acid, and arachidonic acid. However, these fatty acids can be synthesized from linoleic acid if sufficient intake occurs. Linoleic acid should provide about two percent of total dietary calories. Corn, safflower, and soybean oils are high in linoleic acid.

Upper abs—Abdominal muscles above the navel.

Variable resistance—Strength training equipment which can, through the use of elliptical cams and other such technology, vary the amount of weight being lifted to match the strength curve for a particular exercise. Nautilus machines, for example, provide this feature. See *constant resistance* and *accommodating resistance.*

Variable split training—A recent major advance in weight training science that systematizes workout schedules according to the recuperation of individual muscle groups and body parts. This precise method maximizes development by eliminating the effects of overtraining or undertraining. Variable double splits and variable triple splits are also used for multiple daily workouts.

Vascularity—Increase in size and number of observable veins. Highly desirable in bodybuilding.

Vitamin—Organic food substances present in plants and animals, essential in small quantities for the proper functioning of the body. Most are obtained from food.

Vitamin A—A fat-soluble vitamin occurring as preformed vitamin A (retinol), found in animal-origin foods, provitamin A (carotene), provided by both plant and animal foods. Maintains healthy skin, mucous membranes, eyesight, and immune-system function and promotes strong bones and teeth. Vital to the liver's processing of protein. RDA: 5,000 International units. Dietary sources: fish-liver oil, liver, eggs, milk and dairy products, green and yellow vegetables, and yellow fruits.

Vitamin B-complex—A family of thirteen water-soluble vitamins, probably the single-most important factor for the health of the nervous system. They are essential to the conversion of food into energy. When you exercise strenuously, your body quickly burns up its vitamin B supply. A shortage of Bs affects both performance and recovery. High consumption of sugar, caffeine, processed food, and alcohol cause depletion.

Vitamin B$_1$ (thiamine)—Essential for learning capacity and muscle tone in the stomach, intestines, and heart. RDA: 1.4 mg (men); 1.0 mg (women). Dietary sources: brewer's yeast, wheat germ, blackstrap molasses, whole wheat and rice, oatmeal, most vegetables.

Vitamin B$_2$ (riboflavin)—An essential cofactor in the enzymatic breakdown of all foodstuffs. Important to cell respiration, good vision, skin, and hair. RDA: 1.6 mg. Dietary sources: liver, tongue, organ meats, milk, eggs. The amount found in foods is minimum, making this America's most common vitamin deficiency.

Vitamin B$_3$ (niacin)—Essential for synthesis of sex hormones, insulin, and other hormones. Effective in improving circulation and reducing blood cholesterol. RDA: 19 mg (men); 13 mg (women). Dietary sources: lean meats, poultry, fish, and peanuts.

Vitamin B$_5$ (pantothenic acid)—An important stress, immune system, and anti-allergy factor. Vital for proper functioning of adrenal glands, where stress chemicals are produced. Promotes endurance. RDA: 10 mg. Dietary sources: organ meats, egg yolks, whole-grain cereals.

Vitamin B$_6$ (pyridoxine)—Essential for the production of antibodies and red blood cells and for the proper assimilation of protein. The more protein you eat, the more B$_6$ you need! Facilitates conversion of stored liver and muscle glycogen into energy. RDA: 1.8 mg (men); 1.5 mg (women). Dietary sources: brewer's yeast, wheat bran, wheat germ, liver, kidney, cantaloupe.

Vitamin B$_{12}$ (cyanocobalamin)—Necessary for normal metabolism of nerve tissue and formation and regeneration of red blood cells. RDA: 3 micrograms. Dietary sources: animal protein. Liver is the best.

Vitamin C—A critical health-protection nutrient. Body stores are depleted rapidly by exercise and stress. Fortifies the immune system against virus infections, strengthens blood vessels, reduces cardiovascular abnormalities, lowers fat and cholesterol levels, as a natural anesthetic it reduces many kinds of pain, helps detoxify chemical and metal contaminants found in air, water, and food, slows down lactic acid buildup, helps heal wounds, scar tissue and injuries. Necessary in the formation of connective tissue. RDA: 60 mg. Dietary sources: citrus fruits, berries, green and leafy vegetables, tomatoes, potatoes.

Vitamin D—A fat-soluble vitamin, acquired through sunlight or diet. Aids the body in utilization of vitamin A, calcium, and phosphorus. Helps maintain stable nervous system and normal heart action. RDA: 400 International units. Dietary sources: fish-liver oils, sardines, salmon, tuna, milk, and dairy products.

Vitamin E—A fat-soluble vitamin, an active antioxidant that retards free-radical damage as well as protects oxidation of fat compounds, vitamin A, and other nutritional factors in the body. Important to cellular respiration, proper circulation, protection of lungs against air pollution, and prevention of blood clots. Helps alleviate leg cramps and charley horse. RDA: 15 International units (men); 12 (women). Dietary sources; wheat germ, cold-pressed vegetable oils, whole raw seeds and nuts, soybeans.

Warm-up—An essential preworkout routine that prepares the body for strenuous exercise ahead. Warming up generally consists of walking, stretching of major muscle groups, and light, progressive movements that stimulate heart, lungs, and muscles.

Weightlifter's headache—An exertional type of pain which may be due to intense clenching of the jaws during heavy lifts.

Weightlifting—A sport of strength in which athletes compete in defined weight classes to lift the most weight. There are two types of weightlifting competitions: Olympic lifting and powerlifting.

Weight training—Exercise that utilizes progressive resistance movements to build strength. Practiced intensely by weightlifters and bodybuilders in particular and by all athletes interested in developing strength.

Weight training belt—Thick leather belt used to support lower back while doing squats, military presses, dead lifts, bent rowing, etc.

White blood cell—Nucleated cells, originating from the bone marrow, that make up the infection-fighting components of the blood. White blood cells fight infections by producing antibodies, releasing immune factors, or ingesting invading bacteria or viruses.

Yeast—A one-celled fungus used in brewing and leavening bread. Some yeast, such as brewer's yeast, is highly nutritious. Many individuals are allergic to yeast. Candida albicans is a common yeast living within the body which can multiply and produce sickness-causing toxins. Antibiotics, sugar-rich diets, birth-control pills, cortisone, and other drugs stimulate candida growth.

Yerba maté—An extract from an Argentine plant used extensively as a stimulating tea drink throughout the Spanish-speaking world. Contains vitamins B_1, B_2, and C, and a natural substance called mateina, which enhances concentration. Related to caffeine, but without any of caffeine's side effects.

Zinc—Has a significant role in protein synthesis, maintenance of enzyme systems, contractibility of muscles, formation of insulin, synthesis of DNA, healing processes, prostate health, and male reproductive fluid. RDA: 15 mg. Deficiencies are common due to food processing and zinc-poor soil. Excessive sweating can drain up to 3 mg daily. Dietary sources: meat, wheat germ, brewer's yeast, pumpkin seeds, eggs.

Zinc chelate is the element zinc in supplemental form and coated with protein to increase the percentage that can be assimilated by the body.

Deficiency in zinc is associated with anemia, short stature, hypogonadism, impaired wound healing, and geophagia. Zinc salts are often toxic when absorbed by the system, producing a chronic poisoning resembling that caused by lead.

BIBLIOGRAPHY

Allsen, P. E. *Strength Training.* Glenview, IL: Scott, Foresman, and Co., 1987.

American College of Sports Medicine. *Resource Manual for Guidelines for Exercise Testing and Prescription.* Philadelphia: Lea & Febiger, 1988.

Astrand, P. O., and K. Rodahl. *Testbook of Work Physiology.* New York: McGraw-Hill, 1977.

Bentley, S., and F. C. Hatfield. *Toning Your Body.* New York: New Century Publishers, 1982.

Berger, R. A. *Introduction to Weight Training.* Englewood Cliffs, NJ: Prentice-Hall, 1984.

Brooks, G. A., and T. D. Fahey. *Exercise Physiology.* New York: John Wiley and Sons, 1984.

Brunner, R., and B. Tabatchnik. *Soviet Training and Recovery Methods.* San Francisco, California: Sports Focus Publishers, 1990.

Carlotti, P., and D. Gabrielle. *The cellular ageing process and free radicals.* DCI (Sederma, France), February 1989.

Cerutti, P. A. "Prooxidant states and tumor promotion." *Science* 227 (1985): 375–381.

Cooper, P. G., ed. *Aerobics: Theory and Practice.* Costa Mesa, CA: HDL Publishing Co., 1987.

Corbin, C. B., and R. Lindsey. *The Ultimate Fitness Book.* New York: Leisure Press, 1984.

Costes, N. *Interval Training.* Mountain View, CA: World Publications, 1972.

Daugheday, W. H. "The anterior pituitary." In Wilson and Foster (ed.) *Williams Textbook of Endocrinology* (7th ed.), 577–611. Philadelphia: Saunders, 1985.

Davis, Paul O. *The Keiser Manual: A Guide to the Fundamentals of Resistive Training with Keiser Air-Powdered Exercise Machines.* Keiser Equipment Co., 1989.

De Vries, H.A. *Physiology of Exercise for Physical Education and Athletics.* Dubuque, Iowa: Wm. C. Brown, 1980.

DiPasquale, M. *Anabolic Steroid Side Effects*. Ontario: M.G.D. Press, 1990.

————. *Beyond Anabolic Steroids*. Ontario: M.G.D. Press, 1990.

————. *Drug Use & Detection in Amateur Sports*. Ontario: M.G.D. Press, 1984.

————. Update 1, 1986.

————. Update 2, 1986.

————. Update 3, 1987.

————. Update 4, 1987.

————. Update 5, 1988.

Donahue, D. *Treatment of Athletic Injuries*. 3d ed. New York: Saunders, 1978.

Engasser, P. Article on sunscreens. *J. Amer. Derm.*, January 1991: 14.

Fox, E. L. *Sports Physiology*. Philadelphia: Saunders, 1979.

————. *Sports Physiology*. 2d ed. Philadelphia: CBS College Publishing, 1984.

Gaspari, R., with F. C. Hatfield. *Off-Season Nutrition for Bodybuilders*. Newark: New Age, 1987.

Gibson, H. and R. T. H. Edwards. "Muscular Exercise and Fatigue." *Sports Medicine*, March/April 1985, quoting R. T. H. Edwards, "Biochemical bases of fatigue in exercise performance: Catastrophe theory of muscular fatigue" in Knuttgen et al. eds. *Biochemistry of Exercise*. Champaign: Human Kinetics, 1983, pp. 3–28.

Guyton, A. C. *Basic Human Physiology*. Philadelphia: Saunders, 1977.

————. *Function of the Human Body*. Philadelphia: Saunders, 1974.

Hatfield, F. C. *Advanced Sports Conditioning*. Tokyo: Morinaga & Co., 1988.

————. *Aerobic Weight Training*. Chicago: Contemporary Books, 1983.

————. *Anabolic Steroids*. Los Angeles: Fitness Systems, 1982.

————. *Bench Press Training for Powerlifters*. Los Angeles: Fitness Systems, 1982.

————. *Bodybuilding*. Tokyo: Morinaga & Co., 1986.

————. *Bodybuilding: A Scientific Approach*. Chicago: Contemporary Books, 1983.

————. *Bodybuilding for Power*. Los Angeles: Fitness Systems, 1982.

————. *Complete Guide to Power Training*. Los Angeles: Fitness Systems, 1982.

————. *Complete Guide to Strength and Sports Training*. International Sports Sciences Association. Forthcoming.

————. *Complete Guide to Weight Training and Sports Conditioning for Young Athletes*. Chicago: Contemporary Books. Forthcoming.

————. *The Daily Training and Nutrition Planner*. Tokyo: Morinaga & Co., 1987.

————. *Deadlift Training for Powerlifters*. Los Angeles: Fitness Systems, 1982.

————. *Ergogenesis: Achieving Peak Athletic Performance Without Drugs*. Los Angeles: Fitness Systems, 1985.

————. *The Fat Book*. Unpublished manuscript.

————. *Flexibility Training for Sports: PNF Techniques*. Los Angeles: Fitness Systems, 1982.

————. *Guide to Sportsmedicine*. Tokyo: Morinaga & Co., 1990.

————. *Power: A Scientific Approach*. Chicago: Contemporary Books, 1989.

————. *Powerlifting: A Scientific Approach*. Chicago: Contemporary Books, 1981.

————. *The Sports Nutrition Bible*. Tokyo: Morinaga & Co., 1990.

————. *The Squat: Training for Sports and Powerlifting*. Los Angeles: Fitness Systems, 1982.

————. *The Training Bible for Sports*. Tokyo: Morinaga & Co., 1985.

————. *The Training Workbook*. Tokyo: Morinaga & Co., 1989.

————. *Ultimate Sports Nutrition*. Chicago: Contemporary Books, 1987.

————. *Weight Training for Sports*. New York: Sterling Publishers, 1986.

————. *Weight Training for the Young Athlete*. New York: Atheneum Publishers, 1980.

Hatfield, F. C. ed. *Complete Guide to Strength and Sports Training*. International Sports Sciences Association. Forthcoming.

————. *Fitness: The Complete Guide*. International Sports Sciences Association, 1991.

Hatfield, F. C., and J. Comereski. *Sportsmedicine in the Trenches*. Unpublished manuscript.

Hatfield, F. C., and M. Krotee. *Personalized Weight Training for Fitness and Athletics: From Theory to Practice*. Dubuque: Kendall/Hunt, 1978.

Hatfield, F. C., K. Od, and L. Taylor. *The Sports Nutrition Bible & Coloring Book*. Unpublished manuscript.

Hatfield, F. C., with K. G. Saito. *Sports, Fitness and Bodybuilding Curriculum Guide for Coaches*. Tokyo: Morinaga & Co. In press.

Hatfield, F. C., and M. Yessis. *Oxygen: Its Incredible Story*. International Sports Sciences Association, 1991.

Hatfield, F. C., and M. Zucker. *Encyclopedia of Sports Nutrition*. Unpublished manuscript.

————. A series of eighteen manuals on various aspects of sports and fitness nutrition. Los Angeles: Weider Publications, 1990.

Hattinger, T. *Physiology of Strength*. Springfield, IL: Charles C. Thomas, 1961.

Hausman, P. *The Right Dose*. Emmaus, PA: Rodale Press, 1987.

Hill, A. V. and P. Kupalov. "Anaerobic and aerobic activity in isolated muscle." Proceedings of the Royal Society of London: Series B, 1929; 105, 313–328.

Hoshino, T. et al. "Reducing the photosensitizing potential of chlorpromazine with the simultaneous use of beta- and dimethyl-beta-cyclodextrins in guinea pigs." *Archives of Dermatological Research* (Japan) 281 no. 1 1989: 60–5.

Hultman, E., and H. Sjoholm. "Energy metabolism and contraction force of human skeletal muscle in situ during electrical stimulation." *Journal of Physiology* (London), 345; 525–532.

————. "Substrate availability." In H. G. Knuttgen, J. A. Vogel, and J. Poortmans, eds. International Series on Sport Sciences. *Biochemistry of Exercise* (vol. 13, pp. 63–75).

Jensen, C. R., and A. G. Fisher. *Scientific Basis of Athletic Conditioning*. Philadelphia: Lea and Febiger, 1979.

Jones, N. L., N. McCartney, and A. J. McComas. *Human Muscle Power*. Champaign, IL: Human Kinetics Publishers, 1986.

Katch, F. I., and W. D. McArdle. *Nutrition, Weight Control and Exercise*. Philadelphia: Lea & Febiger, 1988.

Kolata, G. "Glaucoma and Cataract: Closing in on causes." *New York Times*, July 12, 1988.

Kremer, J. M. et al. "Fish oil fatty acid supplementation in active rheumatoid arthritis." *JAMA* 1987; 258: 962.

Kronhausen, E., and P. Kronhausen. *Formula for Life*. New York: Wm. Morrow and Co., 1989.

Krotee, M., and F. C. Hatfield. *Theory and Practice of Physical Activity*. Dubuque: Kendall/Hunt, 1979.

Lamb, D. R. *Physiology of Exercise*. 2d ed. New York: MacMillan, 1984.

Lorpela, H. et al. "Effects of selenium supplementation after acute myocardial infarction." (Finland), *Research Community for Chemical and Pathological Pharmacology* August 1989; 65 (2) : 249–52.

Luciano, D. S., J. H. Sherman, and A. T. Vander. *Human Anatomy and Physiology: Structure and Function*. New York: McGraw-Hill, 1983.

Marsa, L. "Oxygen: New Light on the free radicals that cause Ageing." *Los Angeles Times*, August 28, 1989.

Marimee, T. J. "Growth hormone secretion and action." In DeGroot et al. (ed.) *Endocrinology*, vol. 1, 123–132. New York: Grune and Stratton, 1979.

Mathews, D. K., and E. L. Fox. *The Physiological Basis of Physical Education and Athletics*. Philadelphia: W. B. Saunders, 1981.

Mazzurco, P., with F. C. Hatfield. *Exerstyle*. New York: Simon & Schuster, 1985.

McArdle, W. D., F. I. Katch, and V. I. Katch. *Exercise Physiology: Energy, Nutrition and Human Performance*. 2d ed. Philadelphia: Lea & Febiger, 1986.

Meredith, C. "Protein needs and protein supplements in strength-trained men." In Report of the Ross Symposium on Muscle Development. Columbus, OH: Ross Laboratories, 1988.

Morgan, R. E., and G. T. Adamson. *Circuit Training*. London: G. Bell and Sons, 1961.

Morrison, W. L. "Photoimmunology." *Journal of Investigative Dermatology*, 1981; 77:73.

Mukhtar, H. et al. "Inhibitory effects of NDGA on mutagenicity, monooxygenase activities and cytochrome P-450 and prostaglandin synthetase-dependent metabolism of benzo(A)pyrene (BP)." Meeting abstract, Case Western Res. Univ., Cleveland. *Fed. Proceedings* 46, no. 3 (1987): 696.

Niwa, Y. "Lipid peroxides and superoxide dimutase (SOD) induction in skin inflammatory diseases, and treatment with SOD preparations." (Japan) *Dermatologica* 179, (1989), Suppl. 1:101–6.

O'Shea, J. P. *Scientific Principles and Methods of Strength Fitness*. Reading, MA: Addison Wesley, 1976.

Pearl, B., and G. T. Morgan. *Getting Stronger*. Bolinas, CA: Shelter Publications, 1986.

Prentice, W. "Therapeutic Modalities in Sports Medicine." *St. Louis Times Mirror*, 1986.

Prevention Magazine. *The Complete Book of Vitamins*. Emmaus, PA: Rodale Press, 1984.

———. *Future Youth: How to Reverse the Aging Process*. Emmaus, PA: Rodale Press, 1987.

Riley, D. P. *Strength Training: By the Experts*. West Point, NY: Leisure Press, 1977.

Ryan, A. J., and F. L. Allman. *Sportsmedicine*. New York: Academic Press, 1979.

Sharkey, B. J. *Physiology of Fitness*. 2d ed. Champaign, IL: Human Kinetics, 1984.

Shephard, R. J., and K. H. Sidney. "Effects of physical exercise on plasma growth hormone and cortisol levels in human subjects." In Wilmore and Keough (ed.) *Exercise and Sport Science Review*, 1–30. New York: Academic Press, 1975.

Smith, E. L., and R. C. Serfass. eds. *Exercise and Aging: The Scientific Basis.* Hillside, NJ: Enslow Publishers, 1981.

Spande, J. I., and B. A. Schottedius. "Chemical basis of fatigue in isolated mouse soleus muscle." *American Journal of Physiology,* 219 (1970): 1490–1495.

Stone, W. J., and W. A. Kroll. *Sports Conditioning and Weight Training.* Newton, MA: Allyn and Bacon, 1986.

Taylor, C. R. et al. "Photoageing/photodamage and photoprotection." *American Academy of Dermatology* 22, no. 1 (January 1990).

Taylor, W. *Hormonal Manipulation.* Jefferson, N.C., and London: McFarland & Co., 1985.

Taylor, W. *Anabolic Steroids.* Jefferson, N.C., and London: McFarland & Co., 1982.

Wang, S. Y., C. Merrill, and E. Bell. "Effects of ageing and long-term subcultivation on collagen lattice contraction and intra-lattice proliferation in three rat cell types." Massachusetts Institute of Technology, *Mech. Ageing Dev.* 44, no. 2 (August): 127–41.

Westcott, W. L. *Strength Fitness.* 2nd ed. Boston: Allyn and Bacon, 1981.

Williams, M. *Ergogenic Aids in Sports.* Champaign: Human Kinetics, 1983.

Wilmore, J. H. *Training for Sport and Activity.* Boston: Allyn & Bacon, 1982.

Wills, E. D. "Effects of antioxidants on lipid peroxide formation in irradiated synthetic diets." *Int. J. Radiat. Biol.* 37, no. 4 (April 1980): 403–14.

Wright, J. *Anabolic Steroids in Sports.* Sports Science Consultants (Mass.), vol. 1, 1978.

———. vol. 2, 1982.

Yessis, M. *Secrets of Soviet Sports Fitness & Training.* Ontario: Collins Pub., 1987.

Yessis, M., and F. C. Hatfield. *Plyometric Training.* Los Angeles: Fitness Systems, 1986.

INDEX

ABC system of bodybuilding, 35, 42, 44, 263. *See also* Integrated training
Abdominal muscles, 46, 112, 115, 116
Absolute strength, 6–7
Acceleration, 8
Acidosis, 138
ACTH, 250,253
Actin-myosin cross-bridges, 139, 258
Acupressure, 141
Adaption, 281
Addisonic overtraining, 318–19
Adductor muscle group, 74
Adenosine triphosphate (ATP), 9
    breakdown of, 258
    consumption during high-intensity training, 137–38
    effect on muscle growth, 16–17
    regeneration of, 140
ADH (Vasopressin), 253
Adhesions, 14–15
Adrenal cortex, 251
Adrenal hormones, 249, 253
Advertising, 64
Aerobic exercise, 10, 27, 134
Aerobic strength, 6, 9
AIDS, 270
Airola, Paavo, 310
Alcohol, 221, 265–66
Aldosterone, 251
Alfalfa, 284
Allergies, food, 222
Aloe vera, 284
Alternate dumbbell curls, 102, 103
Althea root, 281
American Psychiatric Association, 357–58
Amino acids
    branched-chain, 140, 238, 24
    essential, 237–38
    growth hormone and, 255
Ammonia, 238, 241
Amphetamines, 276, 375

Anabolic steroids, 30–31, 64, 67, 254, 273–74, 374–76
Anadrol 50, 273
Anaerobic strength
    definition of, 137
    factors affecting, 6
    fatigue and, 139
    improving, 140
    nutrition and, 140
Anavar, 273
Anterior deltoids, 111
Antibiotics, 222
Anti-inflammatory drugs, 276–77
Antioxidants, 239, 285–92
Archimedes' principle, 196
Arginine, 255
Arginine/ornithine supplements, growth hormone and, 278
Aristocort, 277
Arms, upper. *See* Biceps; Triceps
Ascorbic acid (vitamin C), 213, 218
Asellincrin, 274
Aspirin, 241, 269–71, 277
Astragalos membranaceus, 284
Atherosclerosis, 211–12
ATP (adenosine triphosphate), 9
    breakdown of, 258
    consumption during high-intensity training, 137–38
    effect on muscle growth, 16–17
    regeneration of, 140
ATP/ADP ratios, 139–40
ATPase, 259
Avena sativa, 282

"B" training, 35–36, 42, 44. *See also* ABC system of bodybuilding
Back
    extensions, 44–45, 100, 101
    lower, 79, 115, 131
    preventing injury to, 118
    target muscles in, 94
    training schedules for, 39–40, 48–49, 60

Baker, Aaron, 346
Baking soda, 141
Barbell curls, 102, 105
Barbell hack squats, 123
Basal metabolic rate (BMR),
    167–69, 182–83, 231–32
Basedowic overtraining, 318–19
Basketball, 143
Batting, 143
BCAAs (Branched-chain amino
    acids), 140, 238, 241
Bear squats, 121
Belly belt (Lumbar Orthopedic
    Repositioning Appliance), 312
Bench dips, 111
Bench press(ing), 44, 84, 88–89
Berberis, 284
Beta carotene. *See Vitamin A*
Beta sitosterol, 241
Beta-endorphins, 278
Betaine, 241
Biceps, 102
    brachii, 75, 102
    exercises for, 45
    femoris, 74
    training schedules for, 39–40,
        48–49, 60
Bicycling, 11
Bilberry, 288, 289
Bioflavinoids, 214
Bio-individuality, 224
Biomechanics (skill) training, 12
Biotin, 213, 217
Black cohosh, 284
Blood
    clotting, 270
    pressure, 267
    herbs and, 281
Blue cohosh, 284
Blue vervain, 282
BMR (Basal metabolic rate),
    167–69, 182–83, 231–32
Body fat percentage, 195–204
    estimating, 196–203
        for men, 197
        for women, 198
    ideals for various sports, 204
Bodybuilding squats, 121
Boldenone, 274
Bones, calcium and, 224
Boron, 220, 241
Box squats, 121

Boxing, 143
Brachialis, 102
Branched-chain amino acids, 140,
    238, 241
Breads and cereals, 176–77
Breathing, proper, 25
Brewer's yeast, 241
Buffers, 140
Burdock, 281, 284
Burnout, 322–28
Bush, George, 301

"C" training, 36, 42–44
Cable crossovers, 44, 90
Cable crunchers, 117
Cable curls, 102, 105
Cable kickbacks, 107, 110
Caffeine, 267–68
Calciferol (vitamin D), 214
Calcium, 218, 224–25
Calf machine, 47
Calf raises, 129–31
Calorie(s)
    burned during various activities,
        233
    estimating need for, 164–65
    -restricted diets, 230
    zigzagging intake, 162, 167–91,
        195
Calves
    exercises for, 47, 74, 129–31
    training schedules for, 39–40,
        48–49, 60
    See also Legs
Cancer
    aspirin and, 270
    smoking and, 267
Capillarization, effect on muscle
    growth, 17
Capsicum fruit, 283
Carbohydrate(s), 162, 208–9
    -restricted diets, 229
    supercompensation, 369–71
    top sources of, 227
Carbo-loading, 369–71
Cardiovascular system, 284, 309.
    See also Aerobic exercise
Cataracts, 270
Catnip, 284
Cayenne, 284
Celery seed, 284
Chaenomeles lagenaria, 284

Chamomile, 284
Chaparral, 284
Chasteberry, 284
Cheating movements, 73, 298–99
Chemotherapy, 141
Chest
  exercises for, 44
  muscles in, 83
  training schedules for, 39–40,
    48–49, 60
  See also Clavicular pectorals;
    Sternal pectorals
Chewing tobacco, 267
Chickweed, 284
Chin-ups (Pull-ups), 98, 99, 106,
  107
Chiropractic care, 11
Cholesterol, 211–12
Choline, 213, 217
Choreography, 339–40
Chromium, 219
Chromium picolinate, 240, 241
Chromium polynicotinate
  (ChromeMate), 240, 241
Churchill, Winston, 301
Ciba Corporation, 325
Cigarettes, 267
Circadian rhythms, 34
Circulatory system, 266
Clavicular pectoralis (upper chest),
  83, 87
Clover, red, 281
Cobalamin (vitamin B_{12}), 213, 215
Cocaine, 375
Codnopsis, 284
Coenzyme B_{12} (dibencozide), 241
Coenzyme Q_{10} (CoQ_{10}), 220–21, 240
Coffee, 221
Colds, 270
Colon, 270, 281
Comerford, Vince, 316
Comfrey, 284
Commonwealth of Independent
  States (C.I.S.), 285
Competition, preparing for, 364–71
Complex carbohydrates. *See*
  Carbohydrates
Complex training, 156–57
Computers, 303–5
Concentration, 18, 353
Concentration curls, 102, 103–4
Concentric strength, 7

Congenital weaknesses, 320
Connective tissue structure, 15
Connelly, Scott, 261
Contest preparation, 364–71
Contraceptives, oral, 223
Contractile cells, 18
Contractile force, 36
Contractile speed, 36
Contraction time, 146
Convenience foods, 222
Cooldown routine, 27, 38
Coordination (skill), 19
Copper, 219, 225
Cornsilk, 281
Corticotropin, 250
Cortisol, 238, 249, 251
Cortisone, 277
Couchgrass, 281
Creatine phosphate (CP), 139
Cresorman, 274
Crew, 143
Crop nutrient losses, 222
Crunchers, 46, 113, 116, 117
Cureton, Thomas K., 292
Curls
  leg, 126–27
  Preacher, 102, 103
  wrist, 112
Cybex Upper Body Exerciser
  (UBE/LBE), 152
Cycle (periodized) training, 31, 33,
  144–45, 148, 157–59, 263
Cycling, 11
Cytomel (T3 thyroid), 275

Dairy products, 176–77, 235
Damiana leaf, 282
Dandelion, 281, 284
Davies, Kevin, 287
Deadlifts, 45, 125, 126
Dean, Ward, 309
Dearth, David, 293
Decadron, 277
Deca-Durabolin, 273
Deep fiber massage, 338–39
Deltoids, 75, 76, 111
DeMey, Barry, 71
Depo-Medrol, 277
Depression, 355–62
Dexadrine, 276
Diabetes, 270
Dianabol, 274

Diet(s)
calorie-restricted, 230
carbohydrate-restricted, 229
effect on growth hormone
production, 256
fad, 222, 228–30
fat-loss, 193, 229
growth hormone production and,
256
muscle-gaining, 178
protein-restricted, 229
See also Fat loss; Nutrition
Dietary supplements. *See*
Nutritional supplements
Digestive system, 221, 266, 284
DiPasquale, Mauro, 272
Dips, 92, 111
Discipline, 41, 347–49
Dr. Squat. *See*Hatfield, Frederick
C.
Donkey raises, 130–31
Drill, 2–3 minute, 155
Drinks
meal-replacement, 239
sports, 240–42
Drug abuse, 247–48, 254, 265–77
alternatives to, 278
myths about, 374–76
testing for, 67
Dumbbell(s)
bench presses, 44, 84–85, 88
curls, 45, 102, 103
kickbacks, 107, 110
lunge walking with, 120
raises, lateral, 76–77
rows, one-arm, 95
Durabolin, 273
Dysthemia, 362

Eccentric strength, 7
Echinacea, 284
Edison, Thomas, 301
Edwards, R. T. H., 322
Eggs, 235
Elbows, 86, 111
Elderly persons, 223
Electrical impedance, 196
Electromechanical fatigue, 325–26
Electrostimulation, 337
Eleutherococcus senticosus
(Siberian ginseng), 241, 281,
282, 284

Elite bodybuilders, training
program for, 48
Emotions, 351–54
Endocrine system, 16, 245–63
Endorphins, 251
Energy
eating for, 205
expended during various
activities, 233
Epinephrine, 251
Equipment, 19, 25
Equipoise, 274
Erector spinae muscle group, 75,
100, 112
Essential amino acids, 237–38
Estrogen, 252
Estrogen blockers, 275
Evening primrose, 284
Exercise(s)
basal metabolic rate and, 231
chest, 44
fat loss and, 181
frequency of, 21
hormonal response to, 253
intensity of, 21
length of sessions, 21
shoulder, 44, 76
technique, 72–73
tolerance to, 331–35
total-body, 131
upper leg, 118
See also Name of body part or
exercise
Exercycle, 134–35
Explosive movements, 8, 42, 131
Extensor muscles, 111, 129
External obliques, 75, 112
EZ curls, 45, 102

Fad diets, 222, 228–30
Failure, fear of, 352
Fat, dietary, 162, 176–77, 209–12
Fat loss
exercise and, 181
herbs for, 284
integrated training and, 180
role of hunger in, 192
role of taste in, 192
timeframe for, 195
See also Zigzagging caloric
intake

Fat-restricted diets, 229
  anaerobic strength and, 139
  antioxidants and, 285
  CP and, 139
  delaying, 140
  high-frequency, 325
  low-frequency, 325–26
  repetitive contractions and, 146
Fatigue, 322–28
Fear, 352
Fenugreek seed, 282, 283
Ferulic acid, 241
FGF (Fibroblast growth factor),
  261
Fiber
  dietary, 227
  muscle, 14–15, 16
Fibroblast growth factor (FGF),
  261
Finger flexion, 112
Fitness and Sports Review, 312
FITT principle, 20–21
Five Rs principle, 20, 21–23
Fleece flower root, 283
Flexors, 111
Flyes, 86–87
Folic acid, 213, 215
Food(s)
  allergies, 222
  consumption log, 166
  glycemic indexes of, 234–35
  processed, 222
  recommended, 176–77
Football, 143
Force, contractile, 36
Forced reps, 73, 294–97
Forearms
  exercises for, 46–47
  muscles in, 75, 111
  training schedules for, 39–40,
    48–49, 60
Franks, B. Don, 26
Free radicals, 285–88
French presses, 45, 106, 107
Front barbell raises, 81
Front squats, 121, 122
Fructose, 208
Fruits, 176–77, 209, 227, 235

Gamma interferon, 270
Gamma oryzanol (Ferulic acid),
  241

Garlic, 220, 284
Gastrocnemius (calf muscles), 74,
  129–31
Genetics, 73
Gentian, 284
Germanium, 221
GH. *See* Growth hormone
Gibson, H., 322
Ginger, 284
Ginkgo, 282, 283, 284
Ginseng, Oriental, 284
Ginseng, Siberian, 241, 281, 282,
  284
Glandulars, 241
Glutathione, 288, 290
Glucagon, 246, 252
Glucose, 208, 240, 278
  hormones and, 246
  polymer drinks, 241
Glum, Gary, 338
Gluteal muscles, 74, 118, 131,
  133–34
Glute-ham-gastroc machine, 100
Glute-ham-gastroc raises, 133–34
Glycemic index, 209, 234–36, 242
Glycogen, 146, 238, 266
Glycolytic sports, 146, 148
Goals, 350
Goldenseal, 281, 284
Gonadotropin, 250
Gotu Kola, 284
Grains, 209, 227, 235
Grip muscles (forearm), 116
Groin muscles, 119
Growth hormone (GH), 248, 250,
  254–56
  releasers, 241
  sauna and, 309
  stimulating, 274, 278
Gymnastics, 143

Habituation, 278
Hack squats, 46, 121, 122, 123
Hammer curls, 102
Hamstring(s), 125
  curls, 46
  explosive high pulls for, 131
  glute-ham-gastroc raises for,
    133–34
  leg curls for, 126–27
Haney, Lee, 302
Hanging leg raises, 116

Hatfield, Frederick C. (Dr. Squat), 119
Hatfield bar, 122
Hawthorn berries, 284
HDLs (high-density lipoproteins), 211,
Head of humerus, 102
Healing, herbal, 281
Health Mate Company, 308
Heart
  alcohol and, 266
  attacks, 269
  rate, 155
  smoking and, 267
  See also Cardiovascular system
Herbs, 240, 279–284
He-shou-wu, 284
hGH. *See* Growth hormone
High jumping, 143
High pulls, 131–33
High-density lipoproteins (HDLs), 211
Hips, 116, 118
Hochstein, Paul, 287
Holistic-sets training ("C" training), 36, 42–44
Hops, 284
Hormones, 245–63
  adrenal, 249
  functions of, 245–53
  glucose and, 246
  response to exercise, 253
  See also Endocrine system; Growth hormone
Horrigan, Joseph, 338
Horsetail grass, 283
Hot beverages, 221
Hultman, Eric, 138, 139
Human chorionic gonadatropin (Pregnyl), 277
Human growth hormone. *See* Growth hormone
Hunger, 192
Hydrangea,281
Hydrogen peroxide, 288
Hydrogenated fats, 210
Hydroxyl radical, 288
Hyper benches, 100
Hypertrophy, 259–61, 263
Hypothalamus, 253, 254
Hypoxia, tissue, 285

ICOPRO (Integrated Conditioning Programs), 66–70
IGF (Insulinlike growth factor), 261
Ilio-costalis, 94
Illinois, University of, 292
Illness, 223
Immune response, 284
Incline bench press, 88–89
Incline dumbbell press, 44, 88
Incline flyes, 87
Injury, 15, 317–20, 352
Inosine, 239–41
Inositol, 213, 217
Insertion point, 73
Insulin, 246, 252, 253, 266
Insulinlike growth factor (IGF), 261
Integrated Conditioning Programs (ICOPRO), 66–70
Integrated training, 41, 50–59, 150–59, 180
Intensity of exercise, 21
Interleukin-2, 270
Intermediate bodybuilders, 49, 60
Internal oblique, 75, 94, 112
International Sports Sciences Association (ISSA), 154, 304–5
International Symposium on Human Muscle Power, 139
Intramuscular pH, 139
Inverted flyes, 82
Iodine, 219
Iron, 219, 224, 225
ISSA (International Sports Sciences Association), 154, 304–5
Issels, Josef, 309

Javelin, 143
Jefferson squats, 121 ·
Jogging, 134
Jones, Arthur, 331
Judo, 143
Jujube, 284

Karate, 143
Katz, Mike, 336
Keystone deadlifts, 126
Kidneys, 252, 253, 266, 281
Kinotherapy, 141
Kola nut, 284

Lactic acid, 285
   anaerobic energy and, 138
   buildup, 140, 146
   effect on muscle growth, 17, 18
   intramuscular pH and, 139–40
   removal during cooldown, 27
Lankford, Alan, 302
Lasix, 276
Lat shrug-downs, 99
Lateral dumbbell raises, 76
Lateral head (triceps), 102
Latissimus dorsi, 75, 94, 97, 99
Law of reversibility, 24
Laxatives, 222
L-carnitine, 241
L-dopa, 274
Leg(s), 46
   curls, 126–27
   extensions, 46, 128
   lower, muscles in, 129
   presses, 122, 124
   raises, hanging, 116
   training schedules for, 39–40,
     48–49, 60
Legumes, 209, 227
Levator anguli scapularis, 94
L-glutamine, 238–39
Licorice, 281, 282, 284
Limit strength, 6, 42145–48
Linea alba, 112
Linea similunaris, 112
Linea transversae, 112
Linear anaerobic strength
   endurance, 9
Liver, 266, 281
Log(s), training progress, 61–63
Lombardi, Vince, 285
Long cable pulls, 44–45, 97
Longissimus dorsi, 94
LORA (Lumbar Orthopedic
   Repositioning Appliance), 312
Low-density lipoproteins (LDLs),
   211
L-tryptophan, 50
Lumbar Orthopedic Repositioning
   Appliance (LORA), 312
Lumbar spine, protecting from
   injury, 126
Lumbar trauma, 311–12
Lunge squats, 119
Lunge walking with dumbbells, 46,
   120

Lunges, side, 119
Lwoff, A., 309

Machine curls, 102
McMaster University (Hamilton,
   Ontario), 139
Macrocycles, 33–34
Macronutrients, 206–12
Macrotrauma,18, 27
Magic circle squats, 121
Magnesium, 218, 225
Mahuang, 241
Manganese, 219, 225
Maria thistle, 288, 289
Marijuana, 375
Marketing tactics, 64
Massage, 141
   deep fiber, 338–39
MCTs (medium-chain
   triglycerides), 210
Meal-replacement drinks, 239
Meals, 164–65, 256
Meat, 176–77, 235
Mechanico-metabolic fatigue, 325
Medial head (triceps), 102
Medicine ball, 154
Medium-chain triglycerides
   (MCTs), 210
Medium-to-high intensity training
   ("B" training), 35–36, 42, 44
Melbourne (Australia), 290
Mesocycles, 33–34, 150
Methandrostenolone, 274
Methamphetamine, 276
Methenolone, 274
Microcycles, 33–34, 37
Micronutrients, 212–14
Microtrauma, 18, 27, 285
Middle deltoids, exercises for, 76,
   78
Midsection, training schedules for,
   39–40, 48–49, 60
Migraines, 270
Milk thistle, 281
Milkweed, 284
Minerals, 140, 224–27, 241
Mitochondria, effect on muscle
   growth,17
Moderate intensity training ("B"
   training), 35–36, 42, 44
Monolift machine, 84
Morant, Johnnie, 381

Motivation,18, 347–49

Movement speed, 37

Mumie, 241

Muscle(s)
caffeine and, 267
fibers,14–15, 36, 259–262, 266
-gaining diet, 178
glycogen in, 238
growth, 6, 14–19, 47, 179
hypertrophy, 259–61, 263
mass, 142, 205, 281
size, recovery time and, 37
structure and function, 74–75,
258–59

Muscle Media 2000 (magazine), 261

Musco MXT, 241

Myofibrillarization, 16

Myosin, 139, 258

Nadroline phenylpropionate, 273

Nandrolone decanoate, 273

Naps, 300–302. *See also* Sleep

Native Americans, 308

Nautilus Fitness Machines, 331

NDGA (nor-di-hydro-guai-aretic
acid), 288, 289

Nervous system
alcohol and, 266
caffeine and, 267–68
hormones and, 246

Neuromuscular reeducation,
338–39

Niacin (vitamin B3), 212, 215

Nicotine, 267

Nolvadex (tomoxifen citrate), 275

Nomogram, 199, 200–201

Non-steroidal anti-inflammatory
drugs, 277

Nonlinear anaerobic strength
endurance,9

Norepinephrine, 251

Nose crushers, 45, 106

Nuclear magnetic resonance
imaging (NMR), 139

Nutrient synergy, 226

Nutrition, 161–83, 205–27
alcohol and, 266
anaerobic strength and, 140
microcycles and, 34
recuperative ability and, 38
See also Caloric intake; Food;
Meals

Nutritional supplements, 12, 34, 38,
163, 214, 221–4, 228–29,
237–43, 305. *See also* Vitamins

Nuts, 209

Obesity, 167–68
factors contributing to, 194
growth hormone and, 278
See also Body fat

Oblique muscles, 115, 118

Octacosanol, 240, 241, 290–92

Olympic Games, 285, 290

Olympic squats, 121

One-arm exercises
bent rows, 45
cable kickbacks, 110
dumbbell kickbacks, 110
dumbbell rows, 95
preacher curls, 102, 103

1-2-3 rule of caloric intake, 163

Onion, 284

Optimum Daily Allowances (ODAs),
215–21

Organic/fatty acid hydroperoxides,
288

Oriental ginseng, 284

Ornithine, 255

Ovaries, 252

Overhead pulley machine, 107

Overhead squats, 121

Overload principle, 23–24, 34

Overtraining, 285, 317–20

Oxandrolone, 273

Oxidized protein, 288

Oxygen, 241, 290
cocktail, 290–92
debt, 138, 146
replacement, 17
therapy, 141

Oxymetholone, 273

Oxytocin, 251, 253

PABA (Para-amino-benzoic acid),
213, 217

Padilla, Danny, 136

Pain,18, 278, 284

Pancreatic hormones, 253

Pangamate (vitamin B_{15}), 213

Pantothenic acid (vitamin B_5), 212,
217

Para-amino-benzoic acid (PABA),
213, 217

Parallel bar dips, 111
Parathyroid, 252
Parmenides, 308
Partial presses, 81
Partial squats,121
Partner-assisted exercise (forced reps), 73, 294–97
Passion, 349–50
Passionflower, 284
Pearson, Tony, 363
Pec deck, 93
Pectorals, 75, 83, 86, 87, 112
Pennsylvania, University of, 167
Periodicity, 31, 305
Periodized (cycle) training, 33, 144–45, 157–59, 263
Peroneus brevis, 129
Peroneus longus,129
Personalized training program, 33
pH, intramuscular, 139
Phosphagens, 9, 16–17, 137–40, 258
Phosphorus, 218, 225
Pitching, 143
Pituitary gland, 248, 250–51, 253–55
Plantain tree, 284
Platform squats, 121
Platz, Tom, 118
Plyo ball, 154
Plyometrics, 10, 150, 156
Polypeptide hormones, 245
Polyunsaturated fatty acid radical, 288
Posing routine choreography, 339–40
Potassium, 220, 225–26
Power (speed-strength), 6–7, 42, 47
Powerlifting, 143
Powerlifting squats, 121
Preacher curls, 102, 103
Pregnancy, 223, 270, 271
Pregnyl, 277
Premenstrual syndrome, 223
Prickly ash, 284
Primobolin, 274
Processed foods, 222
Progesterone, 252
Prolactin, 250, 253
Pronator quadratus, 111
Pronator radii teres, 111
Prostaglandins, 270

Protein
    dietary,162, 165, 206–8, 227, 239, 241
    in muscle tissue, 180
    -restricted diets, 229
Protropin, 274
Pryor, William, 287
Psoas, 112
Psychological strategies, 346–62
Psychotherapy, 141
Psychosis, 360
Pull-ups, 98, 99, 106, 107
Pyridoxine (vitamin B_6), 213, 215

Quadratus lumborum, 94, 112
Quadriceps, 128. *See also* Legs
Quinn, Jim, 244
Quinn, Mike, 160

Radiation, ultraviolet, 341–44
Radio-ulnar pronator muscles, 111
Radio-ulnar supinator muscles, 111
Range of motion, 21–22
Reaction time, 266–68
Reagan, Ronald, 301
Recovery time, 23, 38–39, 329–30
    accelerating, 140
    for major muscles, 40, 41
    mineral balances and, 140
    muscle size and, 37
    sauna and, 310
    training intensity and, 37
Rectus abdominis, 75, 112
Rectus femoris, 74
Red clover,281, 284
Rehmannia glutinosa, 284
Rehydration drinks, 240–42
Renin, 252, 253
Repetitions, 22. *See also* Forced reps
Resistance training, 10, 22
Rest, between-workout, 38. *See also*Recovery time; Sleep
Reverse crunchers, 46, 116
Reverse wrist curls, 46–47
Reversibility, law of, 24
Rhomboids, 94
Rhubarb, 281
Rhythmic cadence, 42
Riboflavin (vitamin B_2), 212, 215
Ritalin, 276

Robinson, Eddie, 29
Rowing, 11
Royal jelly, 241
Running, 10, 143
Russian twists, 46, 115

Safety squats, 46, 121, 313–15
SAID principle, 24
Saint-John's-wort, 284
Salicin, 269–71
Salicylates, 241
Sarsaparilla, 282, 284
Sauna, 255, 308–10
Saw palmetto fruit, 282, 283
Scapular head (triceps), 102
Scar tissue, 14–15
Scott curls (Preacher curls), 102,
    103
Seasonal affective disorder (SAD),
    362
Seated calf machine, 47
Seated exercises
    calf raises, 129
    dumbbell presses, 80, 81
    dumbbell shrugs, 79–80
    French presses, 108
    presses behind the neck, 80
    rows, 96
Selenium, 219, 288
Self-esteem, 352
Semimembranosus, 74
Semitendinosis, 74
Serratus, 76, 94, 112
Sexual dysfunction, 266
Shot put, 143
    Shoulders
    exercises for, 44, 76, 111, 131
    training schedules for, 39–40,
        48–49, 60
Shrug-downs, 99
Siberian ginseng, 241, 281, 282,
    284
Side lunges, 119
Side lunge squats, 121
Sidebends, 46, 118
Singlet oxygen, 288
Sissy squats, 121, 122
Sjoholm, Hans, 138, 139
Skill training, 12
Skin types, 342–43
Skinfold calipers, 199–203
Skinfold measurements, 196

Skullcap, 284
Sleep, 255, 256, 284. *See also* Naps
Smoking, 221, 267
Snuff, 267
Soccer, 143
Sodium bicarbonate, 141
Sodium, 225–26, 249
Soleus, 74
Soleus, 129
Soviet Sports Review, 312
Specific gravity, 196
Specificity principle, 24
Speed, contractile, 36
Speed-strength, 6–7, 42, 147
Spicy foods, 221
Spinalis dorsi, 94
Spironolactone, 276
Splenius capitis, 75
Splenius cervicis, 75
Sports chute, 154
Sports drinks, 240–42
Spotters, 83, 106
Squats
    bear, 121
    bodybuilding, 121
    lunge, 119
    regular, 313–14
    safety, 313
    twisting, 120
Stair climbing, 11
Stairmaster, 134–35
Stamford (Connecticut), 66
Standing calf machine, 47
Standing calf raises, 130–21
Stanzolol, 274
Starches, 209
Starting strength, 8
Static strength, 7
Sternal pectoralis (lower chest), 83,
    87
Sternocleidomastoid, 75
Steroidal hormones, 245
Steroids, anabolic, 30–31, 64, 67,
    254, 273–74, 374–76
Stiff-legged deadlifts, 125
Strength
    aerobic, 9–10
    anaerobic, 6, 8, 137
    definition of, 3–4
    eating for, 205
    explosive, 8
    herbs and, 282

shoes, 131
-to-weight ratio, 144
training, 137–59
Stress, 223, 256, 284
Stretching exercises, 27
Stroke, 269
Stromba, 274
Strydom, Gary, 1
Subclavius, 83
Success
 fear of, 353
 visualizing, 348
Sugar, 208–9, 235
Sunlight, lack of, 224
Suntan, for competition, 341–44
Superoxide anion radical, 288
Supinator longus, 111
Supplements, nutritional. *See*
 Nutritional supplements
Sustanon, 250, 274
Swimming, 10
Symmetry, 336–40
Synthroid (TY thyroid), 275

T-bar rows, 97
Tables of norms, 199, 202–3
Tan, for competition, 341–44
Target muscles
 abdominal, 112
 back, 94
 chest, 83
 forearms, 111
 hips, 118
 shoulders, 76
 upper arms, 102
 See also specific muscles
Targeted-sets training, 35–36, 42,
 44
Taste, 192
Tea, 221
Teasel root, 283
Technique, 72–73
Technologies of training, 10–12,
 303–5
Teenagers, 223
Temperature
 gym, 255, 278
 skin, 267
Tennis, 143
Tensor faciae latae, 74
Terms, training, 7–12
Testes, 252

Testlax (Testolactone), 275
Testosterone, 252, 253, 273, 375
Thermogenesis, 181
Thiamin (vitamin B!), 212, 215
Thor's hammer, 46–47
Thumbless grip, 84
Thyroid, 252–53
Thyroid stimulating hormone
 (TSH), 248–50
Thyrotropin, 250
Tibialis anterior, 74
Tibialis anticus, 129
Tibialis posticus, 129
Tissue hypoxia, 285
Tissue leverage, 14
Tobacco, 267
Tocopherol (vitamin E), 214, 215
Tolerance to exercise, 331–35
Total-body exercise, 131
Training
 belt, 311–12
 growth hormone and, 256
 intensity, 37, 38
 myths about, 376–78
 objectives, 13–14
 periodizing, 157–59
 precontest, 366
 principles of, 20–28
 program(s), 33, 38, 48, 49
 progress logs, 61–62, 63
 schedules, 39–40, 60
 sequences, 152–57
 shell, 31
 strength, 137–59
 techniques, 13–14, 152–57
 technologies, 303–5
 terms, 7–12
Transversalis cervicis, 94, 112
Trapezius muscles, 75, 79, 94, 131
Treadmill, 134–35
Triacana (thyroid), 275
Triceps, 75, 102
 exercises for, 45, 106–7, 109, 111
 training schedules for, 39–40,
 48–49, 60
True squats, 121
TSH (thyroid stimulating
 hormone), 248–50
Twisting squats, 120, 121
Twists, Russian, 115
2–3 minute drill, 155

UBE/LBE, 152
Ulna, 111
Ultrasound, 141, 196
Ultraviolet radiation, 341–44
Underwater weighing, 196
Unilateral exercise, 339. *See also* One-arm exercises
Upper arm. *See* Biceps; Triceps
Upper back,97, 131
Upper body, 157
Upper-leg exercises, 118
Upright rows, for middle deltoids, 78
Urinalysis, 67
Use/disuse principle, 24
Uva ursa, 281

Vaccines, 270
Valerian, 284
Variable split training , 39, 48, 49, 60, 153
Vasopressin (ADH), 253
Vastus lateralis,74
Vastus medialis, 74
Vegetables, 176–77, 209, 227, 235
Versa-Climber, 134–35
Vervain, 284
Visualizing, 348
Vitamin A, 212, 215, 288, 290
Vitamin B_1 (thiamin), 212, 215
Vitamin B_2 (riboflavin), 212, 215
Vitamin B_3 (niacin), 212, 215
Vitamin B_5 (pantothenic acid) , 212
Vitamin B_6 (pyridoxine), 213, 215, 239
Vitamin B_{12} (cobalamin), 213, 215
Vitamin B_{15} (pangamate),213
Vitamin C (ascorbic acid), 213, 218, 288, 290
Vitamin D (calciferol), 214, 215
Vitamin E (tocopherol), 214, 215, 288, 290

Vitamin K, 214, 216

Wadden, T. A., 167n
Warming up, 25-27
Weaknesses, 150, 320–21
Weight change, 170–75
Weight training, 10, 154–55
Weighted dips, 92
Weighted pull-ups, 99
Weightlifting, 143
Wheat germ, 241
Whirlpool, 38
White willow bark, 269–71, 284
Wild yam root, 282
Winstrol, 274
Women
    growth hormone and, 278
    recovery time in, 37
Wood betony, 282
World Bodybuilding Federation, 375
World Wrestling Federation, 375
Wrestling, 143
Wrist curls, 46–47
Wrist muscles, 111

Xu duan, 284

Yarrow, 284
Yellow dock, 284
Yerba maté, 282, 284
Yessis, Mike, 100, 134, 312

Zable, Werner, 309
Zane squats, 121
Zen, 353
Zigzagging caloric intake, 162, 167–91, 195
Zinc, 219, 225
Zuccolotto, Troy, 372